D1087643

BIOLOGICAL PSYCHIATRY

BIOLOGICAL PSYCHIATRY

by

Michael R. Trimble, FRCP, FRCPsych
Consultant Physician to the Department of Psychological Medicine, National Hospital,
Queen Square, London WC1N 3BG UK

and

Raymond Way Senior Lecturer in Behavioural Neurology, Institute of Neurology,
London WC1N 3BG UK

A Wiley Medical Publication

JOHN WILEY & SONS
Chichester · New York · Brisbane · Toronto · Singapore

Copyright © 1988 by John Wiley & Sons Ltd.

All rights reserved.

No part of this book may be reproduced by any means, or transmitted, or translated into a machine language without the written permission of the publisher.

Library of Congress Cataloguing-in-Publication Data:
Trimble, Michael R.
  Biological psychiatry.
  Includes index.
  1. Biological psychiatry. I. Title
[DNLM: 1. Biological Psychiatry. 2. Brain—physiology. 3. Mental
Disorders. WM 100 T831b]
RC341.T73 1987   616.89′07   87–19482
ISBN 0 471 91622 6

British Library Cataloguing in Publication Data:
Trimble, Michael R.
  Biological psychiatry.
  1. Mental illness—Physiological aspects. 2 Psychopharmacology
  3. Psychobiology
  I. Title
  616.89   RC455.4.B5
ISBN 0 471 916 22 6

Printed and bound in Great Britain
at The Bath Press, Avon

To the memory of Raymond Way

Acknowledgements

The author is grateful to a number of colleagues who have read selected pieces of the manuscript, and made helpful comments. These include, Dr German Berrios, Dr Jonathan Brodie, Dr Ray Dolan, Dr Richard Green, Dr Joel Kleinman, Dr Shôn Lewis, Dr Christopher Mace, Dr Mary Robertson, Dr Martin Rossor and Professor Jenifer Wilson-Barnett.

Thanks go to Dr Martin Halliday for assistance with the illustrations of evoked potentials, Dr David Miller and Professor Ian MacDonald for some of the MRI pictures, Dr George Tatler for the plates of the 9800 CT scans and Dr Anthony Pullan for the electronmicrographs.

No book can be completed without secretarial help, and I am indebted to Sarah Presland for preparation of some of the manuscript. My deep thanks go to Barbara Phillips for her help with typing, editing and word processing.

Contents

Preface

In the last thirty years there has been a remarkable explosion of knowledge in medicine, and psychiatry is no exception. Much of the progress is related to the exploration of the biological foundations of the discipline, and this may be referred to as biological psychiatry. It is often said, quite mistakenly, that psychiatrists are unscientific and that psychiatry has made little progress over the years, and in any case lacks an adequate foundation of knowledge. In reality, psychiatry as a discipline is one of the more critical of all in medicine, continually questioning not only its data base, but also its fundamental methodological principles. Further, it has a long and distinguished history of progress, a point of departure for this book.

Thus, Chapter 1 outlines the development of psychiatry from its early origins, noting that it is one of the oldest medical specialties. The emphasis of most practitioners has been to elucidate any underlying pathology that is related to psychopathology, an endeavour that has been highly successful. Although much of this may be more appropriately referred to as neuropsychiatry, it should be recognized that, for example, in the last century, psychopathologists were in the main neuropathologists and vice versa. The reduction in morbidity and mortality of psychiatric patients that followed discovery of the cause and treatment of general paralysis of the insane (GPI) was substantial, and the progress that was made in the first half of this century in relation to treatments such as electroconvulsive therapy had a dramatic impact on the lives of thousands of patients otherwise condemned to long-term institutionalization.

Such progress is often ignored when discussing psychiatry, and emphasis is often given to an alternative stream of thought, one of psychological theorizing, which arose on the neoromantic tide of the turn of the century. This culminated in the psychoanalytic movement, which for a considerable time became synonymous with psychiatry. The point is made, however, that this era has provided psychiatry with a legacy that it does not deserve, the main trend of the tradition for over 2000 years being medical and neuro-pathologically based.

The position today is that these psychological theories of patho-genesis have been overtaken by a wealth of neurochemical and neuropathological hypotheses and findings, especially with regards to the major psychoses. Further, in addition to using knowledge accumulated in cooperation with other disciplines, biological psychiatry now seeks an understanding of psychopathol-ogy using theories and findings often based on clinical observations of patients and their effective treatment with biological remedies. Hence, the importance of the neurochemical era, ushered in by the psychopharmacological discoveries of the 1950s. These have given us not only a completely new image of the brain to work with, but have allowed a more complete understanding of underlying func-tional and structural changes of the brain that accompany psychi-atric illness. Functional, a misused word in the clinical neurosciences, once again may be used in its original sense, to designate a physiological disturbance, rather than as an epithet for 'psychological'. Indeed, with our present knowledge the distinc-tion between 'organic' and 'functional' melts away, stripped of its Cartesian dualism.

In spite of such progress, the very concept of biological psy-chiatry still meets with scepticism in the eyes of many. As we approach the turn of the next century, there may well be a revival of a fin de siècle phenomenon, in which the recent gains will become submerged and lost in a quagmire of new, old or revived psychological theorizing. The reasons for this are not difficult to understand. Thus, biological psychiatry is a complicated subject, requiring in particular an intimate knowledge of the central ner-vous system. Many find such knowledge hard to grasp, and the very pace of discoveries is often bewildering. The principles rely to some extent on diagnosis and measurement of biological variables, yet in the clinical area these are often ignored, thought unneces-sary or counterproductive. This is in spite of them being funda-mental to medicine, and psychiatry being a most important branch of medicine. The latter fact is often trivialized, many, especially of the lay public, but also sadly some practitioners, preferring to deny the medical roots of psychiatry, but in doing so confusing it with psychology.

Biological treatments, in spite of their obvious and proven effi-ciency, are criticized. However, the psychopharmacological revo-lution has given psychiatrists, not for the first time, powerful remedies. The days when multitudes of patients suffered intensely because of lack of adequate treatment are forgotten, and false arguments that compare and contrast psychotherapy to biological treatments are constructed. It is assumed that the use of such treatments implies a lack of interest in patients, and that somehow the doctor is less than adequate for prescribing them. However, in medicine it is obvious that often several approaches to patient care are appropriate and can be applied simultaneously if required. The neurologist or the chest physician know the value of physiotherapy and when it is applicable, and likewise the psychiatrist may recognize the value of other treatments for his patients, in addition to the biological ones. However, the neurologist would not hesitate to prescribe medication to his patient with Parkinson's disease, or the chest physician antituberculous remedies to a consumptive. Indeed, with tuberculosis, the remedies of fifty years ago, which relied mainly on changes in environment and the passage of time, have been superseded by more effective modern treatment regimes, as is the case with many psychiatric illnesses.

One challenge for biological psychiatry is to unite information we now have regarding functional changes in the brain in psychopathology with that which we know about brain–behaviour relationships and brain structure. The latter was of great interest to the neuropsychiatrists of the last century, and has recently been an area of much research, but often referred to as behavioural neurology. This discipline has developed rapidly in the United States of America, and may become seen as a neurological discipline if its relevance for psychiatry is not acknowledged, and the essential value of examining patients with known structural disease for helping to understand the course and development of psychopathology is not appreciated.

In this text I have reviewed a number of key areas of importance for biological psychiatry. A strong emphasis has been placed on the work of Jaspers, and the fundamental distinction between illness, which is related to a process, and development. The whole area of personality disorders is one of continuing disagreement, although as emphasized in Chapter 7 neurochemical and neuropathological substrates of at least some personality traits are being uncovered. However, it is arguable to what extent psychiatrists are an appropriate professional group to deal with personality disorders generally, and their ready acceptance of this in the past has led to a great deal of criticism, not the least being the failure to influence behaviour patterns in ways which the then-accepted theories, predominantly psychoanalytic, predicted they should change with treatment. An alternative argument would be that psychiatrists should deal with illness, not personality problems, for which latter group other agencies in society are readily available as a source of help.

The main diagnostic system used in this book is that of the American Psychiatric Association's DSM III. However, as noted in Chapter 2, classification is in a constant process of change, and is not immutable. However, the DSM III is likely to dominate psychiatric research for many years to come—hence the emphasis. The reader will quickly note the profusion of different terms used in the book for similar states, many of which do not even conform to the alternative ICD system. This is because in quoting papers, the original patient designation used by the authors is selected. Many of the investigations were carried out prior to the introduction of the DSM III, but reclassification of patients would be an inappropriate exercise. It is hoped that the introduction of such systems as the DSM III, and soon the DSM IIIR, will lead to more uniformity of patients included in research populations, making a reviewer's task easier and increasing the validity of any findings.

It is hoped that the two chapters on neurochemistry and neuroanatomy will be of interest, and give an up-to-date account of the state of knowledge. These fields are moving so rapidly that information has a danger of soon being out of date. Nonetheless, it is hoped that areas of importance for biological psychiatry are adequately outlined, and that their inclusion, essential for the text, will increase the reader's interest in exploring some of these areas further.

The main clinical chapters cover the major psychopathologies, notably affective disorders (Chapter 9) and schizophrenia (Chapter 8). Structural disorders of the limbic system are discussed separately (Chapter 6), and individual chapters are devoted to dementia (11) and epilepsy (10). This follows some other psychiatric texts, including in the contents mainly information on the major psychoses, although the neuroses are discussed where relevant (Chapters 7 and 9). These areas of psychopathology have been chosen to reflect subjects of relevance to biological psychiatry, but also relate to the author's interests. Dementia and epilepsy are of growing importance. Patients with dementia, from those with dementia praecox to those with the disorders identified by Alzheimer and Pick, are often assessed and managed by psychiatrists. The recent neurochemical findings, especially in

Alzheimer's disease, and the possibility of replacement therapy to hold the condition for a few years at least have encouraged renewed interest in this area. Epilepsy is included, in part reflecting the author's own area of special interest, but mainly because of the very close relationship between epilepsy and psychiatry that has existed for many years. Epilepsy has a great deal to teach us about the CNS, about psychopathology and about patient management.

There are many topics missing from this book, which no doubt will lead to comment. For example, not discussed are conditions such as alcoholism and the addictions, and eating disorders, the biological bases for which are becoming clarified, and relevant neurochemical and neuropathological findings have been reported. Inevitably, the final size of the volume, as well as the author's personal interests, are responsible for the exclusions. In addition, this volume is a companion to my earlier book *Neuropsychiatry* (Trimble, 1981a). Although there is some overlap, here the data on dementia, epilepsy and biological treatments have been rewritten and updated, and some subjects that may interest the reader, but not included here, may be found there.

Biological psychiatry is such a rapidly advancing field, and the number of papers of relevance so vast, that much selectivity has gone into the choice quoted in this book. Undoubtedly there will be those disappointed that their paper is not quoted, and others who will point to a missing reference of some negative finding not substantiating a claim made in the text. To a large extent I have quoted work that has either been independently replicated or seems to be of interest to the theme of the topic at hand. In several areas, for example the neuropathology of schizophrenia, all the findings consistently show some changes, but there is not exact replication as to the precise changes in all studies. Nevertheless, the combined findings add up to an extremely important conclusion with regards to schizophrenia, namely the obvious, but until recently ignored, relationship of the condition to structural brain lesions.

It is hoped that the text will provide an informative data base for those psychiatrists interested in exploring the biological foundations of their discipline further. It may help to stimulate the interests of students wanting to explore one of the most exciting areas of current research in psychiatry, and may provide those active in the field with ideas for future investigations that will increase our knowledge even further.

MRT, London, 1987

Mental disorders are neither more nor less than nervous diseases in which mental symptoms predominate, and their entire separation from other nervous diseases has been a sad hinderance to progress.

MAUDSLEY (1870, p.41)

CHAPTER 1

Historical introduction

The earliest statement on biological psychiatry is probably attributed to Hippocrates. Born in 460 BC at a time when medicine was beginning to sever its connections with the priesthood and religion, he protested against the a priori speculations of his predecessors and advocated the importance of a naturalistic approach and the value of clinical experience. In his writings on 'The Sacred Disease', the name given by the Greeks to epilepsy, he pointed out that it was no more sacred than any other disease, and 'has a natural cause from which it originates like other affections' (Adams, 1939, p.355). In this dissertation he rails against theological speculations with regards to the causation of disease, describes the appearance of the brain of man, and continues, '. . . and men ought to know that from nothing else but thence (from the brain) comes joys, delights, laughter and sports, and sorrows, griefs, despondency and lamentations. . . . And by the same organ we become mad and delirious, and fears and terrors assail us . . .' (p.366).

Hippocrates used explanations based on the necessity for the correct mixture of various body humors (e.g. phlegm and bile) for health, disease reflecting an imbalance of them. It followed from these ideas that treatment required restoration of the correct balance. Hippocrates also introduced the idea of disease having a longitudinal course—hence his insistence on careful clinical examination and prognosis. Diseases as distinct and static entities were not envisaged. However, the idea that the brain was the central organ in the regulation of man's activities was not fully shared by those who succeeded him, Aristotle and his followers attributing more importance to the heart.

Aretaeus, who lived in the first century AD, in part revived the Hippocratic tradition, emphasizing both clinical observation and prognosis, and made many observations on mental illness. However, his contributions were reflected more in early attempts at differential diagnosis, rather than any new formulations of aetiology. It was Galen, living a century later, whose works were to be so influential over the succeeding centuries. He was especially concerned with the 'temperament' and its biological foundation. This temperament, however, was not viewed as it might be today, in a psychological sense, but as a somatic state. Yellow and black bile, phlegm and blood were the basic constituents, and a categorization of constitutional types was on the basis of relating them to the prevailing humors and their quantities. Galen's conception of disease was, however, different from some of his predecessors, emphasizing diagnosis and the empirical quality of the process. Thus, once the threshold of health had been crossed, disease was established, and from that point it had its own form. He further accepted as aetiological factors both the genetic constituent and external influences. An extract on melancholia from the treatise *De Locis Affectis* illustrates these ideas:

> Black bile arises in some people in large quantity either because of their original humoral constitution or by their customary diet which is transformed into this humor by digestion in the blood vessels. Like the thick phlegm, this heavy atrabilious blood obstructs the passage through the middle or posterior cavity of the brain and sometimes causes epilepsy. When its excess pervades the brain matter itself, it causes melancholy . . . (Siegel, 1973, p.197).

This particular passage also reflects on the relationship between epilepsy and psychiatry, a theme returned to later in this book. In contrast, mania was thought to be an affection of yellow bile, but was a different disease from melancholia since the actions of black and yellow bile were different.

It is generally accepted that after Galen, with a few notable exceptions, and the contributions of the Arab world, that for the next 1300 years medicine abandoned any semblance of a scientific approach, and retreated under the combined influences of theology and demonology.

One of the originators of modern medicine was Vesalius, whose neuroanatomical illustrations in *De Fabrica* of 1543 are superior to anything that had been produced before. Many of his observations contradicted the by now fossilized teachings of Galen, and emphasized the new spirit of empiricism and exploration. Further, such observations were possible only by dissection of cadavers, an exercise still undertaken with great precaution, but nevertheless possible.

The seventeenth century saw a revival of the idea that the brain was the seat of many mental diseases, and the rudiments of present-day localization theories can be found in the writings of several authors. One of the most influential was Thomas Willis, the founder of neurology.

Although his early interests were in chemistry, his medical researches led him to believe that the brain had been inaccurately described. His main neurological contributions were published in 1655 in *Cerebri Anatome* (Dewhurst, 1982a). One of the beliefs held by medieval scholars was that mental functions were localized in the ventricles of the brain, and Willis was one of the contributors who insisted that the substance of the brain itself had specific functions. Animal spirits circulated through the cortex, and the ventricles were more a drain for impurities. The spirits flowed from their store in cortex through medulla and spinal cord to stimulate peripheral nerves and hence movement. Likewise spirits could flow inwards to evoke sensations. Imagination was related to the corpus callosum.

One of his clinical contributions to psychiatry was in relation to hysteria. It was generally considered, and had been so since the Greek times, that this affliction was a disorder of the female reproductive tract, more specifically the uterus. Willis clearly disagreed: 'This passion comes not from the vapours rising into the head from the uterus or spleen, nor from a rapid flow of blood into the pulmonary vessels, but has its origin in the brain itself' (Dewhurst, 1980, p.87).

Interestingly he attributed hysteria to spirits in 'distraction', a similar aetiology being given to epilepsy, although the location in the former was at the beginning of the nerves within the head, and in epilepsy was in the middle part of the brain. This is a further early example of epilepsy and psychiatry being linked through similar pathogenic mechanisms.

Willis also discussed such conditions as delirium, frenzy, melancholia and mania. These latter two were likewise related to disordered animal spirits: 'If either the blood supplies bad material for the spirits, or the digestive operations of the viscera are harmed, men become melancholic . . .' (Dewhurst, 1980, p.126). In mania the spirits 'are obviously restless . . . their force, being widely diffused, passes swiftly into the nerves and muscles . . .' (p.130).

In these extracts it is clear that Willis was one of the first physicians of the new enlightenment to clearly equate mental disorders with brain diseases.

In the eighteenth century, knowledge about the central nervous system increased a great deal. Classification of illness, including psychiatric disorder, was of great concern to many authors (see Chapter 2), and attempts were made to attribute diseases to various localizations of pathology. Morgagni, a pathologist from Padua, in 1761 published his findings of 800 autopsies, and taught that different diseases were due to pathology in different organs. Although such ideas had been steadily fermenting, especially with the elegant anatomical descriptions of Leonardo Da Vinci and Vesalius, this anatomical conception of disease was a new departure for medical thought. Thus, Galen, for example, did not give structures any function. For him function came first, and analysis of vital phenomena started with functions, not structures. In the work of Morgagni, however, localization of pathology became paramount. In psychiatry the inevitable consequence was to seek changes in the brains of psychiatric patients at post-mortem.

At this point it is important to note another shift in the medical conception of disease that was occurring. The earlier idea that disease was related to admixture of the four humors did have rivals; for example that of 'solidism', the concept that disease was due to disorder in the solid parts of the body, rather than its fluids. The shift towards solidism was thus encouraged by these morbid pathological studies. Further, a second dichotomy was emerging with the rise of renaissance science, namely that between the so-called 'iatromechanists' and the 'iatrochemists'. The former were attempting to explain biological activity in mechanistic terms; the latter emphasized chemical changes.

It should be recalled that at this time the ideas of Descartes were fully recognized, and the so-called 'Cartesian dualism' flourished. Descartes, the seventeenth century philosopher, skilfully, with deductive reasoning, was able to philosophically separate mind from body. This allowed examination and speculation about the brain and its relationship to sensation and movement to progress relatively unfettered from the religious domination over anything that had to do with man's mind and hence the soul. Spirits, which as noted formed an important aspect of disease theory from early times, were of fundamental importance in this theme. If, as it seems was essential for successful medical theorizing, the body was to be separated from the soul, for the latter to act on the body some intervening substance was necessary. Spirit filled this role, although it took on many different meanings. With the declining need to discuss disease in relationship to humors and spirits derived from classical antiquity, the Cartesian view allowed a good compromise. The body was viewed as a mechanical device and a permissible area for investigation. The soul was immaterial, and remained the province of theologians. Descartes' view is well summed up with the following quotation:

> . . . Mind can be perceived clearly and distinctly, or suffi-ciently so to let it be considered to be a complete thing without any of those forms or attributes by which we recognise that body is a substance . . . and body is understood distinctly and as a complete thing apart from the attributes attaching to the mind (see Wilson, 1969, p.273).

In this scheme, the body was distinguished by extension in space, and the soul resided in 'a certain very small gland', that which we now refer to as the pineal. Animal spirits were envisaged as radiating through the body in the nerves and arteries to influ-ence the body.

In 1798, Haslam, apothecary to the Bethlem Hospital, at that time situated at Moorfields (the current site of Liverpool Street Station), was one of the first to report an extensive series of post-mortem information on patients with mental illness, and is attributed with the first pathological description of general paral-ysis of the insane. Such investigations were commonplace over the next century, and represent the forerunner of research that still continues today, especially with regard to dementia and schizophrenia.

Other advances in the neurosciences were included in theories of psychopathology. The discovery by von Haller, a leading phys-iologist of the eighteenth century, that muscle possessed the prop-erty of irritability, was utilized by Cullen (see Chapter 2) as an explanation for nervous diseases. Likewise, the theory of reflex action assumed importance. Barely perceived by the mechanistic theories of Descartes, it flowered under the influence of Whytt, whose own experiments demonstrated that only a segment of the spinal cord was necessary for reflex action to occur. He described the pupillary light reflex, and introduced the terms stimulus and response. His book, *On Nervous, Hypochondriacal or Hysterical Diseases*, was probably the first important treatise on psychiatric diseases since Willis (McHenry, 1969). In it he gives a clear defi-nition of the term nervous: '. . .Those disorders may, peculiarly, deserve the name nervous, which, on account of an unusual delicacy, or unnatural state of the nerves, are produced by causes, which, in people of a sound constitution, would either have no such effects, or at least in a much less degree.'

As Hunter and MacAlpine (1963) note, this was replaced by the word neurosis by Cullen some twenty years later.

LOCALIZATION AND MENTAL DISEASE

The nineteenth century saw a rapid expansion of knowledge in medicine, and a continued growth of the anatomicoclinical method. Such an approach was seen especially with the attempts to localize mental functions in the brain (see Figure 1). Apart from the various speculations regarding the origin of the seat of the soul, and the medieval principle of attributing various ventricles certain mental attributes, localization theories such as we are familiar with today did not emerge until the rise of the phrenological movement, the greatest exponents of which were Gall and his collaborator Spurzheim. Gall, who graduated in Vienna in 1781, was interested to know why people possessed various faculties. His main conclusions were that they were innate, and depended on organic substrates which were in the brain (Ackerknecht, 1973). The latter was no longer seen as just a receptacle for sensations, but as the crowning achievement of Homo sapiens. It was conceived of as composed of many different organs, which could be palpated through the scalp. This last contention was the downfall of phrenology, since it quickly became taken up by all sorts of charlatans, and fell into disrepute. Nonetheless, Gall was the originator of modern localization theories, and, for example, suggested the presence of a speech centre, a concept revived later by Broca. Further, he drew attention to the importance of the cerebral cortex for mentation, with neglect of subcortical structures, a state of affairs that persisted until recently (see below).

In contrast to the speculations of Gall, the physiologist Flourens, following animal investigations, concluded differently. He thought the hemispheres of the brain possessed equipotentiality. On account of the unacceptability, on both philosophical and religious grounds, of localization theories, these ideas of Flourens were very popular. However, when Broca presented his findings in 1861, the concept of localization of speech function had already been further suggested by both Bouillard and Dax, and the climate was changing. Broca described eight patients with loss of

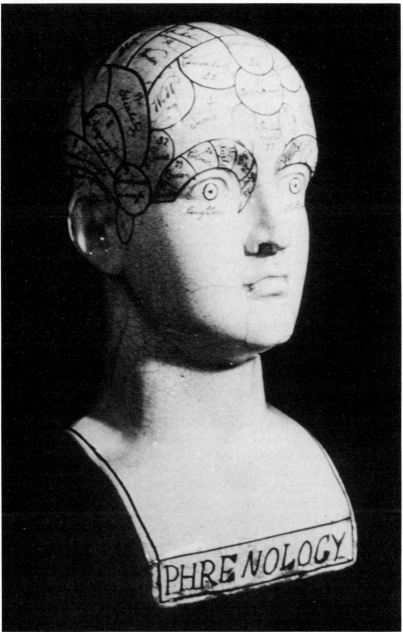

Figure 1. A phrenological bust. The phrenologists unsuccessfully attempted to localize psychological functions in the brain. (From the author's collection.)

speech, noting that all had lesions in the third left frontal convolution.

While now, over a hundred years later, we accept the clinical facts as Broca gave them, the concept of aphasia has altered considerably, and in the intervening years the line of thought attributed to Flourens has not totally subsided. Broca's own statements were met with opposition from several quarters. These included contemporary neurologists such as Marie and Hughlings Jackson, and in this century von Monakow, Lashley, Goldstein and Head. Von Monakow clarified the important principle of diaschisis, namely the idea that regions of the brain distant from the prime area of diminished function may be influenced by a lesion. Common to both von Monokov and Goldstein was the conception that all activities were a manifestation of the entire organism. Others such as Sherrington (1947) stressed the 'integrative action of the nervous system'. These critics wished to know precisely what was localized. Was it, as it appears to be the case, that the area of cortex, for example, that was related to movement of an arm, was the actual site of the volitional activity which resided in an area of its own serving just one function? As Jackson had pointed out, while it may be possible to localize a lesion, this does not apply to a function. They also railed against the extreme proponents of localization whose new phrenology of the brain was leading to the production of brain diagrams in which everything from muscle movements to obesity was allocated a position.

The protagonists of localization theories had support from the elegant experiments of both Fritz and Hitzig (a student of Griesinger and later Professor of Psychiatry at Zurich), and Ferrier. The two Germans noted that stimulation of the cortex of dogs led to the production of contralateral movements, confirmed three years later by Ferrier working at the West Riding Lunatic Asylum. Attempts by Brodmann and Vogt to characterize cortical histological patterns led to the splitting up of the brain into areas, which varied from 19 to 150 depending on the investigator. Attempts were made to relate cortical histology to various functions, culminating in the recent demonstration by Geschwind and Levitsky (1968) of anatomical asymmetry in the left planum temporale of the human brain. This region, an area between the posterior border of Heschl's gyrus, the primary auditory cortex and the posterior end of the Sylvian fissure, is larger on the left side, a feature that can sometimes be seen on computed axial tomographic scans (CT). In psychiatry, the localization ideal reached its zenith with the publications of Kleist.

It is obvious that aphasia was central to these issues. There are cases of aphasia described in the medical literature in the seventeenth and eighteenth centuries, and both Gall and Pinel gave good clinical accounts (Riese, 1959). The studies of Broca initiated a line of literature which sought not only cerebral localization but also lateralization. Broca was unable to explain the coincidence of aphasia and right-sided hemiplegia, although, after consideration of the facts, Hughlings Jackson referred to the left side of the brain as the 'leading hemisphere' for speech, and concluded that there were differences in the functions of the two sides. Laterality differences in relationship to psychopathology, an area of study now actively pursued, underwent a revival in the 1960s with the work of Flor-Henry (1969) in psychotic patients with epilepsy, a disorder that so interested Hughlings Jackson.

It is sometimes forgotten that Freud made significant contributions to the area, both as a neurologist and a neuroanatomist. His monograph on aphasia was only translated into English in 1953 by Stengel. It was an analysis of current concepts of the subject, and his views seemed congruent with those of Hughlings Jackson whom he acknowledged.

PSYCHIATRIC CONTRIBUTIONS OF HUGHLINGS JACKSON

The importance of Hughlings Jackson for psychiatry has been discussed by several authors (Ey, 1978; Dewhurst, 1982b). He was introduced to psychiatry by Daniel Hake Tuke and Thomas Laycock, and early in his training was exposed to psychiatric patients. He had an overriding interest in philosophy, and was appointed assistant physician to the National Hospital, Queen Square, in 1862. He was not a brilliant lecturer, and his writings are not easy to follow. His colleagues apparently considered him to be a genius, and, years later, when a bust of him was unveiled at the hospital, it is said that the great neurologist Gowers remarked, 'Gentlemen, behold the master'. His conception of brain function was based on four ideas, namely the evolution of nervous functions, the hierarchy of functions, the negative and positive symptoms of dissolution and the distinction between local and uniform dissolution.

The nervous system was seen as developing both in space and time, and was not the static organ of the pathologist's specimen. Further, it was hierarchically organized, not merely a collection of reflexes. With any lesion there are two effects, that due to the destruction of tissue, resulting in the negative symptoms, and release due to subjacent activity of other healthy areas of the brain, causing positive symptoms. Acknowledging the work of Bell, who noted that 'in debility the voluntary fails before the automatic' (Taylor, 1958, vol. 2, p.6), and of others such as Laycock, Henry Munro (fifth in a successive dynasty of physicians to practise psychiatry) and Herbert Spencer, he presented his views following observations mainly on patients with aphasia and epilepsy. He discussed mental disorders, and noted that in all cases of insanity the principle of dissolution, the level of evolution that remains and the positive and negative elements need to be considered. In a paper called 'The factors of the insanities' he stated 'In every insanity there is morbid affection of more or less the highest cerebral centres . . . (they) are out of function, temporally or permanently from some pathological process' (Taylor, 1958, vol. 2, p.411), a statement relevant for biological psychiatry. His use of the terms positive and negative symptoms, as a reflection of a mechanism of nervous system function equally applicable to a whole range of conditions, stands in contrast to the recent reintroduction of these expressions into psychiatry, with a more or less descriptive use, and restricted to schizophrenia.

Dewhurst (1982b) assessed Hughlings Jackson's contributions to European psychiatry. Generally his works have been neglected in England, by both neurology and psychiatry. However, his influence on Freud, Ey and on the early thinking of Adolf Meyer, most influential in America for his *Psychobiology*, the use of life charts in the assessment of patients and the conception of 'reaction types', has left many legacies. The medical historian Riese (1954) noted the links between Bleuler's classification of symptoms and Hughlings Jackson's positive and negative terminology, Freud being a possible intermediate link. In France, Ribot, the teacher of Janet, used Jacksonian principles in psychopathology, and Ey combined Freudian psychodynamics with Jacksonian neuro-dynamics in his organodynamic psychiatry (Evans, 1972).

The reintroduction of Hughlings Jackson's terminology into psychiatry, and the continued awareness that strict localization hypotheses are not going to uncover the essential links between the brain and behaviour, will probably mean that the next few years will see a renewed interest in his works, and further adaptation of some of his ideas in psychiatry.

CONTINUED PROGRESS IN BIOLOGICAL PSYCHIATRY

The works of Haslam reflected the beginning of a continuing literature in which the biological foundations of psychopathology were pursued. The main contributions stemmed from England, France and Germany. Reil, who graduated at Halle in 1782 and later went on to be Professor of Medicine in Berlin, introduced the term psychiatry. His adoption of 'vitalism', the concept that there was some natural life force (derived from the animism of Stahl, ideas seen as a reaction to the earlier speculations of the iatromechanists and iatrochemists), which was related to the central nervous system, led him to accept mental diseases as brain diseases. His important contribution was the introduction of psychotherapeutic methods, thought to influence the vital processes in treatment.

The continued influence of romanticism in Germany served to separate psychiatry there from medical progress that was going on in England and France. It was brought to a halt by the appointment of Griesinger as professor in Berlin in 1865. His book, *Mental Pathology and Therapeutics*, was written in 1845, and translated into English in 1867 (Figure 2). His thesis was that insanity is only a symptom, and the brain is the organ that must be diseased in mental illness. He states: '. . .we therefore primarily, and in every case of mental disease, recognize a morbid action of that organ' (p.1). An important tenet, reflecting the essential nature of biological psychiatry is: 'Insanity being a disease, and that disease being an affection of the brain, it can only be studied in a proper manner from the medical point of view' (p.9).

Griesinger recognized both idiopathic and symptomatic causes of mental disease which acted on the brain through changes in circulation, nervous irritation or through disturbed nutrition. After a review of post-mortem studies, including those of Pinel, Esquirol and Chiarugi, he concluded, 'it may be considered a well established fact that the majority of post-mortem examinations of the insane show anatomical changes to exist within the cranium' (p.413).

Griesinger was succeeded by Westphal, who along with Erb described the patellar reflex. Other substantial contributions of German psychiatry in this era come from Meynert, Wernicke,

MENTAL PATHOLOGY

AND

THERAPEUTICS

BY

W. GRIESINGER, M.D.,

PROFESSOR OF CLINICAL MEDICINE AND OF MENTAL SCIENCE IN THE UNIVERSITY OF
BERLIN; HONORARY MEMBER OF THE MEDICO-PSYCHOLOGICAL ASSOCIATION;
MEMBRE ASSOCIÉ ÉTRANGER DE LA SOCIÉTÉ MÉDICO-PSYCHOLOGIQUE
DE PARIS; ETC. ETC.

TRANSLATED FROM THE GERMAN (SECOND EDITION).

BY

C. LOCKHART ROBERTSON, M.D. Cantab.,

MEDICAL SUPERINTENDENT OF THE SUSSEX LUNATIC ASYLUM HAYWARD'S HEATH;

AND

JAMES RUTHERFORD, M.D. Edin.

THE NEW SYDENHAM SOCIETY,
LONDON.

MDCCCLXVII.

Figure 2. Frontispiece to Griesinger's book. A most influential and important landmark in the history of psychiatry. (From the author's collection.)

Kahlbaum and Kraepelin. Meynert, whose work stimulated a whole generation of successors including Freud, contrasted the functions of the cortex and the brain stem, postulating a neuro-physiological foundation of the ego based on the principles of associationist psychology and the presence of different cortical 'centres'. Haemodynamic changes were still a favoured pathogenic mechanism. Wernicke is well known for his aphasiology, and his contributions to the study of chronic alcoholism are recognized in the eponym Wernicke–Korsakov syndrome. Kahlbaum's insistence on the clinical method, and his attempts to clarify disease classification, led to the delineation of catatonia. Later, Kraepelin developed his nosological scheme which has had such a profound influence on psychiatry.

England's representative of this era was Maudsley. He was appointed as medical superintendent to the Manchester Royal Lunatic Asylum at the age of 24, but thereafter returned to London, his posts including Professor of Medical Jurisprudence at University College. His text, *The Physiology and Pathology of the Mind*, was widely read and translated into several languages. It has become one of the classics of English psychiatry. He was no lover of metaphysical speculation or introspection, and some of his theories of pathogenesis have echoes that are heard today. With regards to causation of insanity he stated: '. . . it is easy to perceive how little is taught by specifying a single moral cause, such as grief, vanity, ambition, which may after all be, and often is, one of the earliest symptoms of the disease' (Maudsley, 1868, 2nd ed., p.226).

He acknowledged the frequency of negative pathological changes in post-mortem studies, continuing: '. . . at present we know nothing whatever of the intimate constitution of the nerve element and of the mode of its functional action, and it is beyond doubt that important molecular or chemical changes may take place in those inner recesses to which we have not gained access' (p.428).

Maudsley advocated the need for more research and better education, and in 1907, with the aid of Mott, the pathologist to the London County Asylum, he offered thirty thousand pounds to the London County Council to establish a hospital which was for early and acute cases only, with provision made for pathological and clinical research. Mott's laboratory at Claybury was moved there in 1916, but the hospital was not finally opened until 1923. Mapother was appointed the first medical superintendent, and occupied the first Chair in Psychiatry.

Although German psychiatry, especially the contributors to biological psychiatry (in that era, more properly referred to as 'neuropsychiatry'), was especially dominant in the second half of the nineteenth century, developments in France were somewhat earlier. Pinel's influence was profound, and like many others he had misgivings about philosophy and metaphysics (Pichot, 1983). His line of successors at the Salpêtrière was long and distinguished and included Esquirol, Pinel's favoured pupil; Baillarger, Esquirol's favourite; J-P. Falret, Georget, Felix Voisin, Foville and Calmeil.

Two very important figures in French psychiatry were Bayle and Morel. Bayle, in his doctoral thesis of 1822, related chronic arachnoiditis to dementia paralytica. This ascription of a defined pathology to a common cause of insanity had profound consequences for psychiatry, one of the most important being the reinforcement of somatic theories of mental illness. Further, in later writings, Bayle emphasized the stages of the disease, with a specific form and pattern of development, culminating in dementia. It was not until 1905 that Schaudinn identified the spirochaete in the genital lesions of syphilis, 1906 that Wasserman developed his blood test and 1913 that Noguchi found the organism in the brains of patients with GPI.

Morel, working in the environment of the intellectual and conceptual theories of Darwin, extended the ideas that were germinating from authors such as Pinel and Esquirol on the hereditary factor in mental disease. He defined 'degenerations' as abnormal human types, transmissible by heredity, which eventually burned themselves out. These ideas, at once pessimistic in their conception of psychiatric disease, had a longlasting influence on later theorists. They were continued in France by Magnan, with a Darwinian emphasis, and permeated French psychiatry for several decades. Lombroso took them to Italy, and the ideas of both Kraepelin (who used Morel's term démence précoce in his classification) and Maudsley were influenced by them. In spite of the criticisms that are often brought against these theories, Pichot (1983) refers to them as a turning point; ideas of mental disease that took into account both heredity and environment, and the embodiment of the concept of endogenicity.

THE NEUROSES

Much of the endeavour to uncover the pathological basis of psychiatric illness in the nineteenth century had been related to diseases that today we might refer to as psychotic, or were organic brain syndromes. The neuroses were also studied.

After Cullen coined the term as a synonym for nervous diseases, theories of pathogenesis continued to reflect either disturbed uterine function, abnormal humors, or both. As noted, Willis had made the significant advance of locating the most notorious of the neuroses, hysteria, in the brain, but the rise of anatomicoclinical medicine did little to uncover the origins of the various neuroses.

One attempt was that of Foville, whose view was that the neuroses were diseases localized in the nervous system. This was associated with alteration of brain function (functional), although most authors accepted that, with their techniques, the changes were not to be visualized. Haemodynamic theories and reflex mechanisms were popular explanations for altered neuronal function. The spleen and vapours of the seventeenth century became disorders of the nerves (Whytt), the neuroses (Cullen), and finally, by the beginning of the nineteenth century, emerged as two major disorders, namely hysteria and hypochondriasis.

It was the great French neurologist Charcot who explored the neuroses in detail, in particular hysteria. It is interesting that at this time, the latter half of the last century, neuroses were considered in the province of the neurologist. This in part reflected the fact that most severe pathology was seen in hospitals, and the neuroses presumably, as today, were largely found in out-patients, and tended to be seen by a different group of physicians, usually privately. An example of this was the development in America of the concept of neuraesthenia by Beard, culminating in a book on the subject in 1880, and the interest of Wier Mitchell, one of the earliest and most influential of the American neurologists, in conditions of nervous debility. His 'rest cure' became widely known and used as a treatment for these disorders. Neuraesthenia evolved from ideas such as those of Hall, who in 1850 defined the reflex actions of the spinal cord, applying this to various disease states. The concept of spinal weakness found a counterpart in brain weakness, and hence cerebral neuraesthenia.

Charcot, who was appointed Médecin de l'Hospice de la Salpêtrière at the age of 37, was deeply interested in the neuroses. In an analysis of the patients who were seen at his famous Tuesday clinics, it is estimated that in one academic year the diagnosis of hysteria was made 244 times in 3168 consultations (Guillain, 1959, p.135). It was his belief that the neuroses should be examined and investigated as any other disorder of the central nervous system, and as a consequence he gave elegant clinical descriptions. He described the stigmata noted in hysteria, such as anaesthetic patches, and recorded a whole variety of clinical types. He also felt that pathological principles should apply. Thus, with regards to the symptom of hysterical hemianaesthesia we read: 'Hence it becomes probable . . . that complete hemianaesthesia, with derangements of the special senses—and consequently, such as is presented in hysteria—may, in certain cases, be produced by a circumscribed lesion of the cerebral hemispheres' (Charcot, 1877, p.261).

Charcot experimented with hypnosis, which he felt to induce a pathological state, and made numerous contributions to neurology with original clinical and pathological descriptions, including the delineation of multiple sclerosis. Zilboorg (1941) summed up this era stating:

> The fundamental contribution of the School of the Salpêtrière and its essential historical value lie in the fact that it was the first to capture for psychiatry the very last part of demonological territory, which up to the middle of the 18th Century had belonged to the clerical and judicial marshals of theology and from the middle of the 18th century to the last quarter of the 19th had remained for the most part a no man's land (p.365).

THE TWENTIETH CENTURY

Although the first half of the twentieth century saw an apparent eclipse of progress in biological psychiatry, an undercurrent of ideas and investigations continued which flowered again in the period after the Second World War. Since then, this has provided a new generation of psychiatrists with a wide range of fascinating and important findings, which for the time being places psychiatry once again securely as a medical discipline. This has resulted in part from a vastly increased knowledge of the central nervous system, but three diseases played a prominent and persisting role in the theme, namely syphilis, encephalitis and epilepsy.

A considerable gap in time elapsed from the observations of Bayle to the identification of the spirochaete in the brains of patients with cerebral syphilis. One of the great therapeutic breakthroughs in psychiatry then occurred. It should be remembered that GPI was a frequent diagnosis in mental hospitals, and a cause of severe and often very distressing morbidity. In one report it was estimated that 9 per cent of asylum admissions were for epilepsy, and a similar figure was given for general paralysis (Tuke, 1892, vol. 2, p.1204). Kraepelin reported that in 1913 GPI accounted for from 10 to 20 per cent of all psychiatric admissions in Germany (Pichot, 1983, p.128).

Wagner-Jauregg, observing that the symptoms of some mental patients improved when they had a fever, attempted to induce pyrexia in patients with GPI using malaria. Although no panacea, some were helped by this, their disease process apparently arresting. For this discovery Wagner-Jauregg was awarded a Nobel Prize in 1927, the only psychiatrist as yet to be so honoured. The essence of this discovery was the reversal of the more pessimistic trends that psychiatry assumed, especially under the degeneration theory, which implied that treatment for psychiatric illness was an unrealistic aim and that a downhill progress of disease was inevitable.

The role that encephalitis played in the development of biological psychiatry has yet to be fully appreciated. The most significant contribution initially came from von Economo (1931). He studied with Wagner-Jauregg in Vienna, and towards the end of 1916 he reported on a number of patients who presented with an unusual variety of symptoms which followed an influenza-like prodrome. Some had marked lethargy and disturbance of their eye movements, and on post-mortem examination invariably had inflammation almost exclusively confined to the grey matter of the midbrain. Von Economo defined this as a new entity, previously unrecognized, and referred to it as encephalitis lethargica. It was attributed to influenza pandemics which occurred in the first years of the twentieth century. A wide range of psychopathology was noted in the survivors, including neurotic, especially obsessive–compulsive and psychotic disorders. The importance of this was emphasized by von Economo:

> The dialectic combinations and psychological constructions of many ideologists will collapse like a house of cards if they do not in future take into account these new basic facts. Every psychiatrist who wishes to probe into the phenomena of disturbed motility and changes of character, the psychological mechanism of mental inaccessibility, of the neuroses, etc., must be thoroughly acquainted with the experience gathered from encephalitis lethargica. Every psychologist who in future attempts to deal with psychological phenomena such as will, temperament, and fundamentals of character, such as self-

consciousness, the ego, etc., and is not well acquainted with the appropriate observations on encephalitic patients, and does not read the descriptions of the psychological causes in the many original papers recording the severe mental symptoms, will build on sand (p.167).

The last sentence of the book is 'Encephalitis lethargica can scarcely again be forgotten' (p.167), but this prophesy was to be proved wrong. This elegant work was ignored by a generation of psychiatric theorists, although the viral hypotheses of psychiatric illness has recently been revived. Hunter persistently advocated the importance of encephalitis in psychiatric illness (Hunter and MacAlpine, 1974), and renewed attention to the close links between extrapyramidal disease and psychopathology, as exemplified by encephalitis lethargica. Sacks' (1973) descriptions of the encephalitic patients 'awakened' by the anti-Parkinsonian drug L-dopa gave rich insights into the psychopathology promoted by such brain lesions. The search to identify viruses in the brains of psychiatric patients is once again an active endeavour.

Epilepsy has, and has always had, close links with psychiatry (see Chapter 10). As Hill (1981) commented: 'To the ancient Greeks it was obvious that epilepsy was the most sacred and the most psychological of all diseases. Only a God could throw a sane normal man to the ground, deprive him of his senses, convulse him and then restore him to normality' (p.1).

The links suggested by Galen and Willis already quoted above are two examples of this continuing theme, and Esquirol, Calmeil, J-P. Falret and Hughlings Jackson amongst others established significant clinical associations. Kraepelin, in his *Lectures on Clinical Psychiatry* (1904), included epileptic insanity as a variety of mental illness. Although the suggestion was that of an increased association between epilepsy and psychosis, around the turn of this century an alternative viewpoint was being established, namely of an inverse relationship. Nyirö and Jablonsky (1929), in Hungary, reported that patients with a combination of epilepsy and schizophrenia seemed to demonstrate a decrease of their epileptic attacks when the psychosis emerged. Others, for example Glaus (1931) in Zurich, found only a few cases with the combination, and concluded that schizophrenia had difficulty in expressing itself in the presence of epilepsy. The Hungarian, von Meduna, impressed by the findings of his countrymen and his own pathological findings that suggested different pathological changes in the brains of patients dying with the two disorders, reasoned that if there was an antagonism between schizophrenia and epilepsy, then the artificial induction of a seizure may have a beneficial effect on the psychosis. His initial endeavour was to find a substance that might induce convulsions safely in patients, and he began investigations with camphor injections in animals. The first patient was treated on 10 February 1934, and the effects were dramatic. They have recently been published, as extracts from his autobiography, by Fink (1984):

> This patient had suffered from catatonic stupor for about four years. He never moved, never ate, never took care of his bodily needs, and had to be tube fed . . . . He received five camphor injections and two days after the fifth injection, for the first time in four years, he got out of his bed, began to talk, requested breakfast, dressed himself without any help, was interested in everything around him, and asked how long he had been in the hospital (p.1036).

This was an important event for the history of psychiatry, since von Meduna was still working in a climate which insisted that schizophrenia was an inherited degenerative, hence incurable, disease. He moved on from camphor to pentylenetetrazole, while others used insulin and electricity. Sakel noted that psychiatric symptoms improved in some patients who had coma artificially induced by insulin, although here the emphasis was more on the importance of the hypoglycaemia than on a seizure as the therapeutic factor. Cerletti and Bini introduced electric shock in 1938, and the efficacy of this form of treatment in a variety of conditions was soon reported.

Another bridge between epilepsy and psychiatry emerged around this time, namely the introduction into clinical practice of the electroencephalogram (EEG). The psychiatrist Hans Berger, in a series of publications from 1928 to 1935, made regular observations of the electrical patterns he recorded from the brains of man, but they were largely ignored. However, his claims were vindicated in 1935 when Adrian and Matthews proved that it was possible to detect the brain's electrical rhythms through the intact skull. The identification of temporal lobe epilepsy soon followed, and a new era of investigation and treatment of epilepsy began, including, for the first time, physiological investigations of the links between psychiatric illnesses and epilepsy.

OTHER ADVANCES

In the first part of the century several other significant advances in biological psychiatry occurred. Pellagra was found to be caused by a deficiency of nicotinic acid, and Følling demonstrated amino acid, especially phenylalanine, deficiencies in certain mentally retarded children. Endocrine replacement therapies, for example with thyroxine, became possible. These discoveries and their therapeutic impact were the forerunners of much research that is progressing at the present time on biochemical and metabolic factors in psychiatric illness.

A different line of investigation was initiated by the Portuguese neurologist Moniz. In 1936 he published the results of his neuro-surgical operations in psychotic patients. His preference was for operation on the frontal lobes, an area of the brain then attracting a great deal of interest, especially following the observations of Jacobsen that primates with bilateral frontal lesions underwent marked emotional changes, without apparent loss of intelligence. The procedure of frontal leucotomy was enthusiastically taken up by Freeman and Watts in America, and modifications of the original operation were employed (see Chapter 12).

These advances were made the more possible on account of rapid advancement in the knowledge of the brain's neuroanatomy and neurochemistry. Ramon y Cajal introduced the neurone the-ory in the 1890s, and later Sherrington gave us the word synapse. Pavlov set forward his theory of conditioned reflexes, Hofmann, a chemist from Basle, discovered the psychotropic properties of LSD and the first neurotransmitters were discovered. Dale identi-fied acetylcholine in animals, and in 1936 was able to show it was released following electrical stimulation of the motor nerves. In the 1940s von Euler discovered noradrenaline in the sympathetic nerves. Today a bewildering variety of neurotransmitters and receptors is forming the basis of much research in biological psychiatry.

With regards to brain structure, and the relationship of this to behaviour, Cannon had firmly shown by stimulation and lesion experiments in animals that emotional responses were closely linked to certain brain regions, notably the subcortical structures. In 1937 Papez published his paper 'A proposed mechanism of emotion', in which he laid down a neural basis of emotional expression and described the so-called 'Papez circuit'. This con-cept was elaborated into the 'limbic system' by MacLean, provid-ing psychiatry with what it previously lacked, namely a clear neurological substrate for emotional behaviour and psycho-pathology.

PSYCHOPHARMACOLOGY

Psychiatry, especially since the great discoveries of the early part of this century, has always been a subject dominated by a search for treatments. Although, as with other physicians, psychiatrists always had a vast therapeutic armamentarium from which to offer patients a combination of empirically tried remedies, alcohol and opium were probably the most widely employed.

A turning point in the history of psychopharmacology was the introduction of bromides in the 1860s for the treatment of epilepsy. Locock, obstetrician to Queen Victoria, acting on the knowledge that they somehow interfered with sexual potency, and thinking that epileptic seizures and sexual orgasms were linked, recommended potassium bromide. The treatment was soon acknowledged as beneficial by others including Hughlings Jackson. The bromides became a popular remedy for many conditions in addition to epilepsy, and remained a mainstay of therapy till the barbiturates were introduced for a similar range of problems in the 1920s.

Barbiturates were also used to obtain prolonged narcosis, advocated first by Klasi in 1922, and proved of great value in various forms of abreaction and narcotherapy. This latter mode of treatment, still used in some centres today, owes its introduction to Sargant, who, along with Slater, published the first edition of *Physical Methods of Treatment in Psychiatry* in 1944. Dedicated to Mapother, it outlined the state of the art at that time, therapies included being insulin coma, convulsive therapy, malarial therapy, leucotomy, diet, vitamins and endocrine replacement, and the use of barbiturates, bromide, phenytoin and amphetamines.

Since the end of the Second World War, psychiatry like many other medical disciplines has progressed in an unforeseen yet spectacular way. The trend towards the somatic treatments accelerated, notably since the publication in 1952, by Delay and Deniker, of the results of giving chlorpromazine to psychotic patients. Soon after, Kuhn noted the effects of imipramine, not on psychosis but on depression, and Kline reported the value of monoamine-oxidase inhibitors (MAOI). Lithium was introduced by Cade in 1949, the first prophylactic treatment in psychiatry. 'Librium', the first of the benzodiazepines, was marketed in 1960. The future of biological psychiatry was secure, and the societies followed. The Society for Biological Psychiatry was founded in 1954 and the first World Congress held in 1974.

CONCLUSIONS

This historical account has emphasized the continuing growth of biological psychiatry over two and a half millennia, and certain points can be highlighted. First, there has been a rise of and a continued progress in the anatomicoclinical method, which has had some success in understanding psychiatric illness. The localization hypotheses of mental function have been of value in directing attention to the close links between the brain and some aspects of emotion and cognition, although alternative hypotheses about brain function, such as those suggested by Hughlings Jackson, have importance in order to explore the obvious lacunae of the extreme localizationalist viewpoint.

Secondly, psychiatry has been remarkably successful in combating many of the diseases that were such an important cause of mental illness, such as GPI, epilepsy, severe melancholia, and both vitamin and hormonal deficiencies. The rise of our knowledge about the brain has introduced hypotheses regarding alteration of function in 'functional disorders', and we have a plethora of information on the 'solid' and 'fluid' and the 'mechanical' and the 'chemical' components that have so preoccupied our forefathers. An urgent task at the present time is to unite such information into a cohesive explanation of psychopathology, bringing together our knowledge of the structural and the functional aspects of the brain in health and disease.

Thirdly, in psychiatry, there has been, over the last two hundred years at least, alternating periods with regards to the dominant themes in the literature. The two main streams have emphasized either the tendency to value somatic discoveries, and the search for pathology in relation to psychiatric illness, or have espoused the virtues of psychological enquiry. In the main, these themes have reflected the zeitgeist, with the more Romantic era of the early eighteenth century being replaced by the rise of anatomicoclinical medicine, itself losing favour with the rise at the turn of the twentieth century of the neo-Romantic period. The latter was reflected in the wide popularity of psychoanalysis, and the growing division between neurology and psychiatry. In part it was clear how psychoanalysis was so rapidly accepted. As Maudsley (1868) noted:

> . . . the metaphysician deals with man as an abstract or ideal being, postulates him as a certain constant quantity, and thereupon confidently enunciates empty propositions. The

consequence is, that metaphysics has never made any advance, but has only appeared in a new garb; nor can it in truth advance, unless some great addition is made to the inborn power of the human mind (p.9).

That addition came from the psychodynamic contributions of Freud and his early followers, and offered, in the same way that convulsive therapy was to do a few years later, a new form of therapy for what was considered untreatable. Enthusiasm and optimism reflected by these treatments were important ingredients, which in particular found favour in America. Never impressed by the hereditary models of the Europeans, the country, where a person achieved, not on account of genetic heritage but because of enterprise and hard work, amplified the Cartesian echo, and psychological theorizing regarding the pathogenesis of mental illness became the accepted fashion. The distractions of psychoanalysis for present-day psychiatry cannot be over-emphasized. To base theories today of aetiology, pathogenesis and treatment on ideas that were dominant nearly a hundred years ago makes little sense in view of the increase in knowledge that has accrued since that time. Psychiatry, alone amongst all of the medical disciplines, tenaciously accepts so much of the old dogma, and so reluctantly embraces the new. We still have the situation that often other physicians think that psychiatry involves only enquiry about the mind, abstractly held in limbo, and that most of the advances outlined in this chapter reflect on other disciplines and are not the heritage of psychiatry. As the history of the discipline shows, however, psychiatry is, and has always been, concerned with behaviour in its widest sense, and has continually searched for knowledge of brain–behaviour relationships and the somatic underpinnings of psychopathology.

CHAPTER 2

Concepts of disease and classification

INTRODUCTION

Although it is readily apparent in case conferences, it is often poorly appreciated that our concepts of disease are not immutable, and various models may be proposed. It is customary to assume that disease has some independent existence of its own, visiting our healthy bodies and altering them in some way. Medicine notes these changes, establishes the pattern that they assume, ascribes a diagnosis and prescribes a remedy which will influence the disease process. Earlier theories using this model ascribed disease to the intrusion of spirits and evil forces, often as a punishment for wrongdoing. They were given the most powerful boost by the discovery of microorganisms, and their cure by antibiotics. In many instances, disease is thus seen as having a single cause and, ideally, a single treatment.

In contrast, a number of other concepts of disease may be considered, some of which are of importance for psychiatry. For the Platonics, health was seen as a state of harmony, and loss of this resulted in pain and disease. Since the elements that made up the body were the same as those that constituted the universe, theories of causation were based not on observation, but from the Platonic conception of the universe. An alternative is reflected in those models that assume the existence of disease as an objective reality, and embrace notions not only of aetiology, but also of the nature of the disease and its relationship to the nature of man. In terms of the relationship between the history of man and that of disease, there are various ideas that attribute disease to the increasing or decreasing influence of civilization and the evils of 'modern' society. A forerunner of this view is that of Rousseau, whose dislike for the evils of 'civilization' included the consequent induced diseases. Some current ideas stress the evils of industrialization as both aetiological and pathogenic for psychopathology.

Hippocrates introduced the historical dimension to disease, and the first case histories in medicine were from this era. The disease has signs and symptoms, a beginning, a course, duration and outcome. The step to recognizing diseases as independent entities did not come until the seventeenth century, and the works of Baglivi and Sydenham. They felt that diseases in their natural states were subject to the same laws of observation and description as other natural phenomena. The final step was made by Virchov, who combined his cellular pathology with the new knowledge of anatomicoclinical medicine, completing the notion of disease as a local affection. The search for classification systems as well as aetiology became predominant.

Entwined with the development of the concept of disease as an independent local entity has been the principle of reaction. Sydenham (1740), in spite of his attempts to study the natural history of diseases, recognized this important element: '. . . a disease is nothing else but Nature's endeavour to thrust forth with all her might the morbifick matter for the health of the patient . . .' (p.1).

Thus intrinsic, as opposed to extrinsic, factors assume importance in the pathogenesis of symptoms. The reactions of the organism were seen as healing. An extension of this line of thought is described by Riese (1953):

> A disease is a whole of vital manifestations, elicited by some pathogenic (extrinsic) factor or groups of them, and displayed by organisms whose reactions, though similar in some respects, differ from individual to individual as to the degree but also as to type. More generally speaking, the organism, though diseased, continues to live a life and an evolution of its own. Subsequently, there are as many intrinsic features of diseases as there are diseased individuals (p.39).

This 'biographic' conception of disease stands in obvious contrast to the 'ontological' one, in the sense that it admits only diseased individuals, and not diseases per se. It has had a marked influence in psychiatry. The testimony of individuals, as opposed to clinical observation, assumes with this model an ever-increasing significance. The introspective techniques of the psychoanalytic method took this to its extreme, devaluing diagnosis, elevating the subjective and, in most cases, allowing its practitioners the excuse not even to physically examine their patients! The phrase 'reaction types' became an accepted nomenclature, especially in America, under the influence of both psychoanalytic thinking and the contributions of Adolf Meyer. Extreme conclusions of this stance have been taken by some authors such as Szasz, who would deny the very existence of psychiatric illness.

Finally, the technology of the twentieth century has seen statistics used in attempts to define disease. It was Galton who, in the last century, successfully applied mathematical and statistical methods to measure biological phenomena, and demonstrated how this could also be done for psychological data. The use of statistical models for the definition of normality was adopted by psychiatry, especially for personality disorders, and the development of a large range of rating scales of psychopathology derived from these techniques.

SIGNS, SYMPTOMS, SYNDROMES AND DISEASE

In clinical medicine we recognize two fundamental kinds of data. Symptoms are those complaints of the patient that are spontaneously reported or are elicited by the clinical history. Signs are observed by the physician, the patient, or a friend or relative of the patient, which indicate the presence of some abnormal functioning of one or more body systems. A syndrome is a constellation of signs and symptoms which seem to coalesce to provide a recognizable entity with its defining characteristics. Syndromes may be classified, and are the clinical representatives of illness. The latter infers some biological change or variation of the organism, and the task of medical science has been to explore this. A clear distinction has to be drawn between illness and disease, the former being that which the patient presents with, which only in part represents the expression of disease in any individual. Biological psychiatry attempts to understand psychiatric illness through defining syndromes and ultimately diseases, based on a knowledge of the associated changes of the structure and function of the central nervous system, and their provoking factors.

At the present time, classification of disease in medicine generally represents a pot-pourri of notions, some being defined by symptoms, such as epilepsy, migraine or schizophrenia, others by aetiology such as syphilis, and others by pathology such as Alzheimer's disease. Indeed, with regard to the central nervous system, no attempt has been made to provide a comprehensive classification since that of Romberg in 1853. In general, in medicine progress has led from syndrome delineation and classification based on that to an understanding of pathology and a new classification. GPI is now classified as a syndrome of syphilis. Unfortunately, for many psychiatric syndromes, the underlying aetiology and pathogenesis is unclear, and only relying on syndrome classification has led to a multitude of different systems. As Hughlings Jackson noted (Taylor, 1958), there are two ways to classify flowers—as a gardener or as a botanist. At present we still use the techniques of the gardener, but are progressing towards the position of the botanist.

CLASSIFICATION IN PSYCHIATRY

The two main diagnostic systems in use at the present time are the *International Classification of Diseases* (ICD), which derives from the World Health Organisation, and the American Psychiatric Association's *Diagnostic and Statistical Manual of Mental Disorders*, 3rd edition (DSM III). It is important to emphasize that, although diagnostic fashion changes frequently, some of the categories that we use today were recognized by many earlier generations, and have a degree of constancy over time. Further, the classifications discussed will themselves soon be modified in the light of clinical experience and the accumulation of knowledge, particularly as more biological correlates of clinical syndromes become manifest.

Plato recognized three kinds of madness, namely melancholia, mania and dementia. Madness was equated to loss of reason (Zilboorg, 1941). Personality types, based on the humoral theories, were also recognized by the Greeks. Aretaeus seems to have acknowledged that mania and melancholia were somehow related, recognized that senile mental disorders were distinct and described links between certain temperaments and mental illness.

The first comprehensive classification was that of Cullen (1800), and his works have had an influence to the present day. He divided diseases into four main categories, one of which was the neuroses. A subgroup was the vesaniae, which were disorders of intellectual functions without pyrexia or coma. It included amentia (imbecility of judgement which may be present from birth or come on in old age), melancholia, mania and oneirodynia (disturbed imagination during sleep).

Pinel, who translated the works of Cullen into French, introduced a system of classification including melancholia, mania, dementia and idiotism. In Germany, Griesinger recognized states of mental depression, states of mental exultation and states of mental weakness.

Gradually some newer categories of illness became recognized. J-P. Falret described alternating moods of mania and melancholia (folie circulaire), hebephrenia was described by Hecker in 1871 and Kahlbaum introduced catatonia in 1874. Morel used the term démence précoce for a dementing-like condition that affected young people, which was to reappear later as Kraepelin's dementia praecox.

The origin of the term neurosis has already been noted (p.14). As Hunter pointed out (Hunter and MacAlpine, 1963), the expression largely disappeared from the literature in the nineteenth century, only to reappear with the prefix psycho- and the psycho-analytic speculations of aetiology. The word psychosis seems to have been first used in 1844 by von Feuchtersleben with a rather general meaning (Pichot, 1983), and confusion has surrounded its use ever since.

Kraepelin's textbook of psychiatry went through nine editions, and his views moulded with time and experience. Prognosis was an essential feature of his system, and this was related to diagnosis. Dementia praecox and manic depressive psychosis were his two main groupings, involutional melancholia and paranoia being considered as separate entities. Three forms of dementia praecox were described, namely the hebephrenic, the catatonic and the paranoid. These fundamental categories of psychopathology form the framework of the system in use today. The ideas of the Kraepelinian system were opposed to the unitary psychosis model, and reaffirmed the disease concept firmly for psychiatry.

One more distinction should briefly be discussed, that of the endogenous and the exogenous psychoses. The distinction is attributed initially to Mobius (Lewis, 1971) who introduced a classification based on causes. He distinguished between main and subsidiary causes, and, if the chief factor was seen to be within the individual, it was referred to as endogenous. If it was something which impinged on the individual from without it was exogenous. Bonhoeffer, in 1909, then developed the concept of exogenous reaction types which reflected various ways that the brain responded to injury. This essentially meant organic insults arising from outside the brain, although others extended the concept to include psychological trauma. While the term exogenous is rarely used today, and most of the disorders that it embraced would be subsumed under the organic brain syndromes, endogenous is still popular, although as Lewis (1971) pointed out, it is often merely a cloak for ignorance. Its introduction was strongly linked to the degeneration theory, and Lewis felt its use 'should be openly linked to presumptive evidence of a powerful hereditary factor in causation' (p.196).

KARL JASPERS

Although Jaspers' *Allgemeine Psychopathologie* was first written in 1913, and went through nine editions, the English translation did not become available until 1963. Nonetheless, the influence of his thinking has been widespread, especially in Europe. His ideas came to England with Meyer-Gross, and the writings of such authors as Henderson, Kraupl Taylor, Fish, Anderson, Lewis and Stengel. He was invited to write a treatise on psychopathology, and, recognizing the rise of hermeneutical approaches in psychiatry and the declining influence of natural science, decided to put down the known order of facts. His approach was strongly empirical, in spite of being rooted in the philosophical school of phenomenology.

Influenced by Kant and Husserl, Jaspers developed a method for examining the mental state of another person, which, in its purest form, attempts to delineate psychic events as sharply as possible. Central to his theme is the distinction between psychogenic development and organic process, and the dichotomy between understanding (*Verstehen*) and explanation (*Erklären*), what is 'meaningful' and what is 'causal'.

Some quotations from his book (1963) emphasize these issues:

> Phenomenology . . . gives a concrete description of the psychic states which patients actually experience and presents them for observation (p.55).

> Form must be kept distinct from content . . . from the phenomenological point of view it is only the form that interests us . . . (p.58).

> We differentiate abnormal personality-types that are Anlage-variants, from sick personalities in the narrower sense, where the change has been bought on by a process (p.445).

> We sink ourselves into the psychic situation and understand genetically by empathy how one psychic event emerges from another . . . . We find by repeated experience that a number of phenomena are regularly linked together, and on this basis we explain causally . . . (p.301).

The distinction between what was meaningful and what was causal reflected the 'unbridgeable gulf between genuine connections of external causality and psychic connections which can only be called causal by analogy' (p.301).

Jaspers was clearly opposed to those who confused form and content, and he emphasized how the theories of Freud were only concerned with meaningful as opposed to causal connections. His approach differed from that of Kraepelin in emphasizing a descriptive psychopathology rather than actual diseases. It was continued by Kurt Schneider, who further developed criteria to distinguish development from process. The more recent introduction of such diagnostic tools as the 'present state examination' (PSE) of Wing and colleagues (1974) derive from this approach.

CURRENT CLASSIFICATIONS

The classification schemes in use in psychiatry at the present time are based almost entirely on symptoms. Various operational definitions have been introduced and are widely employed, the basis of which is the completion of a check list of symptoms, signs and historical facts which must be satisfied before a diagnosis is made. The two most popular are the Feighner criteria (Feighner *et al.*, 1972) and the DSM III (American Psychiatric Association (APA), 1980). These are seen in contrast to the more descriptive classifications given in the ICD, the 9th edition of which came into use in 1979. In the section that follows, greater emphasis is given to the DSM III, since, especially in research, it is assuming increasing importance. Although it adopts a multiaxial classification, this is not overemphasized, but it is in keeping with the distinction drawn by Jaspers between personality disorder and psychiatric illness. Axis 1 refers to clinical syndromes, while axis 2 covers developmental and personality disorders. Axes 3, 4 and 5 refer to physical disorders, psychosocial stressors and global assessment of functioning respectively. It is not intended that a comprehensive classification be given here, and attention is mainly paid to the disorders that relate to subsequent chapters.

PERSONALITY DISORDERS

Introduction

We see the personality in the particular way an individual expresses himself, in the way he moves, how he experiences and reacts to situations, how he loves, grows jealous, how he conducts his life in general, what needs he has, what are his longings and aims, what are his ideals and how he shapes them, what values guide him and what he does, what he creates and how he acts (Jaspers, 1963, p.428).

It is thus by the personality traits that we know someone; they are enduring and give an air of predictability to a person. There are two ways of defining an abnormal personality, either by a statistical method or one based on ideal types. Jaspers preferred the former, as did Kurt Schneider (1959) who defined abnormal personalities as those who '. . . suffer from their abnormality or through whose abnormality society suffers' (p.4).

Psychopathic personality

This term was used by Schneider to embrace several differing abnormal personality patterns, but generally now infers antisocial personality traits. In the ICD 9 it is referred to as manifesting mainly as sociopathy, while sociopathic personality or antisocial personality disorder are alternative terms. In Feighner's criteria it is one of the few personality disorders described, suggesting its relatively clear delineation. It is characterized by 'disregard for social obligations, lack of feeling for others, and impetuous violence or callous unconcern' (ICD 9). It usually becomes apparent in early life, often with conduct disorder at school, a continuing history of poor interpersonal relationships, a poor work record and continuing marital difficulties. Drug abuse, alcoholism, pathological lying and prison convictions may be recorded, and sociopaths tend to display more than accepted sexual deviation, somatization and outbursts of physical violence. A characteristic feature is the tendency to remit over the years, either in early or mid adulthood.

Obsessional personality

This is characterized by a lifelong tendency to meticulousness and punctuality. Patients have difficulty in expressing their emotions, and check and re-check their actions. It is better referred to as the anankastic type, which saves confusion with obsessive compulsive disorder. In DSM III it is called compulsive personality disorder.

Hysterical personality

The hysterical personality has links to the sociopathic personality, and in many ways is contrasted with the anankastic. Jaspers (1963) defined the type thus: 'hysterical personalities crave to appear, both to themselves and others, as more than they are and to experience more than they are ever capable of' (p.443). The characteristic traits are excessive dependence; shallow, labile affects; impulsiveness; verbal exaggeration and excessive gestural display; seductiveness in the presence of relative frigidity; and self-dramatization. There is a tendency to take overdoses of medication or make other attempts at self-harm, and there is some association with somatization.

The validity of this category has been established by factor analysis (Lazare *et al.*, 1970), from which studies its traits are clearly distinguished from the anankastic personality. In particular the impulsivity and the tendency to approximate and exaggerate of the hysterical personality stand in contrast to the calculations and deliberations of the ananakast. In contrast to sociopaths who tend to be male, hysterical personalities are commoner in females. There are clear overlaps, both with sociopathic and borderline personalities. DSM III prefers the term histrionic personality disorder to prevent confusion with hysteria.

Borderline personality

This is a new category of disorder, introduced for the first time by the DSM III. 'The essential feature . . . is instability in a variety of areas, including interpersonal behaviour, mood, and self image' (p.321). It was urged on the initiators of DSM III by the psychoanalysts, who had a dynamic formulation of its definition. Associated features include impulsivity, sexual disturbances and transient psychotic episodes. In spite of its recent appearance it has a long tradition, and many clinicians may recognize it and find the category helpful.

Paranoid personality

This type is distinguished by continued suspiciousness, mistrust and excessive sensitivity. Jealousy, transient ideas of reference, litigiousness and a tendency to avoid intimacy are all features, and individuals often take up minor concerns or causes with tenacious vigour, collecting vast amounts of documentary evidence to support them.

Schizoid personality

The features are of people who have little affective or social contact, with a tendency to detachment and eccentricity. While well recognized, the DSM III has split this into three groups, the schizoid, the schizotypal and the avoidant. The schizotypal appears to include 'oddities of behaviour, thinking, perception and speech', and the avoidant emphasizes hypersensitivity and social withdrawal in spite of yearning for acceptance. There are no experimental data at the present time to justify these new categories.

Cyclothymic personality

ICD 9 has a category referred to as affective personality disorder, characterized by a lifelong predominance of mood changes, depressive or elated or both, fluctuating in cycles. It is not included in the DSM III on account of the phenomenological and biological affiliation with the affective disorders.

Neuraesthenic personality

Jaspers refers to people with 'irritable weakness'. There is both an increased sensitivity and an easy fatiguability, often with complaints of exhaustion and minor aches and pains. This is somewhat different from the asthenic personality of ICD 9 which includes 'passive compliance with the wishes of elders and others and a weak inadequate response to the demands of daily life'. There is no equivalent in the DSM III.

Other personality types

In addition to the above groupings which find some concordance in the different systems, various other types are described, although the criteria are often less than clear. The anxious personality defines those who display lifelong anxiety and under stress readily develop anxiety or panic disorder. Narcissistic personality refers to those 'with a grandiose sense of self importance or uniqueness; preoccupation with fantasies of unlimited success; exhibitionistic need for constant attention and admiration; characteristic responses to threats of self esteem; and characteristic disturbances in interpersonal relationships . . .' (DSM III, p.315). Also noted are frequent depressed moods and transient psychotic states. The DSM III includes the categories of the passive aggressive personality, those who habitually express covert aggression, and the dependent personal disorder. The ICD 9 refers to the explosive personality in which liability to intemperate outbursts of anger are seen in people otherwise not prone to antisocial behaviour.

AFFECTIVE DISORDERS

One of the advantages of the DSM III classification of mood disorders is the loss of the distinction between endogenous and reactive depression. Originally the term reactive was introduced to refer to the quality of a depression, reflecting its reaction to environmental circumstances. However, based on Meyerian terminology, some psychiatrists frequently refer to depressive reactions, implying aetiological significance.

Earlier editions of the ICD incorporated various types of depression, including manic depressive reactions, involutional melancholia, neurotic depressive reactions and reactive depressive psychosis. In the ICD 9 there are the affective psychoses, including various manic, manic depressive and depressive subtypes, and under the neuroses is neurotic depression. The latter may also be referred to as depressive reaction or reactive depression. In addition, there is a brief depressive reaction in which the symptoms are closely linked in time to a stressful event. The existence of these different categories arose from the acceptance of the Kraepelinian distinction between dementia praecox and manic depressive illness, and the growing extension of psychiatric practice outside hospitals where it was clear that many people suffered from a type of depression, milder than that referred to by Kraepelin and unrelated to psychosis. Endogenous depression was seen as fundamentally different from the reactive variety, and the latter lost its meaning of a description and became associated with an aetiology. Much time was then spent, and is still spent, on arguments over this dichotomy, some asserting there is only one type of depression, others that there are two. Attempts to settle this issue involved studies of patients' symptoms using such statistical techniques as multiple regression and discriminant function analysis. The main support for a bimodal distribution of symptoms, and hence a distinctive reactive–endogenous dichotomy came from Roth and colleagues at Newcastle (Carney et al., 1965), while a unimodal model was supported by Kendell (1969). What does emerge from studies in this area is that many, using factor or cluster analysis, seem to be able to identify an 'endogenous' group, although few clearly identify a discrete second group corresponding to 'reactive depression'.

In the DSM III, the essential feature of affective disorders is 'a disturbance of mood, accompanied by a full or partial manic or depressive syndrome, that is not due to any other physical or mental disorder' (p.205). Subclassification is into major affective disorders, including bipolar disorder and major depression, specific affective disorders, including cyclothymic and dysthymic disorder, and atypical affective disorders.

Manic disorders are subdivided into mixed, manic or depressed types. Psychotic features are included if present, and two kinds recorded, those that are mood congruent and those that are mood incongruent. The definition of psychotic is given as 'gross impairment in reality testing, as when there are delusions or hallucinations or depressive stupor' (p.214).

Interestingly, the DSM III reintroduces the term melancholia, also as a subcategory of major depressive episode, which is given when there is 'loss of pleasure in all or almost all activities. . .' (p.215) in association with some of the following features: depressed mood, diurnal variation, early morning waking, psychomotor slowing or agitation, anorexia or weight loss and inappropriate guilt. The classification of affective disorders as given by DSM III is shown in Table 1.

The grouping cyclothymic refers to those states where the symptoms are not of sufficient severity or duration to meet the criteria for major depressive or manic episodes, and in dysthymic disorder there is no evidence of hypomanic spells.

A further feature of the DSM III classification is the organic affective syndrome, where the condition is the result of a specific physical disorder in the setting of clear consciousness. The aetiologies given include mood disorder caused by medications such as reserpine, and that associated with endocrine, neoplastic or viral conditions.

One other classification should be presented. The St Louis group refers to primary and secondary affective disorders. The latter is accompanied by some physical illness, or preceded by another form of psychiatric illness (Goodwin and Guze, 1984). It is claimed that this distinction has prognostic and therapeutic

Table 1 DSM III classification of affective disorders

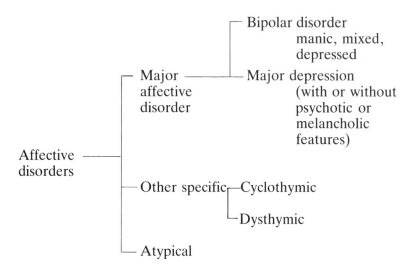

implications, primary affective disorder being associated with periods of normality between attacks and a higher risk of suicide. Winokur further subdivides the primary group into familial, sporadic and depressive spectrum subdivisions (Andreasen and Winokur, 1979).

Clinical features

The essence of the affective disorders is the change of mood. In depressive states the patient loses vitality, ceases to enjoy life and usually admits to a loss of emotional wellbeing. This fundamental change is associated with a change of the whole person, reflected in mood, thought and posture. Concentration difficulties with complaints of poor memory, increased apathy with diminution of movement, and changes of appetite, food intake and sleep patterns are found. Feelings of anxiety and tension are invariably present, and sometimes, in contrast to a psychomotor retardation, an agitation with indecision and excessive motor activity occurs. In its extreme form intense aimless pacing is seen. Loss of energy, fatiguability and tiredness are reported, and many symptoms improve as the day passes.

Some patients do not report or underreport the mood changes, and somatic symptoms are the main complaint. These, referable to any system in the body, easily become the focus of attention both for patient and physician, and may lead both off into excursions involving a multitude of investigations which are usually negative.

Suicidal thoughts and preoccupations are frequent, as are thoughts of worthlessness and guilt. Crying is not always reported, although should always be asked about, especially in males. Irritability and increased hostility, especially towards loved ones, increase tensions at home, as may loss of libido.

Mania, in contrast, is associated with an increased sense of wellbeing and euphoria. Again the process is pervasive and affects thoughts, with a pressure of speech and flight of ideas, and motor activity. Concentration is poor, and patients are easily distractable, and are often irritable. Sleep and appetite are disturbed, some patients sleeping only very briefly and rising early to pursue their manic activities. In more extreme forms the patient may be very restless, have markedly disordered speech with rhyming, punning and word play, and their mood no longer euphoric but dysphoric.

In the depressive and the manic phases, psychotic symptoms may be seen. There is loss of insight—the depressive contemplating imminent death from some dreaded disease, the manic about to spend a fortune he does not possess. Hallucinations and delusions, morbid or magnificent, may occur, nearly always mood congruent. Paranoid states are not uncommon, and their onset should always lead to a search for depressive underpinnings.

SCHIZOPHRENIC DISORDERS

The use of the plural in the heading of this section emphasizes that schizophrenia should properly be viewed as a collection of disorders with differing pathogeneses. This view is not that developed by Kraepelin, who, while acknowledging the differing clinical pictures that may arise, noted the same basic disturbances suggestive of a common underlying process. Bleuler (1911), who introduced the term schizophrenia 'to show that the split of the several psychic functions is one of its most important characteristics' (p.5), extended the range of the psychopathology, and introduced Freudian psychodynamics into his ideas. He suggested that many of the typical symptoms were determined by 'psychic' causes, and distinguished various types including primary, secondary and basic. The symptoms delineated by Kraepelin were mainly secondary, derived by a reaction of the sick mind to the illness, primary ones being directly caused by the disease process. Basic symptoms, present at all times, were alteration of affect and volition, ambivalence and autism. The theory was elaborated further, particularly by Jung, to include the idea that the psychic cause could set an organic process in motion, thus being aetiological. In addition Bleuler considerably widened the boundaries of the disorder to include personality changes and other subtle changes of mental function, atypical manias and melancholias, anergia, obstinacy and moodiness. Simple schizophrenia was added to the classification, which included many of these marginal cases, and the idea of latent schizophrenia was accepted. Bleuler's influence was profound, not only in central Europe, but also in the United States, through the writings of Adolf Meyer.

An important step was taken by Kurt Schneider. Influenced by both Kraepelin and Jaspers, he was especially concerned with symptoms, and was dissatisfied with the way that Bleuler had introduced such concepts as primary and basic ones. He introduced the terms first and second rank, quite different from the divisions of other previous writers. The first-rank symptoms, shown in Table 2, were introduced for pragmatic diagnostic use, and 'if this symptom is present in a non-organic psychosis, then we call that psychosis schizophrenia . . . the presence of first rank symptoms always signifies schizophrenia, but first rank symptoms need not always be present in schizophrenia' (Schneider, 1957, p.44).

Schneider had no presumption of a common structure for these phenomena, although he discussed them in terms of the lowering of a 'barrier' between the self and the surrounding world. Other symptoms were termed second rank, and were considered much less important for diagnosis.

The first-rank symptoms assumed importance for the diagnosis of schizophrenia, especially in the United Kingdom, and were employed widely in research, for example the PSE being biased to detect them for that diagnostic category. Their theme is taken up in a later chapter (Chapter 8), but their influence on the DSM III (see below) is clear.

The work of the various US/UK diagnostic projects which started in the 1960s emphasized the discrepancies between the diagnostic practices of British and American psychiatrists (Kendell, 1975). The hospital-based studies showed how schizophrenia was diagnosed almost twice as often in New York as in London, the opposite being the case for affective disorders. The main problem

Table 2   The first-rank symptoms of Schneider (after Schneider, 1957, p.43)

The hearing of one's thoughts spoken aloud in one's head

The hearing of voices commenting on what one is doing at the time

Voices arguing in the third person

Experiences of bodily influence

Thought withdrawal and other forms of thought interference

Thought diffusion

Delusional perception[a]

Everything in the spheres of feeling, drive and volition which the patient experiences as imposed on him or influenced by others

---

[a]An abnormal significance attached to a real perception without any cause that is understandable in rational or emotional terms.

was the disparity over the classification criteria used for schizophrenia, partly based on the differences between the Bleulerian influences in America and the emphasis on Kraepelin and Schneider in England. Videotape comparisons where then carried out in several countries, which confirmed the US–UK differences, and noted others, for example the tendency of the French to underdiagnose manic depressive illness and of the Scandanavians to use the category psychogenic psychosis.

The International Pilot Study of Schizophrenia was a transcultural investigation of 1202 patients in nine countries including Colombia, Czechoslovakia, Denmark, India, Nigeria and China in addition to the USSR, the USA and the UK (World Health Organisation, 1973). The main rating instrument was the PSE, which was acceptable to the patients and clinicians involved and was shown to possess good reliability. The symptom profiles and the rank order of the most frequent symptoms were similar across countries, and while no single symptom was present in all patients from all cultures, the conclusion was that when psychiatrists diagnose schizophrenia they have the same condition in mind. Lack of insight, delusional mood, ideas of reference, flatness of affect, auditory hallucinations and passivity experiences were commonly recorded and although first-rank symptoms were present in only one-third, when recorded they almost inevitably led to a diagnosis of schizophrenia. The Americans and Russians differed the most, having a broader concept of the condition than the others.

The ICD 9 refers to schizophrenic psychoses as a group in which there is a disturbance of the personality, distortion of thinking, delusions, a sense of outside influence, disturbed perception, an abnormal affect out of keeping with reality and autism. Thought, perception, mood, conduct and personality are all affected by the same illness, but the diagnosis was not restricted to one with a deteriorating course. The main types recognized were simple, hebephrenic, catatonic and paranoid, but latent, residual and schizoaffective types were also included.

The DSM III includes the following as essential features: the presence of certain psychotic features during the active phase of the illness; characteristic symptoms involving multiple psychological processes; deterioration from a previous level of functioning; onset before the age of 45; and duration for at least six months. The full diagnostic criteria are shown in Table 3. Thus, such vague entities as latent schizophrenia are dropped, and appear under the personality disorders in a different guise.

Illnesses of less than six months' duration are classified as schizophreniform disorder, and those after mid life as atypical psychosis. Such Schneiderian symptoms as thought broadcasting, insertion and withdrawal, and delusions of control are specifically associated with a diagnosis of schizophrenia.

Several subtypes are recognized. The disorganized type is characterized by incoherence, an inappropriate blunted affect, associated with mannerisms, social withdrawal and odd behaviour and by an absence of well-systematized delusions. This is equated with the hebephrenia of the ICD 9. In the catatonic type there is marked motor disturbance, sometimes fluctuating between the extremes of excitement and stupor. The paranoid type denotes prominent persecutory or grandiose delusions or hallucinations, with anger and sometimes violence. The undifferentiated type is for those not classified in these groups, and the residual is for patients who have a history of at least one past episode, but have minimal psychotic symptoms in the presence of continued evidence of the illness.

Missing from the DSM III criteria are the motor disorders seen in schizophrenia, which form an integral part of the syndrome, other than the catatonia. These include stereotypes, negativism, automatic behaviour, posturing and catalepsy. Further, tremors,

Table 3   DSM III diagnostic critera for a schizophrenic disorder

A. At least one of the following during a phase of the illness:
1. Bizarre delusions (content is patently absurd and has *no* possible basis in fact), such as delusions of being controlled, thought broadcasting, thought insertion or thought withdrawal
2. Somatic, grandiose, religious, nihilistic or other delusions without persecutory or jealous content
3. Delusions with persecutory or jealous content if accompanied by hallucinations of any type
4. Auditory hallucinations in which either a voice keeps up a running commentary on the individual's behaviour or thoughts, or two or more voices converse with each other
5. Auditory hallucinations on several occasions with content of more than one or two words, having no apparent relation to depression or elation
6. Incoherence, marked loosening of associations, markedly illogical thinking or marked poverty of content of speech if associated with at least one of the following:
    (a) Blunted, flat or inappropriate affect
    (b) Delusions or hallucinations
    (c) Catatonic or other grossly disorganized behaviour

B. Deterioration from a previous level of functioning in such areas as work, social relations and self-care.

C. Duration. Continuous signs of the illness for at least six months at some time during the person's life with some signs of the illness at present. The six-month period must include an active phase during which there were symptoms from A, with or without a prodromal or residual phase, as defined below.

   Prodromal phase. A clear deterioration in functioning before the active phase of the illness, not due to a disturbance in mood or to a substance use disorder and involving at least *two* of the symptoms noted below.

   Residual phase. Persistence, following the active phase of the illness, of at least *two* of the symptoms noted below, not due to a disturbance in mood or to a substance use disorder.

   Prodromal or residual symptoms
1. Social isolation or withdrawal

2. Marked impairment in role functioning as wage-earner, student or homemaker
3. Markedly peculiar behaviour (e.g. collecting garbage, talking to self in public or hoarding food)
4. Marked impairment in personal hygiene and grooming
5. Blunted, flat or inappropriate affect
6. Digressive, vague, overelaborate, circumstantial or metaphorical speech
7. Odd or bizarre ideation, or magical thinking, e.g. super-stitiousness, clairvoyance, telepathy, 'sixth sense'—'others can feel my feelings', overvalued ideas, ideas of reference
8. Unusual perceptual experiences, e.g. recurrent illusions, sensing the presence of a force or person not actually present

Examples. Six months of prodromal symptoms with one week of symptoms from A; no prodromal symptoms with six months of symptoms from A; no prodromal symptoms with two weeks of symptoms from A and six months of residual symptoms; six months of symptoms from A, apparently followed by several years of complete remission, with one week of symptoms in A in current episode.

D. The full depressive or manic syndrome (criteria A and B of major depressive or manic episode), if present, developed after any psychotic symptoms, or was brief in duration relative to the duration of the psychotic symptoms in A.

E. Onset of prodromal or active phase of the illness before the age of 45.

F. Not due to any organic mental disorder or mental retardation.

---

tics and choreoatetosis have all been identified—not as a consequence of treatment but as a part of the disorder (Trimble, 1981a). Further, the emphasis on current or recent symptoms detracts from the essential nature of schizophrenia which, in the majority of cases, pursues a chronic course. The history, typically, is of a patient, who may or may not have demonstrated early developmental language and behaviour problems, who manifests bizarre behaviour in late teens and early adulthood with a loss of academic potential. Initially a bewildering variety of psychopathological states, including anxiety states, manias and depressions, may be recorded, but eventually the longitudinal course becomes apparent and the psychotic symptoms outlined above manifest.

SCHIZOAFFECTIVE DISORDER

Both the DSM III and the ICD 9 have the category schizoaffective, a term that is a source of considerable controversy. It was first introduced by Kasanin to refer to a psychosis with an admixture of affective and schizophrenic symptoms that was precipitated by emotional stress. Sitting between the two Kraepelinian pillars of psychosis, it is not accepted by many, its very existence suggesting a return to a unitary psychosis theory. However, family and genetic data support the concept that some form of schizoaffective subtype exists, but its prognosis is related more to the affective disorders (Procci, 1976). Some use the terms schizodepressive and schizomanic to reflect this.

It may describe the same patients as those referred to as having cycloid psychosis. Leonhard, from whom the idea of bipolar and unipolar disease originated, first published his extensive *The Classification of Endogenous Psychoses* (1979) in 1957. It gave 38 different clinical illnesses, including three types of cycloid psychosis. The features are psychotic episodes which resolve completely, and are associated with confusion and perplexity, mood and motor changes, pan-anxiety and delusions.

PARANOID DISORDERS

The word paranoid has been used in psychiatry for many years, but its meaning has shifted from a general term for madness to a more precise technical expression (Lewis, 1970). Cullen used it as equivalent to vesania, but gradually it assumed the meaning of a primary delusional condition in a setting of clear consciousness. Kraepelin initially classified paranoia as a separate entity from dementia praecox: it represented the insidious development of a delusional system in the presence of an intact personality. He used the term paraphrenia to refer to those who have a paranoid illness developing later than dementia praecox. Lewis (1970), after a careful consideration of the world literature, gave the following definition: 'A paranoid syndrome is one in which there are delusions of self reference which may be concerned with persecution, grandeur, litigation, jealousy, love, envy, hate, honour, or the supernatural, and which cannot be immediately derived from a prevailing morbid mood such as mania or depression' (p.11). He felt that the adjective paranoid could be applied to a personality disorder with similar features, except that dominant ideas should replace delusions.

The ICD 9 includes several categories of paranoid states, and refers to paranoia as a rare chronic psychosis. In DSM III paranoid disorders are characterized by persistent persecutory delusions or delusional jealousy not due to any other mental disorder. This is a more restricted definition, but it does note that the boundaries between it and paranoid personality disorder and schizophrenia, paranoid type are unclear. An acute paranoid disorder, paranoia (at least six months duration) and shared paranoia may also be diagnosed.

NEUROSES

The neurotic disorders of the ICD 9 are in the main included under anxiety disorders in the DSM III, exceptions being some of the affective disorders and hysteria. Some interesting new categories are defined. In particular, panic disorder and post-traumatic stress disorder will be discussed. The word neurosis has been dropped by the DSM III because, in spite of its long history, Freud used the term both descriptively and aetiologically. As the manual is for diagnostic purposes, confusion would arise if a term implying a mechanism was incorporated.

In anxiety disorders, the predominant symptom is anxiety not associated with another psychiatric disorder. The subcategories of the DSM III are shown in Table 4. Hypochondriasis, hysteria and variants such as Briquet's syndrome (somatization disorder) are included under somatoform disorders or dissociative disorders. It can be seen from the table that there are three main subcategories: phobic disorders, anxiety states and post-traumatic stress disorder.

The phobic disorders reflect persistent and irrational fears resulting in avoidance behaviour. Phobias as such are extremely

Table 4   DSM III Anxiety disorders

Phobic disorders

    Agoraphobia with panic attacks

    Agoraphobia without panic attacks

    Social phobia

    Simple phobia

Anxiety states

    Panic disorder

    Generalized anxiety disorder

    Obsessive compulsive disorder

Post-traumatic stress disorder

    acute

    chronic or delayed

Atypical anxiety disorder

---

common, although in the majority they are not disabling. Simple phobias include fear of spiders, thunderstorms, flying, subways, needles and animals. These are usually less socially incapacitating than agoraphobia. In this condition, characterized by a fear of going into crowded places, often combined with a fear of being alone, individuals gradually restrict their activities, until, in its most florid form, they become housebound. They use many techniques to avoid going out, and if they have to venture outside it is invariably with a friend, a spouse or a dog. In one form of the disorder, panic attacks (see below) occur. These may be only on going out, or occur in places such as the supermarket, or they may arise spontaneously at home. This may be in relationship to the thought of going out, or on going near the front door, or may suddenly come on out of the blue. Associated with the agoraphobia there is often a history of an anxious personality, and a tendency to develop affective disorder. It should be noted that agoraphobic symptoms often arise in the setting of a major affective disorder, and in these cases the diagnosis is with the affective disorder.

Social phobia is a fear of embarrassment or humiliation in social situations which thus become avoided as the individual restricts social contacts. There is anticipatory anxiety at the thought of social encounters, often confined to certain situations only, such as eating or speaking in public.

Generally, simple phobias have a better prognosis than others, especially if they start in childhood. Agoraphobia, which is commoner in women, tends to come on in the third or fourth decade of life, and may be very resistant to treatment, not the least problem being the patient's reluctance to leave home to attend the clinic for consultation.

Anxiety states include generalized anxiety disorder, panic disorder and obsessive compulsive disorder. In generalized anxiety the patient has anxiety of at least one month's duration without phobic symptoms or panic attacks. The manifestations of anxiety are multiple, and affect every bodily system. Further, since anxiety is such a common symptom, and many of the symptoms are somatic, many patients with anxiety disorders are misdiagnosed and inappropriately treated, sometimes for many years. Common symptoms include palpitations, sometimes associated with anterior chest pain over the heart; dyspnoea, and a sense of choking or a feeling that the patient will not be able to take in a sufficient breath; dry mouth with unpleasant often metallic tastes and abdominal tension, sometimes associated with nausea or actual vomiting. Others are constipation or diarrhoea; retention of urine or frequency; poor concentration and memory difficulties; dizziness, vertigo, faint feelings, and, on occasions, blackouts which resemble epileptic seizures; increased muscle tone with pain, and tremor; fatigue and loss of energy; and sensory symptoms such as tingling, especially of the hands, diminished vision, or a generalized hyperacusis in which sounds are distorted and magnified, sometimes accompanied by photophobia.

On examination, patients with anxiety show sweating, often have cold extremities, and may show flushing. The resting pulse, respiration rate and blood pressure may be elevated and increased central body movement or restless hand movements with a tremor noted.

The setting up of a separate category of panic disorder in the DSM III has not won universal approval, although in clinical practice patients falling into this grouping are often seen, and readily misdiagnosed. The criteria are shown in Table 5. They stress relatively frequent episodes, of a discrete nature, of panic associated with apprehension and fear. Their paroxysmal nature, their sudden onset and the absence often of any obvious precipitating factor may readily lead to a diagnosis of epilepsy. They often resemble one form of complex partial seizure (see Chapter 10).

A variant of this is the phobic–anxiety depersonalization syndrome in which depersonalization or derealization forms a prominent part of the picture. This is a much more pervasive disorder with generalized anxiety, affective symptoms and a danger of death by suicide. In some patients, between the more extreme manifestations, the depersonalization may persist. When severe it

Table 5 DSM III diagnostic criteria for panic disorder

A. At least three panic attacks within a three-week period in circumstances other than during marked physical exertion or in a life-threatening situation. The attacks are not precipitated only by exposure to a circumscribed phobic stimulus.

B. Panic attacks are manifested by discrete periods of apprehension or fear, and at least four of the following symptoms appear during each attack:
   1. Dyspnoea
   2. Palpitations
   3. Chest pain or discomfort
   4. Choking or smothering sensations
   5. Dizziness, vertigo or unsteady feelings
   6. Feelings of unreality
   7. Paraesthesias (tingling in hands or feet)
   8. Hot and cold flushes
   9. Sweating
   10. Faintness
   11. Trembling or shaking
   12. Fear of dying, going crazy or doing something uncontrolled during an attack

C. Not due to a physical disorder or another mental disorder, such as major depression, somatization disorder or schizophrenia.

D. The disorder is not associated with agoraphobia.

---

may lead patients to feel like automata, or as if they have left their bodies, sometimes with autoscopy. The ICD 9 has a separate grouping for depersonalization syndrome, although the panic and phobias are not a feature.

Post-traumatic stress disorder is a new name for post-traumatic neurosis. This syndrome has a long and distinguished history, and is often referred to as accident neurosis, compensation neurosis or some other variant (Trimble, 1981b). Many physicians come across this in a medicolegal setting, and are familiar with the arguments over the role of financial gain in the production or prolongation of the symptoms. In spite of this being such a common disorder, and costing insurance companies and government administrations millions of pounds in compensation, it has been the subject of little research. The inclusion as a separate group in the DSM III has arisen mainly on account of the growing awareness of long-term psychiatric syndromes that developed following the Korean and Vietnam wars. Although battle neurosis, shell shock and other epithets have been used to describe this condition, American psychiatrists have been concerned in particular to emphasize the growing problem of psychopathology among war veterans, and by redefining the disorder they have succeeded in bringing it to attention (Trimble, 1985). The loss of the handle 'neurosis' will be a relief to those in the courtrooms, where any mention of the term immediately implies, quite incorrectly, malingering. The fact that the clinical picture is similar, whether it is found after a car accident, injury at work, at the battle front or following involvement in some natural disaster like an earthquake, is emphasized by the special category.

The clinical criteria as given are shown in Table 6. The distinction between acute and chronic forms has little validity in practice, and the category does not include a variety of other post-traumatic psychiatric syndromes such as post-traumatic affective disorder or hysteria. There is a requirement for a specific stressor, and the presentation with a combination of anxiety and depressive symptoms. Special emphasis is given to the reexperiencing of the trauma in day dreams, nightmares or by association with an environmental stimulus. In practice, searching for this is most important, and often holds the key to the diagnosis.

Obsessive compulsive disorder

The essential features are the obsessions—persistent ideas, thoughts or images that invade conscious experience against the

Table 6   Diagnostic criteria for post-traumatic stress disorder

---

A. Existence of a recognizable stressor that would evoke significant symptoms of distress in almost everyone.

B. Reexperiencing of the trauma as evidenced by at least one of the following:
    1. Recurrent and intrusive recollections of the event
    2. Recurrent dreams of the event
    3. Sudden acting or feeling as if the traumatic event were reoccurring, because of an association with an environmental or ideational stimulus

C. Numbing of responsiveness to or reduced involvement with the external world, beginning some time after the trauma, as shown by at least one of the following:
    1. Markedly diminished interest in one or more significant activities
    2. Feeling of detachment or estrangement from others
    3. Constricted affect

D. At least two of the following symptoms that were not present before the trauma:
    1. Hyperalertness or exaggerated startle response
    2. Sleep disturbance
    3. Guilt about surviving when others have not or about behaviour required for survival
    4. Memory impairment or trouble concentrating
    5. Avoidance of activities that arouse recollection of the traumatic event
    6. Intensification of symptoms by exposure to events that symbolize or resemble the traumatic event

---

wishes of the patient—and compulsions—repetitive purposeful motor acts. Both the obsessions and the compulsions are somehow alien to the individual (ego-dystonic) and are resisted. Often the thoughts are offensive and repugnant, and the compulsions are senseless stereotyped actions, from which no pleasure is derived, although there is often relief of tension.

Obsessive compulsive disorder is the persistence of obsessions and compulsions, in the absence of other psychiatric disorder, and, as such, is quite uncommon. The contents of the rituals most commonly found are cleaning, avoiding, repeating and checking, and some authors note that the recognition of the senselessness of the phenomena is more relevant than resistance to them (Stern and Cobb, 1978). Variants include the intrusion of vivid imaginary scenes of unacceptable events, ruminations on trivia, convictions of a magical nature (for example that to carry out one act will prevent another), fears of dirt, disease and contamination, and rituals of counting or performing certain acts in specific ways in special order. Although depressive symptoms are common, it is essential to distinguish whether this is secondary, or whether the obsessional symptoms derive from a primary affective disorder in an anankastic personality.

ORGANIC MENTAL DISORDERS

Later chapters of this book consider some of the organic disorders. The DSM III distinguishes between organic brain syndromes and organic mental disorders. The former are subdivided into six categories, namely:
1. Delirium and dementia
2. Amnestic syndrome and organic hallucinosis
3. Organic delusional syndrome and organic affective disorder
4. Organic personality syndrome
5. Intoxication and withdrawal
6. Atypical or mixed

Organic delusional states and affective syndromes are referred to in relevant sections of this book, and have great significance for biological psychiatry. They emphasize that brain dysfunction leads with regular frequency to clinical pictures identical to psychiatric syndromes seen in the absence of evidence of overt brain disease, reflecting identifiable brain–behaviour relationships.

The organic mental disorders are those dementias and deliriums, including the substance-induced acute or chronic disorders, where there is a known or presumed aetiology. Included under this section are the commoner dementias, such as Alzheimer's disease, and diagnoses such as alcoholic hallucinosis or barbiturate intoxication.

FUTURE DEVELOPMENTS

Both the DSM III and ICD 9 will be replaced in the near future. With regards to the DSM III, prior to the introduction of a DSM

IV, a DSM-R (revised DSM III) will be presented. The overall structure of a multiaxial system is the same although mental retardation and pervasive developmental disorders are moved from axis 1 to axis 2. There are minor revisions to the area of psychosis, but more substantial changes for the affective disorders and anxiety disorders. Affective disorder as a term will be replaced by mood (affective) disorders, and the criteria for melancholia eliminate some symptoms but include others, such as complete recovery from a prior episode, absence of personality disorder prior to first episode and a previous good response to somatic antidepressant therapies which have predictive validity for response to treatment.

Agoraphobia with panic attacks will be referred to as panic disorder with extensive phobic avoidance. This recognizes that phobic symptoms are a complication of panic disorder, and means that panic disorder is subclassified in relation to the degree of associated phobic avoidance:

Panic disorder with extensive phobic avoidance

Panic disorder without phobic avoidance

Panic disorder with limited phobic avoidance

The length of symptoms for diagnosis of generalized anxiety disorder will be extended to six months to exclude transient states, and the acute-chronic distinction of post-traumatic stress disorder will be removed.

While the DSM III-R is expected to be published soon, the ICD 10 may not be available and approved until 1993. It is hoped it will have a good deal of conformity with the developing DSM IV.

CONCLUSIONS

It is often thought that classification in psychiatry is an unsatisfactory exercise, and that, as a group, psychiatrists are rarely ever able to agree on a patient's diagnosis. However, one of the most interesting things noted is how some of our categories have been recognized for many centuries, and how classification has been a gradually progressive exercise. Variants of manic depressive illness and dementia have been described since Greek medicine, and the separation of such categories as schizophrenia and affective disorder has evolved after many years of thought, observation and reflection. A major problem has always been the lack of biological indices for psychiatric disorders, although the great progress with such diseases as GPI, pellagra, thyroid and other hormonal conditions cannot be underemphasized. As is noted in later chapters, this trend is continuing with the search for biochemical markers in such conditions as affective disorder, schizophrenia and Alzheimer's disease, such that the DSM IV, when it appears, may contain specific biological indicators of at least some diagnoses. However, in psychiatry, as in most other branches of medicine, we have yet to move from classification based on clinical examination and syndromes to an aetiological one.

The importance for biological psychiatry of both Kraepelin and Jaspers cannot be overemphasized. Kraepelin so clearly helped formulate the recognition of disease entities, yet his views were modifiable by experience as the successive editions of his textbook show. The separation of two main classes of psychosis, one relating to manic depressive illness and the other to dementia praecox, has moulded psychiatric thinking for the rest of this century.

Amongst the many contributions of Jaspers is the acknowledgement of a clear distinction between process and development, between disease and personality. The persisting confusion of these two separable phenomena and the failure to distinguish form from content are the main reasons for the failure of many theories in psychiatry, past and present, to endure and make sense.

The emphasis of the diagnostic classifications given in this chapter has been on the DSM III, although other schemes including the ICD 9 have been included. The DSM III is by no means perfect, yet it has influence both in America and outside. Its emphasis on clarity of the diagnostic process will sharpen the practice of psychiatry, and the use of the DSM III criteria in research will allow a comparison of data from different centres to be made more easily. The multiaxial system partially acknowledges the Jasperian division of process and personality, and the use of both inclusion and exclusion criteria highlights the different categories. However, it will also modify with experience, and the DSM IV will have important new innovations, some of which will hopefully include biological markers, cross-cultural considerations and more attention to the longitudinal development of disease patterns. At present there is no presumption of aetiology inherent in any of the groupings, which has advantages and disadvantages. Benefits include the loss of assumption that the neuroses are linked to unconscious conflict and defence mechanisms, although loss of the term neurosis itself is likely to be only a temporary respite. Its failure to include more pathological and biochemical criteria is a reflection of the uncertainty of such knowledge in psychiatry at the present time, a situation which continued progress in the specialty will overcome. Indeed, it may be hoped that in the future someone, as did Romberg, will attempt a comprehensive classification of all diseases of the nervous system based on biological principles.

CHAPTER 3

Principles of brain function and structure of relevance for psychiatry: (1) physiology and chemistry

INTRODUCTION

It has become fashionable to ascribe much psychopathology to the evils of modern society. Although, as pointed out in the last chapter, this is not a new theme, its resurgence reflects the popularity of the simple. Often imbued with political overtones, and rarely aspiring to scientific insights, such a view of the pathogenesis of psychiatric illness ignores the long tradition of both the recognition of psychopathology and its successful treatment by somatic therapies, referred to in Chapter 1. Further, it does not take into account the obvious fact that the biological heritage of mankind extends back many millions of years. In this and the next chapter, following a brief excursion into evolution, consideration is given to those aspects of the neuroanatomy and neurochemistry of the brain that seem of most importance to those studying biological psychiatry. Most emphasis is given to the limbic system and closely connected structures, since the understanding of these regions of the brain has been of fundamental importance in the development of biological psychiatry. Not only has a neurological underpinning for 'emotional disorders' been established, but much research at the present time relates to the exploration of limbic system function and dysfunction in psychopathology. Although it seems obvious that psychiatrists ought to be interested in the relationship of the brain to behaviour, and have aquaintance with the workings of that organ, it is interesting how often this is ignored both in training and in attempting to understand illness clinically. It would seem an unusual cardiologist that denied the importance of the heart for his discipline, and a dangerous one that had no interest in its structure and function, especially when the prescription of medication with specific cardiological actions was part of his practice.

Although the principle that the brain was the organ that regulated behaviour and emotion was expressed by Hippocrates, the succeeding millenia were unable to grasp this in a meaningful way, and many, even today, seem vigorously to attempt to suppress such a notion. One of the distinguishing features of psychiatry since the 1950s has been to embrace this concept and attempt to bury the Cartesian mantle which so hampered progress.

ORIGINS

It is now generally accepted that man's earliest recognizable ancestors developed in Africa, although the origins recess backwards in time with newer discoveries. One of the contenders seems to be Ramapithicus, a small ape-like creature—an early hominid which was itself the product of 250 million years of mammal and 70 million years of primate evolution. The latter diversified into at least three lineages, one leading to Homo sapiens. The dating of primitive man now stems back some four million years. The development of tool making, increased cooperation in food gathering, the change of diet to a carnivorous one and the agricultural revolution all helped to shape the developing social and biological evolution of mankind.

The first great strides forward to understanding the nature of evolution came in the last century with the writings of Darwin. His book *The Expression of Emotion in Man and Animals* (1889) documented a wide variety of emotional states, their expression and accompanying gestures, and noted the innate or inherited nature of many. Ethology, the science of the biology of behaviour, has introduced us to such concepts as critical periods, those times in ontogeny during which imprinting occurs, the latter being a specific form of learning occurring early in life, resistant to change. Innate releasing mechanisms are sensory mechanisms selectively responsive to specific environmental clues which trigger a stereotyped response, and innate behaviour patterns are those which are genetically determined, and not modified by experience. The ethologists emphasize the biological heritage of behaviour taking an evolutionary perspective. There are many ethologists who have studied the behaviour of man, and psychiatrists who have adopted an ethological approach in their work. Lorenz (1966) emphasized the role of aggression, and Ardrey (1966) that of territory in human behaviour, noting their deep-rooted biological heritage. Bowlby (1975) adopted an ethological approach to the study of infant attachment to, and separation from, parents.

Related to these endeavours are the contributions of anthropology to our understanding of human behaviour and psychiatry. In contrast to the earlier 'functionalist' anthropology of Malinowski, Levi-Strauss (1962) put forward a structuralist view of kinship and social organization, attempting to reveal an underlying order of events. He emphasized the logical properties of human thought and the similarities rather than the differences between the minds of primitive and modern man. This view, that all human behaviour and the human mind have underlying structures which can, by appropriate observation, be derived, stands in contrast to functionalism, which emphasizes psychological explanations of social phenomena. The structuralist approach, which affirms innate mental structures, also attributes to individuals an active role in the construction of their own knowledge. Further, there is an emphasis on the universal similarities among men, and little stress is laid on social differences between cultures in relation to the acquisition of behaviour and knowledge.

Such an approach gains support from the findings that the abnormal behaviour patterns defined by Western psychiatry are to be found all over the world (Foster and Anderson, 1978) and the similarity of psychopathology in many different centres as revealed in the World Health Organization (1973) studies using the PSE for semi-standardized collection of data.

Chomsky developed the structuralist theme for language. He postulated a genetically determined language faculty which specifies a 'certain class of humanly accessible grammars' (Chomsky, 1980, p.35). This view, which implies that the brain possesses innate capacities for language, and also for using knowledge, is at variance with suggestions that the child learns language by imitation of others or by a process of trial, error and reward. In Chomsky's scheme, the development of cognitive structures should be studied from the same perspective as somatic structures, attempting to understand their general properties, their place in a system of structures and their genetically determined basis. One of his most powerful pieces of evidence is the remarkable speed with which children learn language, and the incompatibility of learning theory and behaviouralism with the linguistic abilities of the child acquiring language. Interesting support for the idea that the brain possesses innate language facilities comes from the now-acknowledged lateralization of many language functions to the dominant hemisphere, and the demonstration that asymmetry of the left temporal lobe can be seen in man. Thus, Geschwind and Levitsky

(1968) noted that the left Sylvian fissure was longer in most brains and that the area between the posterior border of Heschl's gyrus (which contains the primary auditory cortex) and the posterior end of the Sylvian fissure is larger on the left. These differences are seen at post-mortem, on CT scans, and, based on endocasts, were probably present in Neanderthal man. Further, they are probably accompanied by cytoarchitectonic differences, and may be observed in the brains of closely related primates, the great apes (Le May and Geschwind, 1975).

GENETICS

Modern genetic theories are based on knowledge of the deoxy-ribonucleic acid (DNA) molecule, its spontaneous and random mutations and the recombination of its segments. DNA is composed of two intertwined strands (the double helix) of sugar–phosphate chains held together by covalent bonds linked to each other by hydrogen bonds between pairs of bases. There is always complimentary pairing between the bases such that guanine pairs with cytosine and adenine with thymine. This pairing is the basis of replication, and each strand of the DNA molecule thus forms the template for the generation of another. On the DNA strand are many specific base sequences that encode for protein construction. Thus proteins are chains of amino acids, and one amino acid is coded by a triplet sequence of bases (the codon).

In the synthesis of protein, ribonucleic acid (RNA) is an intermediary. RNA is almost identical to DNA, except that uracil replaces thymine, the sugar is ribose, and it is single stranded. Thus an RNA molecule is created with a complimentary base sequence to the DNA (messenger RNA). Transfer RNA attaches the amino acids to messenger RNA, lining up the amino acids one at a time to form the protein. The transfer RNA achieves this by having an anticodon at one end to attach to the messenger RNA and the amino acid at the other.

Much is now known regarding the various sequences of bases that form the genetic code. There are twenty amino acids that are the universal constituents of proteins, and 64 ways of ordering the bases (Wolpert, 1984). Most amino acids are represented by more than one triplet, and there are special sequences for starting and stopping the code. Although originally it was thought that the only direction of information flow was from DNA to RNA to protein, investigations with malignant cells have shown that some tumour

RNA viruses (retroviruses) may be incorporated into the host DNA.

The genetic programme is determined by DNA, and at various times in development, and in daily life, various genes will be turned on or off depending on the requirements of the organism. There is a constant interplay between the genetic apparatus and chemical constituents of the cell cytoplasm, and activation of genes by signals from such elements as hormones may not be an immediate sequence of events.

In the human cell there is one DNA molecule for each chromosome, and there are some 100 000 genomes on 46 chromosomes. These are divided into 22 pairs of autosomes and the sex chromosomes XX for females and XY for males. The genotype reflects this genetic endowment, and the phenotype is the appearance of the organism at any particular stage of development. If an individual has two identical genes at the same locus, one from each parent, then he is referred to as a homozygote; if they differ he is referred to as a heterozygote. If a heterozygote develops traits as a homozygote, then the trait is called dominant, and in medicine there are many diseases for which the genetic evidence suggests dominant inheritance. If traits are recessive then the trait will only be expressed if the gene is inherited from both parents. Dominant traits do not skip a generation, appearing in all offspring with the genotype.

Many conditions where some genetic element is suspected do not have these classical modes of inheritance, and polygenetic inheritance is suggested.

In modern genetics, restriction enzymes are used to split the DNA into base sequences which can be identified by gene probes—DNA fragments that are radioactively labelled and used to identify the presence of particular genes. Restriction fragment length polymorphisms are DNA fragments produced by the use of restriction enzymes, which differ in length between individuals. They may be used as genetic markers for inherited diseases if they are linked to a gene thought to be abnormal and responsible for that condition. Families in which several members have the condition in question are examined, and the restriction fragment length polymorphisms are probed to search for those present only in the afflicted individuals. When found, the chromosome on which the abnormal gene resides can be identified, and the linked marker, which may even be the gene itself, used to detect genotypes likely to become phenotypes.

HLA ANTIGENS

It is well known that it is difficult to transplant body tissue from one individual to another, and that there are inherent mechanisms for the recognition of self from non-self. This has stimulated much research into the mechanisms of graft rejection, and the genetic and immunological basis for it. Histocompatibility antigens were identified and consequently histocompatibility genes. Although much of the early work was done on rodents, human leucocyte antigen (HLA) was discovered in the 1950s. The HLA complex has been shown to consist of a system of closely linked genes. The association of these to many biological phenomena has been studied, including the individual's susceptibility to develop various diseases.

The HLA complex is to be found on the short arm of chromosome 6 (Zaleski *et al.*, 1983) and is classified on the basis of structure and biological products.

BRAIN CHEMISTRY AND METABOLISM

In order to function adequately, the brain requires energy which is derived from the catabolism of the food we eat. The major nutrient for the brain is glucose, which, in the process of oxidization to carbon dioxide (CO_2) and water gives up energy. This process results in the formation of adenosine triphosphate (ATP) from adenosine diphosphate (ADP). In the course of energy use through cellular transport and biosynthesis the ATP is degraded to ADP (see Figure 1).

The oxidation of one molecule of glucose generally gives 36 to 38 moles of ATP (Siesjo, 1978). It is obvious that ATP has a central role in cellular metabolism, being the product of oxidation and the substrate for further chemical reactions requiring energy. Its structure is given in Figure 2. It is composed of a nitrogenous base (adenine), a five-carbon sugar and attached phosphate groups; it is one of several triphosphonucleotides in the cell that yield energy.

As noted, the main energy requirements are those of cellular transport mechanisms and biosynthesis. The former includes the movement of both charged and uncharged particles across cell membranes and the transport of molecules intracellularly. Biosynthesis involves the formation of simple and complex moleculeswhich are required for cellular function, in addition to such energy storage molecules as glycogen.

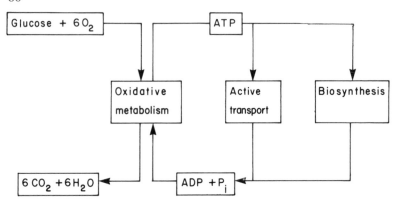

Figure 1. Showing the generation of ATP by means of oxidative metabolism with glucose as substrate. Oxidation of 1 mole of glucose yields 36–38 moles of ATP. (After Siesjo, 1978. Reproduced with permission.)

A related molecule is adenosine 3,5-monophosphate (cyclic AMP) which has one phosphate molecule and forms a ring structure with links between the sugar and phosphate molecules. It is formed from ATP in a reaction that utilizes adenyl cyclase as a catalyst. It is activated by adrenaline, and is known to be involved, via the intermediary phosphorylase, in the activation of glycogen. Further, cyclic AMP appears to act as an intermediary in many other cellular reactions, including those stimulated by hormonal or neurotransmitter stimuli (see below).

Chemical reactions in the body are facilitated by enzymes, some of which themselves are activated by coenzymes which transfer atoms or groups of atoms from one molecule to another. Since the quantity of active enzyme present is the essential ingredient that determines the rate of a biochemical reaction in the presence of appropriate substrates, activation and inhibition of enzymes regulate the metabolic activity of cells. One method of inhibition of a particular metabolic reaction is by feedback from a resulting metabolite (feedback inhibition).

THE METABOLISM OF GLUCOSE

Glucose and glycogen catabolism result in the production of ATP via the well-known tricarboxylic acid (Krebs) cycle (see Figure 3). Glucose is first phosphorylated by hexokinase to yield glucose-6-phosphate. This is converted, via the several intermediary steps of glycolysis, to lactic acid. This yields two molecules of ATP thus:

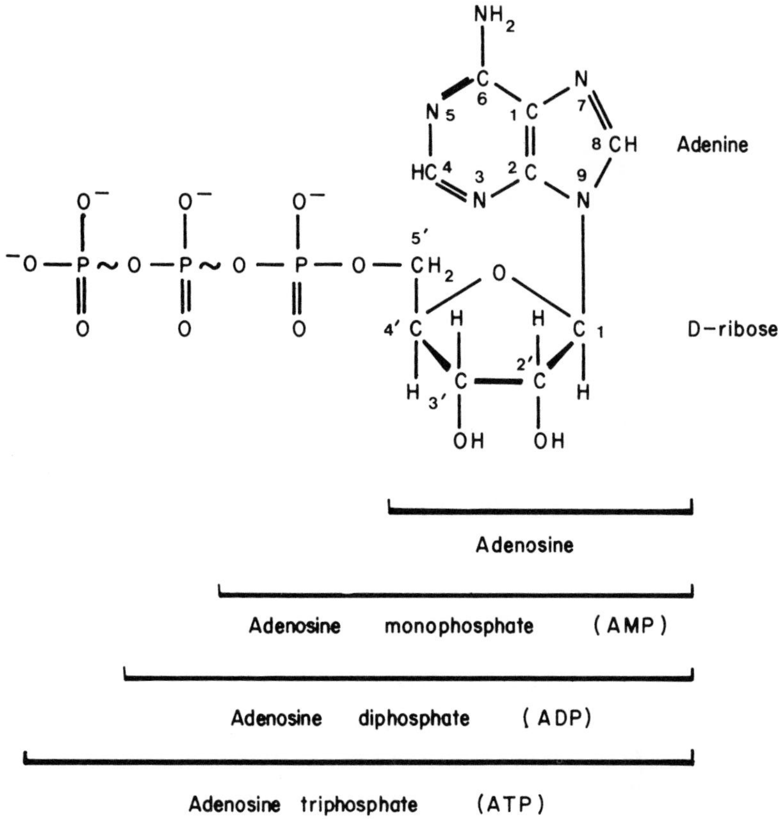

Figure 2. Structure of adenosine, and adenosine mono-, di- and triphosphate. (After Siesjo, 1978. Reproduced with permission.)

Glucose + 2 ADP + 2 phosphate → 2 lactic acid + 2 ATP
+ 2 water

Lactic acid is converted to acetyl-coenzyme A via pyruvic acid, and the former is oxidized by the tricarboxylic acid cycle to citrate and ultimately oxaloacetate, which itself is incorporated with acetyl-coenzyme A to yield citrate. Hydrogen atoms which are generated react with oxygen to form water, and further molecules of ATP are generated. Since other products of digestion undergoing catabolism also utilize the tricarboxylic acid cycle, it represents a final common path, and almost two-thirds of all energy released in the breakdown of food occurs during the reactions of this cycle.

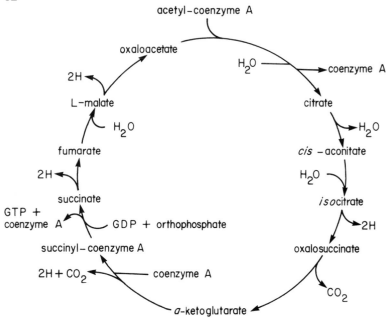

Figure 3. The tricarboxylic acid cycle

PROTEINS AND FATTY ACIDS

While glucose is the most important food involved in metabolism, proteins and fatty acids are also involved. Protein is broken down to amino acids, which can be oxidized through the tricarboxylic acid cycle. Degradation reactions common for several amino acids include deamination, in which an ammonia group is removed, transamination, in which there is exchange between amino and ketonic acids of amino and keto groups, and decarboxylation, with the giving up of a carbon dioxide radical. Only some amino acids are broken down for energy, others being involved in the synthesis of neurotransmitters, and most to the building of proteins.

There are only a limited number of amino acids in living cells, some of the most important being shown in Table 1.

Fats are hydrolysed to free fatty acids and glycerol. The fatty acids are chains of carbon atoms terminated with a carboxylic acid (—COOH) group. Glycerides are esters (compounds formed by the interaction of an acid and an alcohol) of fatty acids and glycerol, and phospholipids are esters of fatty acids and alcohol, the latter containing a phosphate group. Sphingolipids have the base sphingosine instead of glycerol, and sphingomyelines contain

Table 1 Some essential amino acids

Histidine
Arginine
Ornithine
Valine
Methionine
Lysine
Phenylalanine
Tyrosine
Tryptophan
Homocysteine
Cysteine
Glycine
Amino butyric acid

---

choline. The cerebrosides and gangliosides are sphingolipids with a hexose, and in the case of the gangliosides, a polyhydroxy amino acid. All of these are found in abundance in nerve tissue.

CELL MEMBRANES

Neurones, in common with other cells, are bounded by a membrane. It is now known that this is a continuous double structure with two electron-dense layers separated by an interzone. The thickness is approximatly 100 Å, and similar membranes are seen in the cell forming, for example, the endoplasmic reticulum or the mitochondria (see Figure 4).

They are mainly formed from lipids (whose central components are fatty acids) and proteins. One end is hydrophilic and the other hydrophobic, which align to form a structure suggested to look like that shown in Figure 5. The inside is hydrophobic, and proteins seem embedded in the structure, carrying out such functions as aiding active transport, forming the structure of receptors and enzyme activity. Channels in the membrane are thought to be protein aggregates, and they help regulate permeability. These are either active, which can be open or closed, or passive, which remain open all the time. Active channels may be influenced by various stimuli including electrical or chemical ones such as the neurotransmitters.

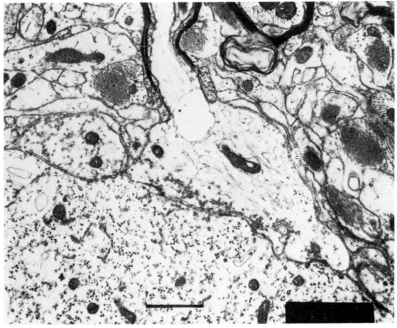

Figure 4. This shows a myelinated afferent nerve fibre synapsing onto a motor neurone. Note the flattened presynaptic vesicles; neurofibrils of the cytoskeleton and a mitochondrion in the centre. To the right is a presynaptic membrane density. (Because of the orientation of the preparation, the synaptic cleft is not shown.) (Supplied and reproduced with permission by Dr A. H. Pullen, Sobell Department of Neurophysiology, Institute of Neurology.)

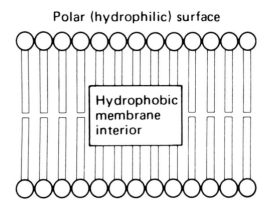

Figure 5. A schematic representation of a cell membrane. (From Shaw et al., 1982. Reproduced by permission of Butterworth & Co.)

In order that the cell is excitable a potential difference across it must exist (polarization). This membrane potential is positive on the outside and negative on the inside. It is due to electrolyte differences on the two sides of the membrane, and in most neurones is in the region of 50–60 mV. This is referred to as the resting potential, and to generate the action potential the membrane must be depolarized by alteration of the ion distribution on the two sides of the membrane.

There are four main ions in the cells: sodium (Na^+), potassium (K^+), chloride (Cl^-) and organic anion (A^-). Sodium and chloride are at lower concentrations on the inside of the cell; the other two have higher concentrations. At rest the potential is maintained by the action of the sodium pump which, at the expense of energy, forces the sodium out and draws the potassium in. The resting potential acts as the energy store of the cell, and neuronal action is dependent on it. The electrical signals of the nerve cells result from a change in the resting potential with alteration of the distribution of ions on either side of the membrane.

The action potential is generated by depolarization, during which sodium flows into the cell and, with slight delay, the potassium moves out. This process is initiated by the opening of the sodium channel, allowing sodium to flow in, a process that opens more sodium channels. Then, as sodium channels begin to close the potassium voltage-regulated gated channels begin to open and repolarization occurs. The sodium and potassium changes during the action potential are shown in Figure 6, and the resulting phases of the action potential are shown in Figure 7.

These action potentials are generated by such stimuli as synaptic transmission, and propagation of the current along the membrane proceeds as adjacent portions of the membrane become depolarized by electronic conduction. Generally the larger the diameter of the axon of the cell, the more rapid the current flow; however, in myelinated axons (see below), where the resistance at the nodes of Ranvier is low compared with that at the internodes, current travels along intracellular fluid from node to node, a process referred to as saltatory conduction. Following the action potential there is a brief refractory period during which the sodium channels are returning to their closed state.

Although the most important ions for the generation of the action potential are sodium and potassium, others exert influences such as calcium and magnesium.

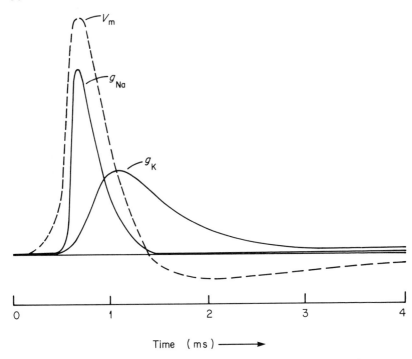

Figure 6. Showing the changes in sodium and potassium during the action potential. V_m = membrane potential signal. Reprinted by permission of the publisher from Kandel and Schwartz. Copyright (1981) by Elsevier Science Publishing Co.

SYNAPSES

The main link between one neurone and the next is via the synapse, and in the human central nervous system transmission is mainly chemical. However, it is recognized that electrical synapses occur (bridged junctions) with only small gaps (around 20 Å) separating the presynaptic and postsynaptic membranes and identifiable channels between them (Makowski *et al.*, 1977). In contrast, chemical synapses (unbridged junctions) have a larger gap (200 Å), the synaptic cleft, and specialized vesicles are identifiable in the presynaptic terminals (see Figure 8). Information flow across the electrical synapse is more rapid than across chemical junctions, although the latter are more flexible.

Postsynaptic potentials are either inhibitory (IPPS) or excitatory(EPPS). The former prevent the initial area of the axon from reaching the threshold required to generate an action potential (hyperpolarization) by increasing the influx of potassium and chloride. These IPSPs can summate either temporally or spatially, and

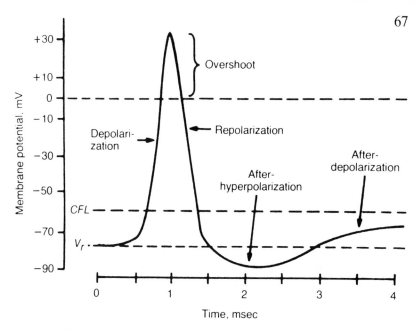

Figure 7. Showing the action potential and its phases. V_r = resting membrane potential, CFL = critical firing level. (From Mann, 1981. Reproduced by permission of Harper & Row.)

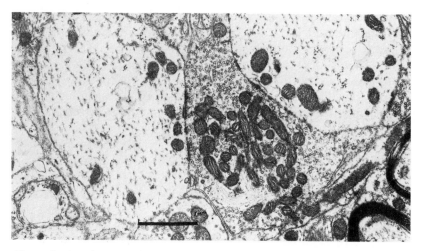

Figure 8. An electron micrograph of a synapse. (See also Figure 4.) Note the mitochondria in the centre. Pre- and postsynaptic membrane densities can be seen with a synaptic cleft in between. (Supplied with permission from Dr A. H. Pullen, Sobell Department of Neurophysiology, Institute of Neurology.)

interact with EPSPs to determine the ultimate excitability of the postsynaptic cell. The EPSP results from an influx of sodium via chemically gated channels, and the spike discharge is generated not at the postsynaptic membrane, but at the axon hillock which has a low electrical threshold (see Figure 9).

In addition to these postsynaptic events, presynaptic factors which control transmitter release also affect postsynaptic activity. These include presynaptic inhibition or facilitation via activity in synapses on the presynaptic boutons (axo-axonic synapses) and ionic influences such as calcium (Ca^{2+}) influx. The presynaptic terminals come from interneurones, and they provoke an EPSP or IPSP in the terminal of the afferent nerve fibre. In the case of inhibition, this partial depolarization reduces the amplitude of the oncoming afferent action potential. Since the transmitter release is proportional to the amplitude of the action potential, less transmitter is released and a smaller EPSP results in the postsynaptic cell. Although first discovered in relation to spinal cord afferents (Frank and Fuortes, 1957), this form of inhibition has been shown to exist in many CNS areas. Varieties of presynaptic connections are shown in Figure 10. Where the neurone has receptors to its own transmitter on these terminals they are called autoreceptors.

Calcium has been shown to be essential for transmitter release (del Castillo and Katz, 1954). During depolarization of the presynaptic terminal the calcium channels open and calcium moves into the cell. This allows the presynaptic vesicles that contain neurotransmitters to bind to releasing sites on the postsynaptic membrane (Katz and Milendi, 1967). Control of calcium currents by presynaptic receptors is thought to be an important mechanism of their action.

RECEPTORS

In recent years much attention has been paid to the structure and function of receptors. These are proteins to which transmitters bind, and are located on the outer surface of the cell membranes. A variety of receptors have been characterized, and they can be identified experimentally by the binding of specific agents. As a general model it is thought that there are two components to the receptor, the binding component and the ionophore (Schwartz, 1981). The neurotransmitter is thought to bind to form a transmitter–receptor complex, which changes its conformation, opening

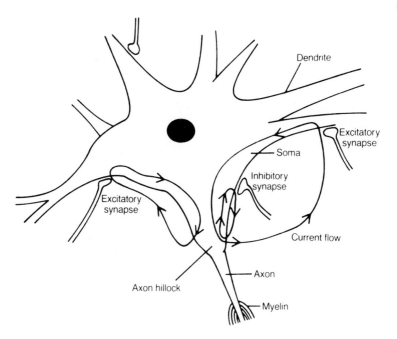

Figure 9. Showing current flow at synapses. The spike is thought to be initiated at the axon hillock. (From Mann, 1981. Reproduced by permission of Harper & Row.)

up the ionophore and allowing ion exchange to occur with consequent changes of the membrane potential. Some ionophores are specific for chloride or sodium, others are less selective. This mode

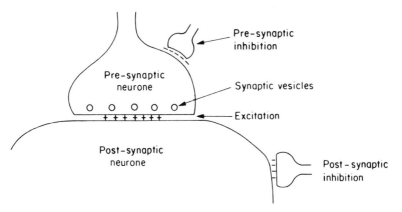

Figure 10. Showing pre- and postsynaptic neurones, and the synaptic cleft schematically. (From Trimble, 1981a. Reproduced with permission.)

of action is only one mechanism of receptor activity. An alternative is by interaction of the transmitter and receptor to provoke alteration of intraceluar metabolism by the stimulation of second messengers. Specifically adenylate cyclase is activated, producing cyclic AMP. This in turn activates a protein kinase, and hence a protein. This is thought to occur with such neurotransmitters as adrenaline, noradrenaline, dopamine, serotonin, histamine and substance P. Gamma amino butyric acid (GABA), glutamate and aspartate probably act by changing ionophore configuration, and acetyl choline employs both (Mann, 1981).

The intricacies of the second messenger system have been worked out in more detail (see Sulser, 1984). This involves an intermediary, G protein (nucleotide regulatory protein) which has binding sites for guanine nucleotides and which binds with the transmitter–receptor complex. A GTP binding site is exposed on the G protein and displacement of GDP by GTP alters the conformation of the G protein. It dissociates from the activated receptor to reveal an adenylate cyclase binding site. G protein now links with the adenylate cyclase, activating the cyclase and leading to cyclic AMP formation. The G protein then returns to its original state, inactivating the adenylate cyclase, and with dissociation of the transmitter the receptor also resumes its original state. An important feature of this system is the amplification whereby each activated receptor protein stimulates many molecules of G protein, which in turn activate many molecules of adenylate cyclase, each one further generating many cyclic AMP molecules. The resulting protein kinase activates enzymes, including membrane phosphorylases which influence the permeability of the neuronal membrane to ions, and thus alters its responsiveness. Some of these steps are outlined in Figure 11 (a) and (b).

In addition to the action of cyclic AMP in the phosphorylation of proteins, calcium is also involved as a second messenger since some adenylate cyclase is dependent on calcium for its action. A calcium binding protein, calmodulin, appears to mediate calcium-dependent events including the phosphorylation of protein and release of neurotransmitters from synaptic vesicles.

At the present time many different receptors have been classified and subclassified, although there is not universal agreement. It should be noted that, when receptor binding studies are presented, usually either receptor agonist affinity or receptor number are referred to. Receptor reactivity, a third but crucial variable, is

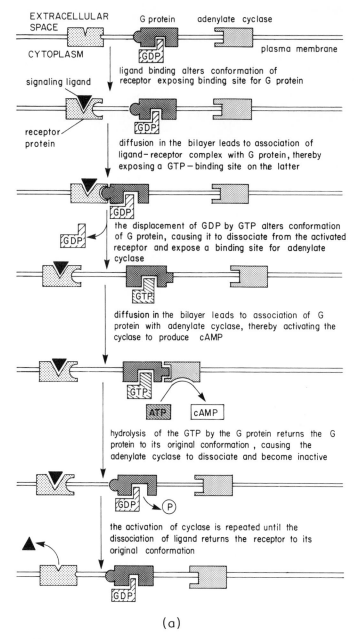

Figure 11(a). A proposed model of receptor and a secondary messenger system. A key feature is the amplification. The activation of the cyclase and production of cyclic AMP are outlined. (From Sulser, 1984. Reproduced with permission.)

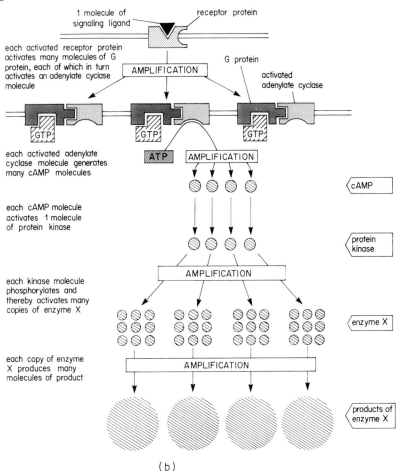

Figure 11(b). A proposed model of receptor and a secondary messenger system. The amplification is presented. (From Sulser, 1984. Reproduced with permission.)

poorly investigated owing to the limitations of in vivo techniques. Some of the more relevant ones for psychiatry are now presented.

Dopamine

There is great controversy over the number of and siting of dopamine receptors. Reflective of similar arguments that clinicians have over the classification of depression or schizophrenia, the number of subtypes of the dopamine receptor varies from one to seven or more. Generally, however, there is agreement that there are at least two, one of which acts through the adenylate cyclase system (see Table 2).

The D-2 receptors are labelled by butyrophenones, and are the only class found in the pituitary. They are adenylate cyclase independent and found in abundance in the striatum. Here they are postsynaptic to dopamine terminals. All the behavioural and antipsychotic effects of dopamine can be explained through action of the D-2 receptor. D-1 receptors are also found in the striatum, but also occur in the substantia nigra. Sulpiride and related drugs seem to be relatively specific D-2 antagonists.

The situation is confused further by the use of terms such as excitatory and inhibitory dopamine receptors (Cools, 1981), and the postulated existence of D-3 and D-4 receptors, not linked to adenyate cyclase and possessing different pharmacological properties to the D-2 receptor (Creese, 1982). In some terminologies, the D-3 receptor is presynaptic.

Table 2   Different classes of dopamine receptors

	D-1	D-2
Agonist affinity	Low	High
Butyrophenone affinity	Low	High
Adenylate cyclase	Stimulation	?Inhibition
Location	Striatum	Striatum, pituitary
Functions	Release of parathyroid hormone	Inhibits pituitary hormone release; dopamine mediated behaviour
Antagonists	Thioxanthines, butyrophenones	Thioxanthines, sulpiride

Adrenoceptors

In the same way that dopamine receptors can be subdivided, so can those for several other neurotransmitters. The adrenoceptors are divided into alpha-1, alpha-2, beta-1 and beta-2 subgroups. Alpha-1 receptors are postsynaptic, and alpha-2 are both post- and presynaptic. At the presynaptic location they are involved in noradrenaline release, and their postsynaptic role is undetermined. Relatively selective agonists and antagonists have been defined for all subtypes (see Table 3). The beta receptors are associated with adenylate cyclase, while alpha receptors are not. The beta-1 receptors are predominant in the cortex, limbic forebrain and striatum, while the cerebellum has almost exclusively beta-2 receptors (Nahorski, 1981).

Serotonin (5-HT)

Two serotonin receptors are now recognized: 5-HT$_1$ and 5-HT$_2$. They are labelled by radioactive serotonin. However, three subtypes of the 5-HT$_1$ receptor have been defined, referred to as A,B and C respectively, which are identified by different ligands (a compound that binds selectively to a receptor which can be, but does not have to be, the relevant neurotransmitter). The 5-HT$_2$ receptors are labelled by such substances as radioactive ketanserin, the serotonin antagonist, and spiperone, and are thought to be more involved with some of the behavioural effects of serotonin (Leysen, 1984). In addition to being present in brain, especially the frontal cortex, they are present on platelets.

Table 3   Agonists and antagonists of adrenoceptors

	Alpha-1	Alpha-2	Beta-1	Beta-2
Agonists	Adrenaline Noradrenaline Methoxamine Phenylephrine	Adrenaline Clonidine	Adrenaline Isoprenaline Noradrenaline	Adrenaline Isoprenaline Salbutamol Terbutaline
Antagonists	Phenoxybenzamine Phentolamine Prazosin	Yohimibine	Practolol Atenolol Metoprolol Propranolol	Propranolol

GABA

The GABA receptor has been shown to be closely associated with the benzodiazepine receptor. A proposed model is shown in Figure 12 (Braestrup and Nielsen, 1982). The molecular complex floats in the lipid plasma membrane, and when activated the chloride channels are opened. GABA and chloride seem to interact with the benzodiazepine binding sites, enhancing the benzodiazepine binding (Iversen, 1983). GABA-A and GABA-B sites have now been identified (Bowery *et al.*, 1984). The former have bicuculline and picrotoxin as antagonists, enhance the binding of benzodiazepines and barbiturates and link to chloride channels. GABA-B receptors are selectively activated by baclofen, may decrease the inflow of calcium, but are not linked to the benzodiazepine receptor. In many brain regions both receptor subtypes are found, such as in the cortex, although in others, for example the interpeduncular nucleus, the greatest concentration is of GABA-B (Bowery *et al.*, 1984).

Other receptors

Many other receptors have been identified in the central nervous system, although their functional significance is in some cases unknown. One particularly important group is peptide, especially

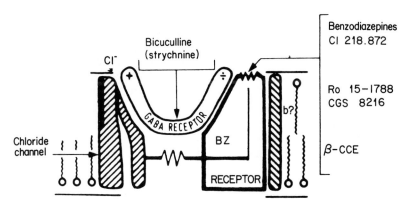

Figure 12. A proposed model of the GABA-benzodiazepine receptor. The GABA-activated chloride channel floats in the lipid-plasma membrane. (From Braestrup and Nielsen, 1982. Reproduced by permission of *The Lancet*.)

endorphin, receptors. At least five opiate receptor subtypes have been identified, mu, delta, kappa, epsilon and sigma, as have receptors for encephalins, substance P, prolactin and other peptide and non-peptide neurohormones such as steroids. Histamine receptors, with two subtypes H-1 and H-2, adenosine receptors, acetylcholine nicotinic (for which D-tubocurarine is an antagonist) and muscarinic (atropine is the main antagonist) subtypes, and even receptors for imipramine are described.

NEURONES

The main types of cells in the central nervous system are the neurones and the glial cells. The neurone has dendrites, an axon, the soma or cell body, and sites for synapses (see Figure 13). Essential metabolic molecules are synthesized in the soma and transported to other regions of the neurone. The difficulty of moving products down the long axon is accomplished by a microtubular system composed of a protein called tubulin. The larger axons are surrounded by a myelin sheath which aids the speed of electrical conduction.

The glial cells vastly outnumber the neurones, and while they play a structural supportive role, they are also involved in metabolic processes and the manufacture of myelin. Five types are identified: astrocytes, oligodendrocytes, microglia, Schwann cells and ependyma cells which line the inner surface of the brain.

The synaptic region of the neurone is highly specialized for the storage and release of neurotransmitters. The latter are contained in storage vesicles along with ATP and proteins, and are here protected from breakdown from intracytoplasmic degradation enzymes. Release of the transmitter into the synaptic cleft is by exocytosis, and quanta of transmitter are shed into the synaptic cleft. This process requires calcium, which interacts with presynaptic release areas facilitating fusion between the vesicle and cell membranes. The interaction of transmitter with receptors then takes place, and IPSP or EPSP are generated. The synaptic contacts can be to an opposing soma (axo-somatic), dendrite (axo-dendritic) or axon (axo-axonic), and the position of contact has relevance for the postsynaptic effect: the nearer to the axon hillock the greater the effect.

NEUROTRANSMITTERS

Several years ago, a section on neurotransmitters would be short, and contain reference to only a few substances known to be

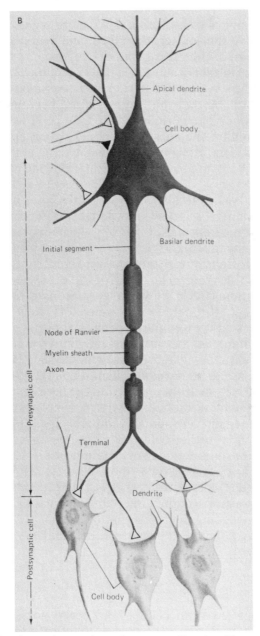

Figure 13. Showing various regions of neurones. Reprinted by permission of the publisher from Kandel and Schwartz. Copyright 1981 by Elsevier Science Publishing Co., Inc.

involved in chemical transmission. Now there are many transmitters and putative transmitters described, and the potential for the future expansion of the list is great.

A neurotransmitter is a substance that is manufactured by a cell, released into the synaptic cleft in response to stimulation and has a specific effect on another cell. In the central nervous system this cell is a neurone, but peripherally it may be a secretory cell. Further, to qualify, the substance should, when applied experimentally, mimic the effect of the natural release, and some mechanism should be available to remove it from the synaptic cleft (Schwartz, 1981).

Although it was generally understood that one neurone used only one transmitter, it is now known that two transmitters can be identified in some neurones, especially the coexistence of a peptide and an amine together (see below). Further, while the criteria given for neurotransmitter status have been identified, the situation is not so discrete. Thus it is possible to see all levels of chemical communication between cells from direct neurone–neurone contact, through to neurosecretory cells that release neurohormones either into the hypophyseal portal system which influences pituitary cell output or directly into the circulation via the posterior pituitary gland (neurohypophysis). Receptors for some neurotransmitters have been identified in the brain, and the possibility of feedback from release into the peripheral circulation exists. Finally, as in the autonomic system, neurones make contact with adrenal medulla cells, directly influencing hormonal output.

The situation is further complicated by the concept of neuromodulators. Thus, the action of neurotransmitters is considered to be brief and to operate over a short distance. However, some neurotransmitter candidates, especially the peptides, lead to longer alterations of synaptic tone, thus modulating the environment of other ongoing neurotransmitter events.

Of the many potential transmitters, the synthesis of a few key ones is described.

Acetylcholine

This is synthesized from choline and acetyl coenzyme A, the reaction being catalysed by choline acetyltransferase. Following release into the synaptic cleft, it is broken down by acetylcholinesterase. It is the main transmitter used by motor neurones in the spinal cord and is the transmitter for all preganglionic autonomic neurones and for postganglionic parasympathetic neurones. In the central nervous system it is found in high concentration in the caudate nucleus and hippocampus, and an ascending cholinergic system has been defined innervating the thalamus, the striatum, the cerebellum, the limbic system and the cerebral cortex.

GABA

GABA is synthesized from L-glutamate utilizing the enzyme glutamate decarboxylase (GAD). It is metabolized by GABA transaminase to glutamic acid and succinic semialdehyde, which, following oxidation, enters the citric acid cycle. The highest concentrations of GABA are in the substantia nigra, the globus pallidus, hippocampus and the hypothalamus. In the spinal column it is in the spinal grey matter. It is an inhibitory transmitter, and antagonists such as bicuculline provoke convulsions. It is one of a group of amino acid transmitters that have a ubiquitous distribution, some of which serve as substrates in metabolic cycles. These include glycine, beta-alanine, glutamate and aspartate. Glycine is thought to be an inhibitory transmitter in spinal cord interneurones, while glutamate and aspartate are excitatory.

Serotonin (5-HT)

This is one of the amine neurotransmitters; others include dopamine and noradrenaline. It is synthesized from tryptophan under the influence of the enzyme tryptophan hydrolase, which converts it to 5-hydroxytryptophan. This is decarboxylated to serotonin. It is metabolized to 5-hydroxyindole acetic acid (5-HIAA) by the enzyme monoamine oxidase.

The main nucleus containing serotonin is the raphe nucleus of the brainstem, from which fibres ascend and descend to influence many areas of the brain, especially the neocortex, limbic system, thalamus and hypothalamus.

Catecholamines

These are metabolized from tyrosine. Conversion to DOPA occurs under the influence of tyrosine hydrolase. DOPA is then decarboxylated to dopamine. In the presence of dopamine-beta hydrolase this is converted to noradrenaline. In a few areas, N-methylation of the latter results in adrenaline.

Breakdown involves two main enzyme systems: monoamine oxidase and catechol-O-methyl transferase. The former acts mainly intraneuronally, the latter in the synaptic cleft. The main metabolite of dopamine is homovanilic acid (HVA), while noradrenaline breaks down to vanillomandelic acid (VMA) and methoxyhydroxyphenylglycol (MHPG).

Noradrenaline is the transmitter at postganglionic sympathetic neurones, but in the brain the main synthesizing neurones are in the brainstem, in the locus coeruleus and related nuclei. The ascending neurones terminate widely to influence cerebral cortex, limbic system and hypothalamus. Dopamine derives from nuclei in the brainstem, but its output is more restricted than noradrenaline or serotonin. In particular, it involves the striatum and limbic system. It is of interest that the cortical dopamine projections in primates suggest a functional specialization. The major influences are motor rather than sensory; sensory association areas more than primary regions; and auditory association over visual association areas (Lewis, 1986).

Peptides

In recent years a large number of peptides have been recognized that may have a central role, either as neurotransmitters or as neuromodulators. A list of these is given in Table 4, although at present the evidence that many are actually transmitters awaits confirmation. Most peptides are formed by cleavage of larger precursors and a family tree can be constructed as in Figure 14.

An interesting feature of the peptides is their wide distribution throughout the body, identical ones being found, for example, in the gut and the brain. These include cholecystokinin, vasoactive intestinal peptide (VIP) and gastrin. In view of their increasing importance, some are described in more detail (Snyder, 1980).

Enkephalins

These were the first morphine-like (endorphin) substances to be discovered in the brain, being penta peptides. They were shown to possess opiate-like activity, along with other peptides such as beta-endorphin and dynorphin. Enkephalin neurones and opiate receptors have been identified in the limbic system and striatum, and

(a)

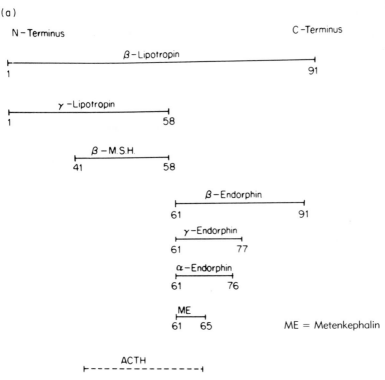

(b)

Tyrosine − Glycine − Glycine − Phenylalanine − Methionine

Figure 14. (a) Beta-lipoprotein and some peptide derivatives. (b) Amino acid sequence of metenkephalin.

receptors in such areas as the hippocampus, nucleus accumbens, thalamus and amygdala. They occur in several areas of the spinal cord including the substantia gelatinosa. Beta-endorpin distribution is more restricted, the highest concentration being in the pituitary, which structure is almost devoid of enkephalins. Mu receptors are more related to sensory events, being found in cerebral cortex, whereas the limbic system has an abundance of delta receptors.

Neurotensin

This is found in high concentrations in the hypothalamus, basal ganglia and the amygdala. It inhibits neuronal firing in the locus coeruleus, where neurotensin is abundant. Receptor sites in the brain are widespread.

Substance P

This occurs in dorsal root ganglia with terminals in the substantia gelatinosa, a region of the spinal cord thought to be involved in the pain pathways. It is found in high concentrations in the striatal–nigral system, the habenula, the amygdala and the bed nucleus of the stria terminalis.

Cholecystokinin

This is found in high concentrations in the cortex, this and VIP being brain peptides well represented with cells in the cortex. It is found in the hypothalamus, and terminals are in the amygdala. It also is seen in the periaqueductal grey region and, like substance P, in the dorsal root ganglia cells.

VIP

Highest levels are found in the cerebral cortex, and terminals containing it are identified in the amygdala and the hypothalamus.

Table 4   Potential peptide neurotransmitters

ACTH	Liprotropin
Angiotensin	LHRH
Bombesin	Alpha-MSH
Bradykinin	Motilin
Calcitonin	Neuropetide Y
Carnosine	Neurotensin
CCK (cholecystokinin)	Oxytocin
Dynorphin	Prolactin
Beta-endorphin	Secretin
Met-enkephalin	Somatostatin
Leu-enkephalin	Substance P
Gastrin	TRH
Glucagon	Vasopressin
Growth hormone	VIP
Insulin	

In the body it has several functions including vasodilation and enhancing lipolysis and pancreatic secretion.

Angiotensin

This has for some time been known to be involved in vasoconstriction and sodium regulation by the kidney. It is found centrally in several regions including the hypothalamus, and many angiotensin receptor sites have been identified. Complimenting its peripheral action, it is involved in the central regulation of drinking.

Releasing factors

These are found in the median eminence of the hypothalamus, and pass through the portal capillaries to influence hormonal release from the anterior pituitary. They include thyrotropin releasing hormone (TRH), a tripeptide, the majority of which is found outside the hypothalamus. Somatostatin inhibits growth hormone release, and is found in the amygdala, hippocampus and cortex, with terminals in these sites and in the striatum. Luteinizing hormone-releasing factor (LHRH) stimulates LH and FSH release, and is found primarily in the hypothalamus.

Other central peptides

The posterior pituitary hormones oxytocin and vasopressin seem to have a central role with pathways projecting to some brainstem and limbic system structures. Adrenocorticotrophic hormone (ACTH) is found throughout the brain, especially in the hypothalamus, thalamus, periaqueductal grey and reticular formation.

Some of the differences between the peptide transmitters and the more classical ones are summarized by Hokfelt *et al.* (1980) and shown in Figure 15. In particular, peptides are produced in the cell soma and not synthesized at synaptosomes as are other transmitters, and there are no re-uptake mechanisms back from the synaptic cleft. This may be compensated for by their effective action at much lower concentrations, their more prolonged action and intermittent rather than tonic release.

INTERRELATIONSHIPS AMOUNG TRANSMITTERS

Dale's principle, namely that one neurone synthesizes and releases only one neurotransmitter, has had to be modified in the light of

84

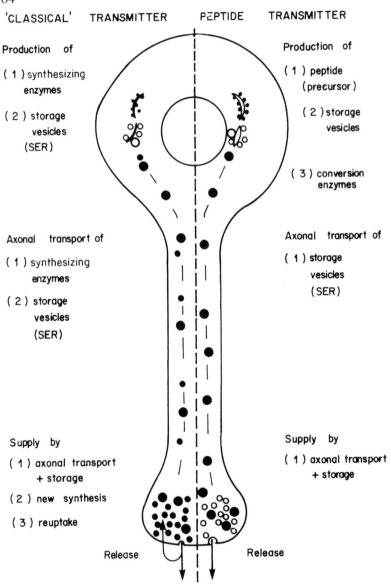

'CLASSICAL' TRANSMITTER   PEPTIDE   TRANSMITTER

Production   of

(1) synthesizing
      enzymes

(2) storage
      vesicles
      (SER)

Production   of

(1) peptide
      (precursor)

(2) storage
      vesicles

(3) conversion
      enzymes

Axonal   transport of

(1) synthesizing
      enzymes

(2) storage
      vesicles
      (SER)

Axonal   transport of

(1) storage
      vesicles
      (SER)

Supply   by

(1) axonal transport
      + storage

(2) new synthesis

(3) reuptake

Supply   by

(1) axonal transport
      + storage

Release   Release

Figure 15. Some differences between peptides and classical transmitters. (Reprinted by permission from Hokfelt *et al.*, *Nature*, **284**, p.516. Copyright © 1980 Macmillan Journals Limited.)

recent data. Although it has been known for some time that certain neurones probably released both acetylcholine and noradrenaline, the coexistence of peptides and other neurotransmitters has been reported for several neurone groups. A list is shown in Table 5. However, not all neurones possessing one classical transmitter contain the same peptide, and vice versa. The functional significance of such arrangements has been a matter of speculation. For example, in one group of neurones from sympathetic ganglia involved in sweat gland secretion, both acetylcholine and VIP are present (Hokfelt *et al.*, 1980). It is suggested that the VIP may be the mediator of vasodilation aiding the acetylcholine primed secretion. A further example is the coexistence of CCK in a subpopulation of dopamine neurones. These are mainly in the substantia nigra and related ventral tegmental area (VTA), and project to the limbic forebrain (Hokfelt *et al.*, 1980).

Other examples of interaction include the influence of monoamine release by peptides, such as the association between substance P and dopamine, the former acting as an excitatory transmitter for some dopamine neurones (Iversen and Iversen, 1981), or peptides interacting with peptides as in the case of opiate receptors located on substance P terminals.

TRANSMITTER DISPERSAL

Following interaction with the postsynaptic cell, transmitters are either broken down by enzyme systems in the synaptic cleft or

Table 5   The coexistence of classical and peptide transmitters

Transmitter	Peptide	Location
Dopamine	Enkephalin	Carotid body
Dopamine	CCK	Ventral tegmental area
Noradrenaline	Somatostatin	Adrenal medulla
Noradrenaline	Enkephalin	Adrenal medulla
Noradrenaline	Neurotensin	Adrenal medulla
Serotonin	Substance P	Medulla oblongata
Serotonin	TRH	Medulla oblongata
Adrenaline	Enkephalin	Adrenal medulla
Acetylcholine	VIP	Autonomic ganglia, sweat glands

taken back up by the neurone for degradation or re-use. Some are lost by simple diffusion away from the cell. The intracellular enzymes, monoamine oxidase and catechol-O-methyl transferase are of importance for the amine transmitters, and the major extra-cellular mechanism for the degradation of acetylcholine is acetylcholinesterase.

CHAPTER 4

Principles of brain function and structure of relevance for psychiatry: (2) anatomy

INTRODUCTION

Understanding of brain structure and interrelationships between different brain regions has expanded a great deal in the past few years. This progress has stemmed from a renewed interest in brain–behaviour relationships from psychiatrists, neurologists and behavioural psychologists, and the advancement of techniques for staining neurones and fibre tracts. The latter endeavour has essentially resulted in the emergence of an entirely new map of the brain, and a multitude of neuronal interrelationships are now known which forms a basis for speculation about and correlation with behavioural repertoirs.

It is not intended here to cover these developments completely, and this chapter concentrates on those areas of most importance to biological psychiatry. In particular, it covers the limbic system, the basal ganglia and the thalamic connections. In essence the behavioural correlates relate to the control of emotion, motor behaviour and sensation respectively, although frontal, parietal and related cortex are referred to in relevant sections.

It should be understood that it is not the intention to suggest that these various systems, including the limbic system, somehow act independently and are separate from the rest of the brain. The failure of theories of strict localization of function to adequately explain behaviour, especially with regard to psychiatry, has already been mentioned, and to renew localization theories with respect to 'systems' would also likely fail. In action the brain is holistic, and any suggestion that one function is discretely localized to a single locus or group of neurones does not make sense. To repeat, it may be possible and is clinically helpful to localize lesions, but not functions. This is not to deny that there are regions of maximum vulnerability within the brain, disruption of which provokes or obliterates certain behaviour patterns, and it is in this context that the various systems described here are discussed.

THE LIMBIC SYSTEM

Willis, in his *Cerebri Anatome*, referred to an area of the brain around the brainstem as the cerebri limbus, and Broca (1878) defined the comparative anatomy of a region of cerebral cortex which included the hippocampus and parahippocampal gyrus, sub-callosal gyrus and cingulate gyrus as 'le grand lobe limbique'. Although primarily an anatomical definition, he noted the close connection of this to the olfactory apparatus, which led to the adoption of the term rhinencephalon. This name, and the association with olfaction, remained in use until the mid part of this century when the concept of the limbic system was elaborated in the writings of Papez (1937), Yakovlev (1948) and MacLean (1970). Papez laid down a neurological substrate for the emotions, and defined the so-called Papez circuit. This was composed of the neuronal elements shown in Figure 1. He drew attention to the activities of the medial cortex, with the hippocampus and cingulate cortex participating in hypothalamic activity, contrasting this with the general sensory activities of the lateral cortex linking with the dorsal thalamus.

Yakovlev and Maclean adopted an evolutionary perspective to the development of both behaviour and its neural representations. Yakovlev noted how the behaviour of vertebrates differentiated into three spheres of movements, namely visceral motility, the motility of the outward expression of internal states and the motility of effectuation, that is the animal impressing itself upon the world, creating change in the world. These behaviours had neuroanatomical correlates as the neuroaxis developed from a cylindrical hollow to a three-tiered system. The innermost system was composed of diffuse short neurones which integrated the energy needs of the organism and maintained homeostasis. The intermediate system, which included limbic structures, was more external, more myelinated and more clearly differentiated into nuclear areas. This integrated axial and essentially postural motility of the outward expression of emotional states. The most exterior system, appearing only in mammals, consisted of well-myelinated neurones with cells of origin in the cerebral cortex which connect with long axons to the anterior horn cells of the spinal cord. Yakovlev commented: 'The intrinsic synaptic surface of the neuroaxis and the behaviour of vertebrates and man evolve thus from within outward as a stereodynamic unity' (p.329).

MacLean reemphasized the development of limbic structures in mammals, and the associated behaviour changes. Thus reptiles

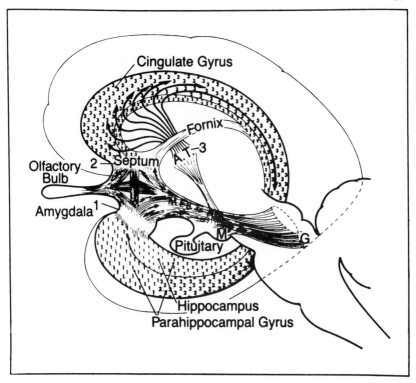

Figure 1. An anatomic framework for considering functions of three main sub-divisions of limbic system. Cortical sectors of three divisions are indicated by overlying small numerals, while associated nuclear groups are correspondingly identified by large numerals. AT = anterior thalamic nuclei; G = tegmental nuclei of Gudden; HYP = hypothalamus; M = mammillary bodies; MFB = medial forebrain bundle. (From MacLean, 1970. Reproduced with permission.)

have large olfactory bulbs and long narrow hemispheres, but the 'limbic lobe' is found in mammals. It has a common structure and is divided into two, the archicortex, so called because it is the first type of cortex to differentiate, and the mesocortex, which is intermediate in structure between the archicortex and neocortex. These non-neocortical areas of cortex are collectively referred to as allocortex. In man, on account of the migration of the temporal lobes posteriorly, inferiorly and then anteriorly, and the large increase in size of the corpus callosum, much of the archicortex lies folded and buried in the medial temporal lobe in the hippocampus. In contrast to the neocortrex, the limbic cortex has rich connections with the hypothalamus and the central grey regions of the midbrain, and, further, the limbic system structures all show a low seizure threshold.

The structures that comprise the limbic system vary, depending on the literature source. MacLean stressed the common link to the hypothalamus, and included the hippocampal formation, the amygdala, the septum, the habenula, some thalamic nuclei, parts of the basal ganglia and the gyrus fornicatus (gyrus cinguli, retrosplenial cortex and the parahippocampal gyrus). Further included were the large interconnecting pathways such as the medial forebrain bundle (MFB), stria terminalis, fornix and the mammillothalamic tract (see Figure 1 and Table 1).

Table 1   A list of limbic system structure (from Trimble, 1981a)

Gyri: Subcollosal G	Nuclei: Amygdaloid N
Cingulate G	Septal N
Parahippocampal G	Hypothalamic N
Hippocampal	Epithalamic N
formation	Anterior thalamic N
Dentate G	Mammillary bodies
Indusium griseum	Habenula
Subiculum	Raphe N
Entorhinal area	Ventral tegmental
Prepiriform cortex	area
Olfactory tubercle	Dorsal tegmental N
	Superior central N

Pathways: Fornix
Mammillothalamic tract
Mammillotegmental tract
Stria terminalis
Stria medullaris
Cingulum
Anterior commissure
Medial forebrain bundle
Lateral and medial longitudinal striae
Dorsal longitudinal fasciculus

The inclusion of other structures has been discussed further by Nauta and Domesick (1982). Thus the posterior orbitofrontal cortex and the temporal pole, which project to the amygdala and hippocampus, may be included, as may some subcortical structures linked by reciprocal pathways. These include the nucleus accumbens, a striatal element, and such midbrain structures as the ventral tegmental area (VTA) and the interpeduncular nucleus. The inclusion of the latter has led to the designation of a midbrain limbic area, the mesolimbic system. These, and other realignments to the original anatomical definitions of the limbic system, have arisen in part from the extensive developments of new methods of anatomical research, including newer staining techniques, immunofluorescence using monoclonal antibodies specific for various neurochemicals, autoradiographic tracing methods and the ability to label cell bodies retrogradely with horseradish peroxidase. The latter is injected into a structure, absorbed by the axons, and travels retrogradely towards cell bodies and is identified after death by special staining. In autoradiographic tracing, tritiated labelled amino acids are injected into the neural structure of interest, which absorbs them and uses them in the manufacture of proteins which are then transported down the axon and later identified by the exposure to a photographic emulsion.

Amygdala

This is found in the depth of the medial temporal lobe, medial to the inferior horn of the lateral ventricle. Various subdivisions of its nuclei have been suggested, most recognizing a basolateral and a corticomedial group. The basal nucleus has a high acetylcholine content and projects to the basal nucleus of Meynert, which (see below) provides a widespread cholinergic influence on the cerebral cortex.

The main afferent and efferent pathways traverse the stria terminalis, and the ventral amygdalofugal pathway. The latter is a longitudinal association bundle linking to the ventral striatum (see below) and the medial frontal cortex. There is also a medial amygdalohypothalamic bundle going to the lateral hypothalamus and, via the MFB, to the brainstem, and the uncinate fasciculus that projects to the frontal cortex. The connections to the brainstem come almost exclusively from the central nucleus, the fibres ending in several structures that serve autonomic and visceral

92

functions. These include the catecholamine and serotonin brain-stem nuclei, the VTA and the substantia nigra, the central grey, the dorsal nucleus of the vagus and the nucleus of the solitary tract. The basolateral area has cortical and ventral striatal links, and the basomedial group connects to the hypothalamus. In the cortex, amygdaloid fibres are found in the orbital and medial frontal lobe, the rostral cingulate gyrus and most of the temporal lobe (Price, 1981).

The connections of the amygdala to the hippocampus are primarily via the entorhinal cortex (see below), which is a major source of hippocampal afferents. Those to the hypothalamus may influence the control of pituitary hormone release, especially the projections to the ventromedial nucleus, which itself projects to the arcuate nucleus. Some of these connections are shown diagrammatically in Figure 2.

GABA is an important inhibitory transmitter in the amygdala, and other neurotransmitters identified in it include acetylcholine, histamine, dopamine, especially in the basolateral and central nuclei, noradrenaline, serotonin and peptides such as substance P, metenkephalin, somatostatin, VIP and neurotensin (Ben-Ari, 1981).

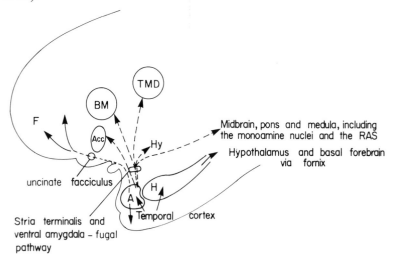

Figure 2. Showing some of the afferent and efferent projections of the amygdala. Note the extensive inputs from the temporal cortex and widespread influence on a number of important areas from the frontal cortex to the brainstem. A = amygdala; Acc = nucleus accumbens; BM = basal nucleus of Meynert; F = frontal and cingulate areas; H = hippocampus; Hy = hypothalamus; TMD = mediodorsal nucleus of thalamus.

Hippocampus

The hippocampal structures are closely linked to the septal nuclei, sometimes referred to as the septohippocampal system. The expansion and development of the human brain leads to separation of these two structures, but in lower animals they are closely linked. Gray (1982) likens this to a pair of joined bananas, where they join being the septal area, and progression from anterior to posterior is accompanied by the structures spreading laterally as they descend into the temporal lobes. The main fibre systems connecting the two are the fimbria and the fornix, and the two hippocampi are interconnected by the hippocampal commissures.

The structure of the hippocampus displays a constant architectural pattern, and three main divisions are recognized. These are the fascia dentata, Ammon's horn and the subiculum. This is shown in Figure 3.

The fascia dentata consists of a compact layer of granular cells that form a U-shape and embraces the pyramidal cells of Ammon's horn (see Figure 4). The latter is sometimes subdivided into four areas, CA1 to 4, the CA1 area in man being particularly prominant and susceptible to damage by anoxia (an alternative name is Sommer's sector). The subiculum is a transitional structure between CA1 and the parahippocampal gyrus (see Figure 3). On sections it is found where the neat structure of Ammon's horn breaks down as it merges with the six-layered neocortex, and is an exit region for many hippocampal efferents.

The laminar organization of the hippocampus is derived from its regular cell layers, notably the pyramidal cells, granular cells and the interneuronal inhibitory basket cells. Essentially the circuit of information flow is from the entorhinal cortex to the dentate gyrus, then from CA3 to CA1 and the subiculum. The latter feeds into the fornix.

The main neurotransmitter associated with inhibition in the hippocampus is GABA, but the structure receives dopaminergic, serotoninergic and noradrenergic afferents. Peptides such as VIP, CCK, neurotensin, somatostatin, substance P and metenkephalin have been identified in the hippocampus (Roberts et al., 1984).

The parahippocampal gyrus

This structure is of central importance in the limbic system. It is adjacent to the hippocampus and covered by the entorhinal cortex.

94

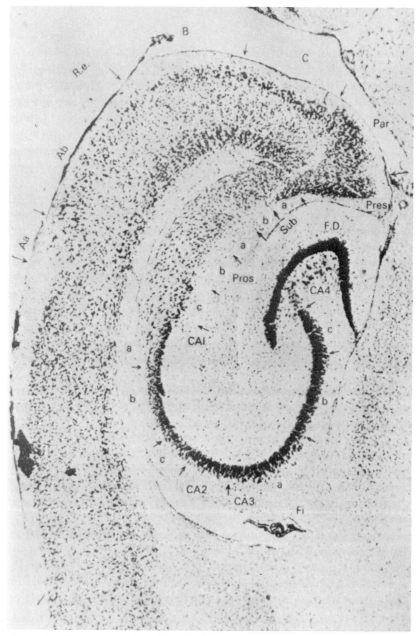

Figure 3. Horizontal section through the hippocampus. Re = entorhinal cortex; Par = parasubiculum; Pres = presubiculum; Sub = subiculum; FD = fascia dentata; Pros = prosubiculum. Note the three-layered (CA1–CA4) hippocampal structure. (From O'Keefe and Nadel, 1978. Reproduced with permission.)

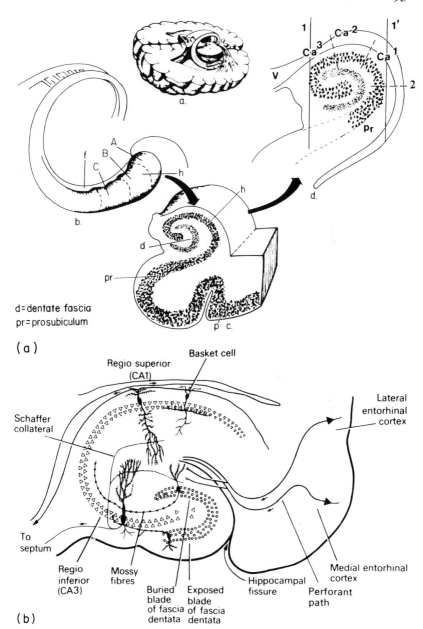

d = dentate fascia
pr = prosubiculum

(a)

(b)

Figure 4 (a) Showing the hippocampus within the hemispheres and after dissection. (From Kovelman and Scheibel, 1984. Reproduced with permission.) (b) A schematic representation of hippocampal connections. (From O'Keefe and Nadel, 1978. Reproduced with permission.)

Because it shares with the latter only poorly defined cortical layers, it has been referred to as schizocortex (split cortex). In Brodmann's system, the entorhinal cortex is represented by area 28 (see Figure 5). It has extensive projections to the hippocampal formation via the perforant pathway and, most importantly, cortical afferents from many cortical sites. Thus, the association cortices project to this region, providing a direct limbic system input of visual, auditory and somatic information. Further, as noted, the amygdala, with its strong hypothalamic connections, projects to the entorhinal area such that the hippocampus receives, via the parahippocampal gyrus, multimodal sensory information derived from the external and internal world.

The subiculum also projects to the parahippocampal gyrus, and the latter in turn has widespread limbic and association cortical projections in frontal, parietal, temporal and occipital lobes (see Figure 6; van Hoesen, 1982).

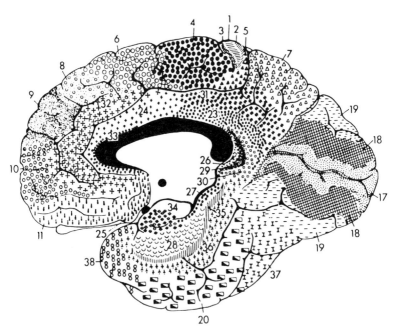

Figure 5. Showing Brodmann's areas. The prefrontal cortex is represented by numbers 9–15, 46 and 47. Area 46 is seen on the lateral surface, while 13, 14, 15 and 47 are on the orbital surface.

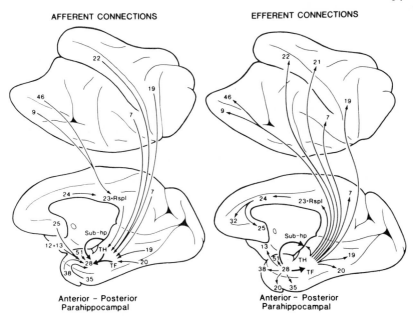

AFFERENT CONNECTIONS

EFFERENT CONNECTIONS

Figure 6. Showing the cortical connections of the parahippocampal gyrus. (From van Hoesen, 1982. Reproduced with permission.)

The septal area

The septal nuclei are situated below the corpus callosum, ventrally bounded by the olfactory tubercle and the nucleus accumbens. The lateral boundary is made by the lateral ventricle, and the caudal boundary by the third ventricle and hypothalamus (see Figure 7). In man, the dorsal part is elongated by the development of the corpus callosum to form the septum pellucidum which forms a glial and fibre attachment to the corpus callosum.

The septal area is usually subdivided into medial and lateral groups, and the medial septal area is further divided into the medial septal nucleus and the nucleus of the diagonal band of Broca. Both contain acetylcholine, and project to the hippocampus and entorhinal cortex via the fimbria and fornix. The lateral nuclei receive hippocampal afferents mainly from CA3 and the subiculum. Since the lateral and medial septal nuclei interconnect, a functional circuit is derived as follows:

Hippocampus–lateral septum–medial septum–hippocampus

Also shown in Figure 7 are the bed nucleus of the stria terminalis, which receives amygdala projections, and the substantia innominata.

98

The septal area receives rich monoamine projections, especially dopamine from the VTA via the MFB. VIP, CCK, somatostatin, metenkephalin, neurotensin and substance P are all found in the septum.

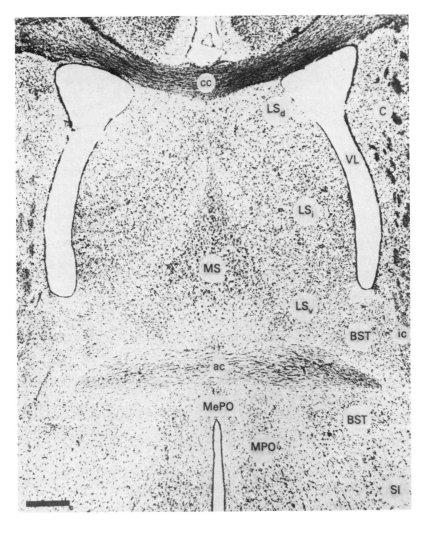

Figure 7. Showing the septal area. BST = bed nucleus of stria terminalis; C = caudate nucleus; LS = lateral septal nucleii; MePO = median preoptic nucleus; MPO = medial preoptic nucleus; MS = medial septal nucleus; VL = lateral ventricle; ac = anterior commissure; SI = substantia innominata; cc = corpus callosum. (From Swanson, 1978. Reproduced with permission.)

The cingulate gyrus

This runs dorsal to the corpus callosum, following a C-shaped curve as it progresses posteriorly. The anterior cingulate region is the area outlined by Brodmann as areas 23, 24, 25, 31 and 33 (see Figure 5). The retrosplenial region is Brodmann's 26, 29 and 30, and here the cingulate gyrus becomes narrow and continuous with the lingual gyrus, a dorsal extension of the parahippocampal gyrus. The cingulate cortex is continuous with the frontal cortex anteriorly, is rich in dopamine fibres and contains CCK and opiate receptors.

Hypothalamus

The hypothalamus, positioned dorsal to the pituitary gland, is a site of convergence for much limbic system activity. Posterior to it are the mammillary bodies, and anteriorly are the optic chiasm and the preoptic area. The descending fornix divides the hypothalamus into medial and lateral areas. The medial border of the medial hypothalamus is formed by the third ventricle, and several nuclear groups are defined (see Figure 8). The suprachiasmatic nucleus is thought to be a regulator of rhythmic activity, a sort of biological clock. The axons of neurones from the supraoptic and para-ventricular nuclei are neurosecretory fibres travelling mainly to the posterior pituitary gland. The lateral area contains many fibres of passage of the monoamine brainstem and midbrain nuclei trav-elling with the MFB, but the fornix, stria terminalis and the mam-millothalamic tract connect anteriorly, and the mammillotegmen-tal tract and dorsal longitudinal fasciculus posteriorly.

Several of the hypothalamic nuclei secrete neuropeptides, some of which are releasing hormones. These are released into the hypophysial portal blood vessels which carry them to the anterior pituitary where they stimulate or inhibit various pituitary hor-mones. A list of some of these and the accompanying releasing hormones is shown in Table 2.

The neurohormones typically are released in a pulsatile fashion. They are found in brain areas other than the median emminence and also influence the pituitary gland via secretion into the CSF. The extrapituitary influence is exerted on limbic system structures, thalamus, the periaqueductal grey region and the brainstem catecholamine nuclei. A list of peptides found in the hypothala-mus, as yet without known function, is shown in Table 3.

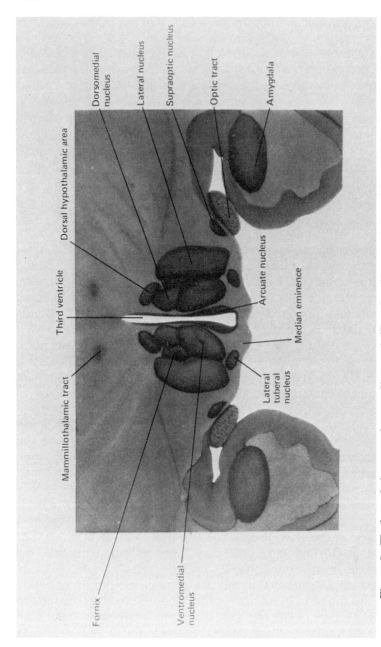

Figure 8. The hypothalamus and some of its nucei. (Reprinted by permission of the publisher from Kandel and Schwartz. Copyright 1981 by Elsevier Science Publishing Co., Inc.)

Table 2   Hypothalamic releasing and inhibiting factors and pituitary hormones

Neurohormone	Pituitary hormone
Thyrotropin releasing hormone	TSH, prolactin
Corticotropin releasing hormone	ACTH, beta-endorphin
LH/FSH releasing hormone	LH, FSH
Growth hormone releasing factor	Growth hormone
Prolactin releasing factor	Prolactin
Melanocyte stimulating hormone (MSH) releasing factor	MSH
Prolactin inhibitory factor (PIF)	Prolactin
Somatostatin	Growth hormone, TSH
MSH inhibiting factor	MSH

Monoamine transmitters are also present in the hypothalamus, some of which impinge on the median emminence to influence hormone release. These are shown in Table 4.

Of importance is the intrahypothalamic dopamine pathway with cell bodies in the arcuate and ventromedial nuclei. Here the dopamine is thought to inhibit prolactin release, dopamine being prolactin inhibitory factors (PIF).

ASCENDING AND DESCENDING LIMBIC SYSTEM CONNECTIONS

Knowledge of the anatomy and functional unity of the limbic system has altered radically in recent years. It is now known that a

Table 3   Some hypothalamic peptides

Bombesin	Neurotensin
Bradykinin	Angiotensin
Calcitonin	Leuenkephalin
Glucagon	Metenkephalin
Insulin	Beta-endorphin
Lipotropin	Gamma-endorphin
Secretin	VIP
Substance P	CCK

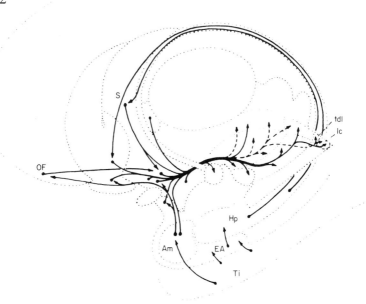

Figure 9. The medial forebrain bundle. OF = orbitofrontal cortex; lc = locus coeruleus; S = septum; tdl = nucleus tegmenti dorsalis lateralis; EA = entorhinal area; Am = amygdyla; Ti = temporal cortex; Hp = hippocampus. (From Nauta and Domesick, 1982. Reproduced with permission.)

'limbic forebrain–midbrain circuit' exists which unites the mono-amine- and peptide-rich zones of the midbrain with rostral structures such as the hippocampus, amygdala and the septal area, and a limbic midbrain area has been defined in the paramedian zone of the mesencephalon (Nauta and Domesick, 1982). The main connecting structure is the MFB (see Figure 9), a poorly defined fibre system with a loose arrangement, characteristic of brainstem reticular formation. It receives contributions from such structures as the septal nuclei, hypothalamus, olfactory tubercle, substantia innominata, nucleus accumbens, amygdala, bed nucleus of stria terminalis and the orbitofrontal cortex. Caudally it projects to the VTA, the interpeduncular nucleus, the raphe nuclei, the locus coeruleus and the midbrain reticular formation. Its further descent to autonomic and spinal nuclei has already been noted.

The stria medullaris, which carries fibres from limbic forebrain structures and the globus pallidus (see below), projects to the habenula nuclei, paired structures found at the caudal end of the midbrain which connect with the raphe nuclei.

The ascending components of this limbic forebrain–midbrain circuit arise from the VTA, the raphe nuclei and the locus

Table 4 Possible role of brain neurotransmitters in regulation of anterior pituitary secretion

Neurotransmitter	Corticotrophin (ACTH)	Growth hormone (GH)	Prolactin	Gondadotrophins (LH/FSH)	Thyrotrophin (TSH)
Dopamine	−	+−	−−	+−	+−
Noradrenaline	−−	+ +	+−	+	+?
Serotonin	+−	+ +	+ +	+−	+−
Acetylcholine	+ +	0	−	+	?
Histamine	+−	?	+−	+−	+−
γ-Aminobutyric acid (GABA)	−	+	−	+	−

+ = stimulation; − = inhibition; 0 = no apparent regulation; ? = unknown regulation. The net responses shown here do not reflect precisely the intricate mechanisms which operate but are based on numerous and often conflicting data in the literature and should not be considered conclusive. Also differences between mammalian species are often observed.

β-Lipotrophin is not included since at the present time neurotransmitter regulation of the secretion of this hormone is uncertain.

(Reproduced by permission of Croom Helm Ltd from Bennett and Whitehead, 1983.)

coeruleus. The VTA occupies the basomedial midbrain, dorsal to the substantia nigra, and is continuous rostrally with the lateral hypothalamus. It borders on the ventral periaqueductal grey substance, the dorsal raphe nuclei and other nuclei of the limbic midbrain (see Figure 10).

The main ascending connections to the limbic forebrain (see Figure 11) are from the dopamine-rich cells which innervate the

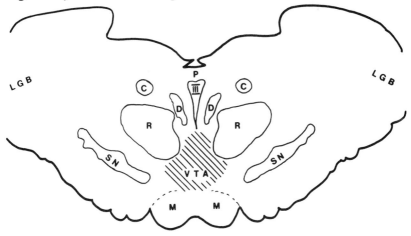

Figure 10. Showing the location of the ventral tegmental area in the midbrain. C = nucleus of Cajal; D = nucleus of Darkschewitsch; LGB = lateral geniculate body; M = mammillary bodies; P = posterior commissure; R = red nucleus; SN = substantia nigra; VTA = ventral tegmental area.

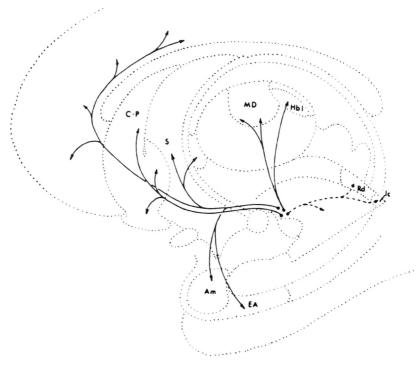

Figure 11. The ascending components of the dopaminergic projections from the VTA. CP = caudatoputamen; S = septal area; MD = mediodorsal nucleus of thalamus; Hbl = habenula; Am = amygdala; EA = entorhinal area; Rd = dorsal raphe nucleus; lc = locus coeruleus. (From Nauta and Domesick, 1982. Reproduced with permission.)

nucleus accumbens, olfactory tubercle, amygdala, entorhinal area, frontocingulate cortex and septal area. The catecholamine nuclei are found in relatively discrete areas of the brainstem, and were first identified using fluorescent histochemical techniques. On the basis of animal work they have been designated as A1, A2, . . . up to A13 (Ungerstedt, 1971), and those arising from the substantia nigra and the VTA are referred to as A9 and A10 respectively. From these the majority of dopamine neurones that project to the limbic system and striatum arise (the so-called mesolimbic system). Using this terminology, the locus coeruleus is A5 and A6.

In a similar fashion the serotoninergic neurones are confined virtually to the brainstem raphe nuclei. Some of these relationships are shown in Figure 12.

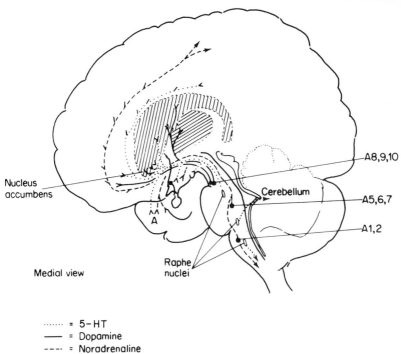

Figure 12. Some monoamine pathways in the brain. A = amygdala; hatched area = caudate nucleus/putamen.

More recently it has been appreciated that the A10 projection also innervates the striatum and the thalamus and has connections with the locus coeruleus and raphe nuclei, although not all paths are thought necessarily to be dopaminergic (Nauta and Domesick, 1982).

In contrast to the relatively restricted termination areas for the dopamine neurones of A9 and A10, the ascending catecholamine neurones distribute widely, exerting a tonic modulatory influence on many cortical neurones. 5-HT distribution is intermediate, being more extensive than that of dopamine and projecting to the hippocampus and amygdala, parahippocampal gyrus, habenula, thalamus and cortex.

THE BASAL GANGLIA

This term usually refers to the caudate nucleus, putamen and globus pallidus but may also include the subthalamic nucleus and the substantia nigra. Although the amygdala is closely related developmentally, it is usually referred to as part of the limbic system. The striatum refers to the caudate nucleus and putamen, divided as they are by the internal capsule. In lower animals the separation is less complete, and the structure is referred to as the caudatoputamen. The caudate nucleus is a large curved nucleus which adheres throughout its length to the lateral ventricles, anteriorly being continuous with the putamen. The putamen and globus pallidus are referred to as the lenticular nucleus.

The afferent connections to the striatum are from the cerebral cortex, thalamic nuclei, the substantia nigra, the amygdala and the raphe nucleus. The most investigated is the nigrostriatal projection, mainly on account of its obvious association with Parkinson's disease. There is a nigrostriatal dopamine system originating in the pars compacta of the substantia nigra (A9), but an extensive striatal projection also derives from the related A10 area. The corticostriate connections come from nearly all regions of the neocortex, projecting onto the striatum topographically. The thalamostriate connections come from non-specific cell groups.

Efferents pass via the globus pallidus, some fibres traversing this, establishing a direct striatonigral connection. The striatopallidal projection is rich in enkephalin, and the striatonigral in substance P. The striatonigral fibres synapse on the dendrites of dopamine neurones in the pars reticulata, forming a nigro–striatal–nigral loop. These connections are shown in Figure 13.

Other peptides and neurotransmitters related to these structures include the GABA-dominated striatonigral link; the presence of

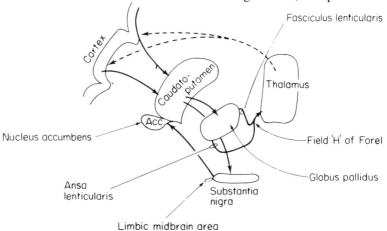

Figure 13. Main fibre connections of the basal ganglia.

enkephalin-like, substance P and CCK immunoreactivity in the substantia nigra; and acetylcholine, enkephalin, neurotensin, somatostatin, substance P and opiate binding in the striatum (Graybiel, 1984). The large corticostriate projection is thought to be glutaminergic.

The efferent connections of the globus pallidus travel through the ansa lenticularis to the subthalamus and thalamus, the habenula, and midbrain tegmentum. Several neuronal loops are thus identified:

Substantia nigra–caudate–substantia nigra

Globus pallidus–thalamus–(putamen)–globus pallidus

Globus pallidus–habenula–raphe nucleus–striatum–globus pallidus

Further, since the thalamus has efferents to the cortex, there is a further circuit:

Cortex–striatum–globus pallidus–thalamus–cortex

THE VENTRAL STRIATUM AND 'LIMBIC STRIATUM'

The anatomy of the basal forebrain and its relationship to behaviour has been reevaluated in recent years, and much attention has focused on dopamine-rich structures lying ventral and medial to, and associated with, the head of the caudate nucleus. One such structure is the nucleus accumbens. This, together with the closely associated olfactory tubercle, has been referred to as the ventral striatum, in contrast to the dorsal striatum, the structure of which has already been discussed above.

Its caudal boundary with the bed-nucleus of the stria terminalis is difficult to establish, but anteriorly it extends into the ventromedial portion of the frontal lobe, and it lies lateral to the septal region (White, 1981). Heimer *et al.* (1982) referred to this complex of olfactory tubercle and nucleus accumbens as the ventral striatum to emphasize its close anatomical, developmental and structural relationship to the striatum. Both receive a dopaminergic input from VTA (Anden *et al.*, 1966) and have limbic system connections. In particular, the ventral striatum receives projections from the hippocampus via the fornix, the amygdala and frontal cortex, this allocortical input contrasting with the neocortical dorsal striatum connections (see Figure 14).

Thus, as a generalization, most afferents to the nucleus accumbens come from the limbic system. Others come from the thalamus and hypothalamus.

Substance P, enkephalin and CCK are found in both ventral and dorsal striatum, while VIP, TRH and neurotensin are found mainly in the nucleus accumbens. Other peptides located in the nucleus accumbens include somatostatin and MSH (Johannsson and Hokfelt, 1981). There are also high concentrations of acetyl-choline, glutamate and GABA.

Some of the contrasts between the dorsal and ventral striatum are shown in Table 5.

As fibres leave the nucleus accumbens they project to a rostro-ventral extension of the globus pallidus referred to as the ventral

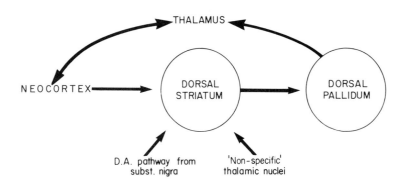

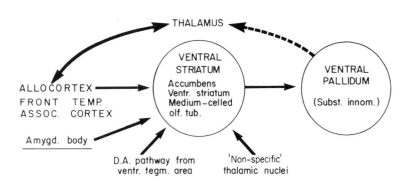

Figure 14. Showing the different connections of the dorsal and ventral striatum. Note the predominant limbic connections with the latter. DA = dopamine.

Table 5   Some contrasts between the dorsal striatum and ventral striatum

	Dorsal	Ventral
Dopamine projection	Mainly A9 (substantia nigra)	Mainly A10 (VTA)
Cortical afferents	Limbic and neocortical	Limbic
Main efferents	Dorsal pallidum (globus pallidus)	Ventral pallidum

pallidum. This region is also referred to as the substantia innominata, an area rich in acetylcholine and substance P. It forms part of the basal nucleus of Meynert. The ventral pallidum projects to the mediodorsal nucleus of the thalamus, which in turn projects to the prefrontal, limbic and cingulate cortices (Heimer *et al.*, 1982). Thus the circuit:

Limbic cortex–ventral striatum–ventral pallidum–thalamus–limbic cortex

is a counterpart to the other cortical–striatal loop noted above.

Other projections are to the subthalamic nucleus, substantia nigra, amygdala, habenula and the VTA. The cholinergic cells project to the medial regions of the cerebral cortex and amygdala.

Nauta has repeatedly emphasized the cross-talk between the limbic system and the basal ganglia (Nauta and Domesick, 1982). This is of great importance for biological psychiatry, not the least because of the close links between motor and emotional behaviour (Trimble, 1981a). Direct connections exist between the hippocampus, amygdala, cingulate cortex and the ventral striatum, and the habenula has both limbic and pallidal afferents. Hypothalamic MFB efferents impinge on the VTA and substantia nigra. Further, indirect links by way of the substantia nigra and raphe nucleus exist, both being influenced by the descending fibres of the MFB and fasciculus retroflexus. In contrast connections in the opposite way, from striatum to limbic system, are limited.

One further point of anatomical interest is that three limbic projections converge on the anterior ventral component of the striatum, namely the dopaminergic fibres from the VTA, the projection from the amygdala and fibres from the frontal cortex.

THALAMUS AND FRONTAL CORTEX

The thalamus is usually considered to play a key role in the transmission of somatic sensory impulses on their way to the cerebral cortex. It is composed of three main nuclear groups, the medial, lateral and anterior. The ventral posterolateral nucleus conveys medial lemniscal and spinothalamic infomation to the primary and secondary sensory cortical areas; the basal ganglia afferents project mainly to ventrolateral, ventroanterior and so-called intralaminar nuclei (located within white matter laminae that transect the thalamus)—these thalamic nuclei also receive cerebellar projections; and reciprocal connections with the frontal cortex are made by the ventral anterior and mediodorsal nucleus, the anterior nucleus connecting to the cingulate gyri as part of the Papez circuit. The reticular formation, that loosely assembled, closely packed network of neurones in the brainstem, activates many thalamic fibres, and continues by relay and direct connection to influence all fields of the cortex.

The frontal lobes are anatomically represented by those areas of cortex anterior to the central sulcus, including the main cortical representations for the control of motor behaviour. The term prefrontal cortex designates the most anterior pole, an area sometimes referred to as the frontal granular cortex or the frontal association cortex (see Figure 5). One definition of the prefrontal cortex is that region which receives projections from the mediodorsal thalamic nucleus (Fuster, 1980). These are topographically organized such that the medial part of the nucleus projects to the medial and orbital frontal cortex, and the lateral to the lateral and dorsal cortex. The medial thalamic area receives afferents from the mesencephalic reticular formation, and the amygdala, entorhinal and inferior temporal cortex, whereas the lateral nuclear area only has afferents from the prefrontal cortex (Fuster, 1980).

Other important prefrontal connections are made by the mesocortical dopamine projections from VTA. Unlike the subcortical dopamine projections, these neurones lack autoreceptors (Bannon *et al.*, 1982). Further links are to the hypothalamus (the orbital frontal cortex alone in the neocortex projects to the hypothalamus), the cingulate gyrus, the amygdala, hippocampus, and retrosplenial and entorhinal cortices. On the basis of primate data,

Nauta (1964) suggested that the orbital frontal cortex made connections with amygdala and related subcortical structures, whereas the dorsal cortex links more to the hippocampus and parahippocampal gyrus. Certainly there seems to be a comparable circuit to the Papez circuit, but based on the amygdala instead of the hippocampus; thus:

Amygdala–thalamus (mediodorsal nucleus)–orbitofrontal cortex–inferior temporal cortex–amygdala

In the same way that sensory information from primary sensory cortex, after passing to adjacent secondary areas, cascades to the anterior temporal areas (Jones and Powell, 1970), the prefrontal cortex is also a projection area for extensive somatic, auditory and sensory information.

The prefrontal cortex has efferents to, but does not receive afferents from, the striatum, notably to the caudate nucleus, globus pallidus, putamen and substantia nigra.

A final point is that the area of the prefrontal cortex that receives the dominant dorsomedial thalamic nucleus projection overlaps with that from the dopaminergic VTA.

THE CEREBRAL CORTEX

The phylogenetically older area of cortex, the allocortex, has already been discussed in some detail. This is intimately related to the control of emotion and behaviour. However, the neocortex, while equally important in the overall functioning of the brain for the individual, relates less to complex, complete behavioural actions, and on stimulation or lesioning tends to provoke more limited, circumscribed changes of sensation or movement. As it was relatively accessible to the exploring electrodes of the early investigators, much more became known about its structure and function than that of the buried limbic system structures. Further, the deficits that arise with areas of destruction and the identification of these lesions by clinical testing led to the successful growth of neurology, and its increasing separation from psychiatry.

It is generally known that the human neocortex has expanded in development, being some 156 times greater than that of some of the primitive insectivores, early primate ancestors. It is identified by its six-layered structure, and has been divided into various areas dependent on microscopic differences, such as those described by

Brodmann (see Figure 5). In addition to the frontal lobe already discussed, three others are defined in relation to surface markings, namely the temporal, parietal and occipital cortices. It possesses a large number of association fibres that link areas of the same hemisphere and commissural fibres that link homotopic areas of both hemispheres. The largest collection of these is the corpus callosum.

The layer closest to the pia mater contains mainly dendrites of the deeper lying cells. The pyramidal cells, with long axones that traverse the internal capsule to form part of the pyramidal tract, are found in layer 5. It is the granular cells of layer 4 that mainly receive the thalamic sensory afferents, and this layer, in contrast to layer 5, is best developed in primary sensory cortices.

The primary sensory somatocortex is located posterior to the central sulcus in the postcentral gyrus, equivalent to Brodmann's areas 1 to 3. More posterior, corresponding to areas 5 and 7, is the somatic sensory association area. The auditory cortical areas are in the superior temporal gyrus (Brodmanns 41 and 42), and the visual ones are the striate cortex (area 17, the primary visual cortex) and areas 18 and 19, the visual association areas.

The main motor cortex is situated in the precentral gyrus, immediately rostral to the central sulcus (area 4), its main afferents coming from area 6, adjacent to it, which itself receives prefrontal projections. Area 8, another region anterior to the precentral gyrus, is referred to as the frontal eye field, and on stimulation eye movements are provoked.

It is now known that the cerebral cortex has a columnar arrangement, which has functional significance. The cortical neurones form connections within a column, but also ramify with cells in adjacent columns. This arrangement allows for an amplifying effect on afferent impulses, in the motor cortex permitting sufficient neurones to discharge for movement or in the sensory cortex to distinguish two closely related stimuli. Further, by allowing for the development of positive feedback loops and inhibition of neighbouring columns, the columns are self-excitatory, sharpening their effect by surround inhibition. In the visual cortex, columns of orientation selective cells have been identified, many of which are developed and present at birth.

A large proportion of intrinsic cortical neurones are GABAergic, many of which receive thalamic synapses. Cortical peptides include somatostatin, VIP, CCK and neuropeptide Y. In the cortex, cholinergic neurones have been shown to contain VIP

(Parnavelas, 1984). The noradrenergic innervation of the neo-cortex is extensive and tangential to the columnar arrangement. The fibres run longitudinally through the cortical grey matter and branch widely, thus affecting activity over wide areas of cortex. In contrast, some peptides, such as VIP, exert specific local effects, possibly complimentary in terms of information processing, with the influence of monoamines.

THE CEREBELLUM

This structure lies posteriorly, over the brainstem, and its cortex is divided into the central vermis and the cerebellar hemispheres. It receives afferents from both peripheral sense receptors and sensory and motor cortices, and projects to the thalamus, spinal cord and the same areas of cortex. Recently, direct influences of the cerebellum on limbic system structures have been reported, notably at the septal region and the amygdala. These may be mediated via the fastigial nucleus of the vermis (Heath *et al.*, 1978).

SOME RELATIONSHIPS BETWEEN BRAIN STRUCTURE AND FUNCTION AND BEHAVIOUR

The preceding sections have outlined some of the important elements of brain structure and chemistry that underpin our more elaborate knowledge of the relationship of the brain to behaviour. Since it is suggested that the brain is the organ that regulates our behaviour, and that disturbances of that organ will be reflected in behaviour change, and further that psychiatry is the study of abnormal human behaviour, then it is clear that seeking changes of brain function and structure in the presence of psychopathology is of fundamental importance to the discipline. It has further been emphasized that the limbic system and related structures form the main neuronal areas of interest. Before proceeding to examine changes in various psychiatric conditions, some of the data from animal investigations, particularly where they may compliment human studies, are reviewed.

Although as noted the expansion of the cerebral cortex has been a distinguishing feature of the brain of man, the limbic system has likewise developed. Thus, the septum is 4.8 times, the hippocampus 4.2 times (CA1 = 6.6) and parahippocampal gyrus 5.5 times greater in size than the insectivore equivalents. In contrast the olfactory bulb and cortex are much less developed, being only 3 and 33 per cent respectively of their equivalent volume (Stephan, 1975).

MacLean (1958) emphasized that the frontotemporal pole of the limbic system was primarily concerned with functions that regulate self-preservation and that stimulation leads to two main types of responses, namely licking, chewing and other oral activities, and sniffing, searching and anger. In contrast, the cingulate gyrus and septum are involved with preservation of the species as seen in grooming and sexual activity. Further, he has emphasized a triad of behaviours, namely nursing, play and the isolation call which are basic for mammalian family life, noting the growth in size of limbic system structures in mammals as such social bonding behaviour develops phylogenetically. Ablation of the cingulate gyrus thus leads to a deficit in maternal behaviour and play, and stimulation of the anterior cortex leads to vocalizations in animals and in man.

The role of the hypothalamus in regulating eating and drinking has been well investigated. Destruction of the ventromedial nuclei result in hyperphagia, and the lateral hypothalamus, aphagia. Stimulation led to the opposite. In part the effects are due to alteration of activity in fibres of passage passing through the region, and it is now known that dopamine projections from substantia nigra are involved. An interesting observation is that CCK, injected in small amounts both intraperitoneally or intraventricularly, leads to satiety in hungry animals. Another example of the central and peripheral action of a peptide neurohormone is in the regulation of drinking. The hypothalamus contains cells sensitive to osmotic signals and sodium levels. However, angiotensin 2, the active form of angiotensin, peripherally causes vasoconstriction and renal sodium retention, and centrally it stimulates drinking. Findings such as these emphasize how the brain is a target organ for hormones released peripherally and centrally, and may explain the presence of central receptors that bind hormones, especially in limbic and hypothalamic structures.

The increasing relevance of peptides becomes clearer as peptide circuitry is worked out. This is similar to the catecholamine systems, originating from a few discrete sites but influencing wide areas of the brain. Thus the central nervous system peptides can be divided into two groups depending on the origin of their cell bodies (Roberts *et al.*, 1984). One group derives from the hypothalamus, the other has extrahypothalamic as well as hypothalamic neurones. The origin of some of these is indicated in Table 3. The hypothalamic ones project to a variety of structures including the limbic forebrain, the amygdala, the thalamus and the VTA. These are areas of confluence of much neuronal information, where they may exert great influence over several systems at the same time. In contrast, the extrahypothalamic ones are less diverse, with local projections and longer fibre bundles suggesting more specific functions.

Some other specific roles for peptides can be defined. Thus substance P is thought to be involved with sensory transmission, being present in the dorsal roots of the spinal cord. Afferent fibres are seen in the substantia gelatinosa, an area known to be linked to pain perception, and in other areas related to pain such as the pain fibre receptive region of the trigeminal nuclear complex (Iversen and Iversen, 1981). Release of substance P leads to intense pain. Enkephalin has been shown to exist in proximity to substance P neurones, and opiates inhibit the release of substance P. This suggests functional links between this peptide, opiates and pain appreciation.

Significant observations of brain–behaviour relationships were reported by Kluver and Bucy (1939), following the placement of bilateral lesions in the temporal lobes of monkeys. As a consequence the behaviour of the animals changed totally. They became tame, with loss of fear and aggression, hypersexual, and demonstrated excessive oral exploration of their environment. They also displayed a visual agnosia. Since the lesions removed the uncus, amygdala and part of the hippocampus it was reasonable to assume that the intactness of these structures was a prerequisite for the organization and control of mood, sexual behaviour and visual perception (Koella, 1982).

Aggression

The relationship of the amydala to aggression seems well established, although a reciprocal link with the hypothalamus and frontal cortex seems important. Thus, following on from the Kluver–Bucy experiments, Schreiner and Kling (1956) tamed various aggressive feline species with bilateral amygdala lesions, an effect abolished by additional lesions in the ventrolateral hypothalamus. Aggression can be provoked by stimulation of the amygdala, hypothalamus and the area around the fornix in the diencephalon, and hypothalamic elicited aggression can be inhibited by stimulation of the ipsilateral frontal cortex (Siegel *et al.*,

1975). Delgado (1966), using implanted intracerebral multilead electrodes to stimulate various regions of the brain in monkeys, also recorded aggressive responses from the ventral posterolateral nucleus of the thalamus and the central grey area. By studying behaviour in a colony under various conditions of stimulation, he reported that the aggression artificially provoked by stimulation was indistinguishable from spontaneous aggression. Rosvold *et al.* (1954) demonstrated how amygdala lesions lead to loss of dominance in a social heirarchy.

Adamec, based on studies with kindling, introduced the concept of 'limbic permeability'. Thus kindling is an experimental procedure in which small, brief, high-frequency currents are passed across electrodes in an area of brain. At first no effects are seen, but after several trials, usually given on a daily basis, an after-discharge develops, and behaviour changes are seen. As the process continues, eventually the animal will have, in spite of still receiving subthreshold doses, a generalized seizure. The associated changes in brain physiology, as yet unidentified, are long-lasting, and the animal remains susceptible to a seizure on passing the current for a considerable time. Kindling is best from limbic system structures, but can be obtained from the neocortex. It has not been achieved from brainstem or cerebellar stimulation.

Adamec and Stark-Adamec (1983) used cats to kindle lasting behavioural changes, notably aggressiveness or defensiveness. Limbic permeability, the degree and facility of seizure propagation from limbic to hypothalamic areas, could be related to these behaviour changes.

The literature on the role of various transmitters in aggressive behaviour is confusing and highly species dependent. It is further complicated by the differing models of aggression involved. Generally, depletion of serotonin and GABA, and increasing cholinergic or catecholaminergic drive facilitate aggressive behaviour. Tricyclic antidepressants and monoamine oxidase inhibitors (MAOI) are likewise facilitatory (Eichelman, 1979), as are hormonal influences such as the increase in aggression associated with testosterone.

In summary, while the spontaneous display of aggression is obviously dependent on environmental stimuli from many sources, the central roles of the amygdala and hypothalamus in its neural organization seem established from animal studies. In as much as the amygdala receives cortical sensory information from temporal structures, its role as a gate to the limbic system through which threatening stimuli may be evaluated, which has major outflows to the hypothalamic and limbic forebrain structures, may be suggested (Herbert, 1984). Further, the catecholamine influences from midbrain nuclei could influence the potency of the gate, modulating the threshold of incoming stimuli.

Anxiety and the septohippocampal link

Gray (1982), on the basis of extensive animal experiments, has postulated the existence of a behavioural inhibition system which modulates anxiety responses. The neural counterpart of this is the septohippocampal circuit, and anxiolytic drugs are thought to act by inhibiting this system. Briefly, lesions of the septal area or the hippocampus lead to a pattern of behaviours similar to that seen after giving anxiolytic drugs, and stimulation of the septal area the opposite. The septohippocampal system, as noted, forms an extensive interconnected neural network, and in Gray's theory it acts, with the associated Papez circuit, as a comparator, generating predictions about anticipated events and matching them to actual events. Mismatch allows the behavioural inhibition system to dominate, interrupting behaviour and generating a search for alternatives by increased arousal and attention. Gray also discusses the role of ascending monoaminergic systems, especially noradrenaline and serotonin which modulate information flow into the hippocampus. In his system the prefrontal cortex is a comparator for motor programmes, and in man is a route for verbal influences over septohippocampal functions and a possible neurological substrate of obsessive symptoms.

Other functions assigned to the hippocampus, in the light of electrophysiological stimulation and lesion experiments, mainly relate to memory. Although severe memory problems after hippocampal destruction were first defined in man, animal studies produced conflicting data. Several competing theories now exist, although all ascribe to the hippocampus a role in higher cognitive function. One suggestion is that it is involved in the construction of spatial maps (O'Keefe and Nadel, 1978). An alternative is that it subserves spatial memory. Its precise role in human memory is unclear, and relates either to the consolidation of short-term memory or the retrieval of information once remembered.

There is substantial evidence that the hippocampus is involved in neuroendocrine regulation. Thus it binds more corticosterone than any other brain region, a pattern extending along the septotemporal axis. Further, fornix lesions interfere with normally observed corticosteroid responses, and ACTH can modify hippocampal responses (Issacson, 1982). This may explain the postulated effects of peptide fragments such as ACTH 4 to 10 on learning and extinction in animals (de Weid, 1974).

The septal area is also involved in a variety of behavioural responses. Lesions here initially lead to irritability and hyperreactivity, and, as with the amygdala, may lead to changes in the threshold for aggression and dominance, depending on the species and the status of the individual. Of most interest, however, has been the observation that stimulation of this area appears to produce rewards. Olds and Milner (1954) referred to this, and other sites from which the same effect could be produced, as 'pleasure centres'. The most active sites were along the path of the MFB, and were related to dopaminergic and/or noradrenergic activity. It has been suggested that this reward system may play a role in memory consolidation (Routtenberg, 1979). Pleasurable responses are obtained in humans from septal stimulation, and spike and slow wave discharges are recorded there during orgasm (Heath, 1972).

Sexual behaviour

The changes in sexual activity first seen with the Kluver–Bucy syndrome were confirmed in other species. The amygdala seems to be important in its regulation. The hypersexuality induced by amygdala destruction can be reversed by septal lesions (Kling *et al.*, 1960), supporting the role of the latter in pleasurable sexual experiences. Penile erection in monkeys can be seen after stimulation of the septum (MacLean and Ploog, 1962), and electrical activity is recorded here in female rabbits and man with orgasm (Sawyer, 1957; Heath, 1972). The hypothalamus is clearly involved in sexual behaviour, and lesions in the anterior hypothalamus prevent the hormonal activation of sexual activity (Heimer and Larsson, 1966). There are many steroid binding sites in hypothalamic regions that interact with systemic hormones to modulate behaviour, further interrelated with the influence of monoamine and peptide systems (Herbert, 1984).

Arousal, sleep and the reticular activating system

Arousal and consciousness are related to the tonic control of the ascending reticular activating system (RAS), extending from the medulla upwards to the thalamus. On stimulation of this area there is desynchronization of the electroencephalogram (EEG) and behavioural arousal. Lesions in this area lead to permanent sleep, although regions within it, such as the median raphe, when destroyed lead to a state of permanent insomnia. Thus, the homogeneous mass of reticular neurones referred to originally as the RAS has now been shown to contain in it many different neuronal groups, including the long ascending monoamine and peptide pathways, and nuclei sensitive to sensory information from the cardiovascular and respiratory system. Some of its efferents descend to the spinal cord, influencing motor neurones and sensory afferents. Thus, the RAS receives input fibres from adjacent ascending and descending tracts and nuclei, the hypothalamus, limbic system and cortex, and moderates arousal, conscious activity and sleep–wake cycles.

Parahippocampal gyrus

The entorhinal cortex may be viewed as the great gate through which neocortical information reaches the hippocampus and thence other limbic system structures.

There is clear evidence that this region has access to specific sensory and multimodal sensory representations. The links with the amygdala, and hence the hypothalamus and forebrain limbic structures, implies it is a meeting point for internal and emotional data with current and past sensory information. The traffic is two way, however, both from sensory cortex to the limbic system, and vice versa, allowing for limbic influences on sensory experiences.

Motion, emotion and motivation

An early attempt to understand the neurological underpinnings of emotional experience was that of Papez, although knowledge of the limbic system has developed substantially since he described his circuit. MacLean elaborated further on the behavioural relationships derived from comparative and clinical data, emphasizing the rise of social bonding relating to increasing limbic system size and complexity. The most significant advances in this field have derived from the anatomical observations of the close links between the limbic system and the basal ganglia, and the role of the latter in motivation. Thus, traditionally the basal ganglia have been viewed as solely related to motor behaviour. However, emotional display involves motor patterns (hence e-motion), motor abnormalities are seen in patients with psychiatric illness as a part of their symptomatology (Trimble, 1981a), motor disorders are frequently associated with psychopathology (Trimble, 1981a), and movement and emotion are linked in common speech (hence 'a moving experience').

Nauta (Nauta and Domesick, 1982) has drawn attention to the areas of limbic–striatal integration. Iversen (1984), following observations of alteration of behaviour after stimulation or lesion of either the ventral or dorsal striatum, has emphasized how the the former is related to sensorimotor integration of interoceptive information. Damage here leads to impairment of organized motivational behaviour such as exploration of novel environments. In this scheme, the dorsal striatum is seen as involved with neocortically derived motor behaviour, and the ventral striatum is related to emotional arousal. The nucleus accumbens is central, receiving connections from amygdala and hippocampus, and midbrain limbic areas. It projects to the ventral pallidum, and hence, in association with neocortical–globus pallidus efferents, influences motor behaviour. These striatal structures have been suggested to be filters of limbic and cortical information permitting appropriate signals to gain access to motor pathways (Mogenson *et al.*, 1980). The role of dopamine is crucial here. Not only are its influences greater on information derived from association cortices, but different populations of dopamine-related hormones exist. The meso limbic–prefrontal system lacks autoreceptors, has a higher cell firing rate than the other dopamine neurones and is the only one to show an increased turnover in response to stress.

In addition, the limbic system influences the RAS and its nuclear structures, thus ultimately affecting visceral motor neurones and the spinal cord. RAS activity is further transmitted to the cortex via thalamic relays. There are also hypothalamic and substantia innominata–cortical relays, all of which, associated with the ascending monoamine cortical afferents, influence cortical information in a non-specific way. Some of the behaviours that relate to limbic system structures as discussed are shown in Table 6.

The limbic system could be viewed as a neural mechanism that not only monitors the sensory processes of the cerebral

Table 6 Some limbic system structures and their behavioural influence

Cingulate:	Maternal behaviour, play, vocalization
Hippocampus:	Memory, anxiety
Amygdala:	Fear/anxiety, aggression, sex, mood
Septum:	Pleasure
Hypothalamus:	Eating, drinking, sex, aggression, hormonal control
RAS:	Arousal, sleep–wake cycle
Entorhinal:	Memory, sensory integration
Ventral striatum:	Motivation

cortex, but can also reach out and intervene in these processes. . . the limbic system affects not only. . . the organism's visceral and endocrine functions and its motivational state, but also the sensory and associative mechanisms involved in its perceptions and ideational processes (Nauta and Domesick, 1982, p.201).

CHAPTER 5

Investigations

It is not intended in this chapter to outline the basic or essential features of the neuropsychiatric examination, nor to discuss various methods that are available for the quantification and documentation of the mental state. Accounts of these are given elsewhere (Trimble, 1981a; Roberts, 1984). Here some of the more important clinical investigation techniques are presented, including an account of some of the newer methodologies such as magnetic resonance imaging (MRI) and positron emission tomography (PET).

The importance of careful history taking in the evaluation of patients cannot be overemphasized in psychiatry, as in other branches of medicine. This should, where possible, extend to third party accounts of the patient's behaviour, and in particular must concentrate on change of behaviour. An understanding of the more regular patterns of the patient's activities is derived from information about his past, including those of any previous change in behaviour which has led to psychiatric referral. Genetic diatheses must be sought by careful questioning. The essence, however, is the delineation of change—the identification of the point in time that a process intervened. Personality, its style and development, has to be dissociated from process. The manifestations of the latter are then analysed for their form, noting the problems that occur if form and content are confused. Diagnosis proceeds, as indicated in Chapter 2, through documentation of psychopathology, the combination of signs and symptoms, and the application of some recognized nomenclature. As in medicine generally, the essential point of the initial patient evaluation in psychiatry is to draw up a differential diagnosis so that a plan of investigation and treatment can be initiated.

In the clinical setting, the initial diagnostic process should be accompanied by a search for aetiology and if possible an understanding of pathogenesis. As noted, many of the conditions that once formed a significant part of psychiatric practice have now a clarified disease base, often associated with structural brain change. However, the fact that the signs and symptoms of psychiatric illness are reflections only of disturbed brain function, and alteration of function arises either from intrinsic alteration of function (functional disorder) or as a consequence of structural change (structural disorder), requires us to examine the central nervous system (CNS) in our patients.

The development of the clinical examination has arisen from the need to detect altered brain function in patients, especially in view of the difficulties in examining the brain itself, in vivo. In the past the prime aim of neurological examination was to uncover an inequality on one or other side of the body, which reflected the presence of focal pathology. The simple fact that many patients with localized structural disease present with psychopathology, which often is identical in phenomenology to the presentation of functional disease, makes physical examination in pychiatric practice an important part of any patient evaluation. Further, although the detection of lateralizing signs is important, physical examination may reveal many other aspects of the patients' life-style and state of health.

A revolution occurred with the introduction of techniques for investigating brain structure and function in vivo that could extend the routine physical examination. First came the electroencephalogram (EEG) in the 1940s, followed by the development of evoked potential investigations. With regards to imaging, although the first radiographs were produced at the end of the last century, and both pneumoencephalography and cerebral angiography were used widely in this century, it was the introduction of computed axial tomography (CT) that has had such a profound impact on the clinical neurosciences. Thus, for the first time, a relatively non-invasive, safe and repeatable technique for examining the brain was available. Unlike the complicated nuances of the angiogram, where detection of pathology often rested on the subtle detection of change in the patterns of the cerebral arterial or venous tree, assessment of the CT scan required mainly knowledge of neuroanatomy. The inexpensive generation of such images permits its use in the evaluation of psychiatric patients, and many would consider access to a CT scan essential for investigating psychopathology.

A further development, especially in the past decade, has been the assessment of hormones by techniques widely available in most laboratories. Because some of these, notably cortisol abnormalities, seem to relate to some psychopathologies and others may provide a 'window' into limbic and hypothalamic function, their use in biological psychiatry is growing.

CLINICAL INVESTIGATION

Since psychiatry is a branch of medicine, it is reasonable to offer to psychiatric patients the same facilities for medical investigation as they would expect from other specialists. In particular, their clinical evaluation should always be accompanied by appropriate laboratory tests, many of which are routine. Thus all patients should have assessment of their basic haematology profile, an ESR measurement and certain biochemical tests. The latter include urea and electrolytes, and liver function tests. The latter are important since alcohol intake is usually underestimated, and may be significant in the patient's pathology. If alcoholism is suspected, estimation of red cell transketolase activity may be of value. It is still wise to test the patient's syphilis serology.

Routine skull and chest X-rays are not now recommended unless there is a suspicion that they may be revealing. In in-patients, Larkin (1985) made the point that unexpectedly abnormal chest X-rays came from patients over 55, while skull films were unrewarding in any age group.

Measurement of vitamin B_{12} and folic acid status, thyroid function studies and blood glucose are often indicated, and in cases of 'funny turns' an extended glucose tolerance test is often done. On occasion, rarer investigations will be indicated such as measurement of plasma and urine osmolality, tests for LE cells and antinuclear factors, further endocrine evaluation, and tests for infectious mononucleosis or other disorders such as brucellosis.

Urine investigations include screening for drugs if any state of intoxication is suspected, ruling out infections, especially in the confused elderly, and rarely testing for urinary catecholamines in suspected phaeochromocytoma or searching for metachromatic material in suspected cases of metachromatic leucodystrophy. Testing for porphyrins when porphyria is suspected still occasionally yields rewarding results.

In therapy, serum level monitoring of certain drugs has now become routine, especially for lithium and anticonvulsants. Antidepressant monitoring can be of value, especially if a patient is responding poorly to good oral doses of the drug. Low levels may indicate a rapid metabolism or poor compliance. In addition, measurement when there is a complaint of toxic side effects on small doses may allow the physican to determine if this may be related to unexpectedly high levels, especially helpful in the elderly who often show reduced clearance of drugs. Serum alcohol or barbiturate levels are helpful in cases of dependence, or suspected dependence.

One neuropeptide that is useful to assess is prolactin. This is elevated by drugs that block dopamine receptors, and thus may be helpful in detecting compliance in patients on neuroleptic drugs. Although there is tolerance to the initial higher levels of prolactin over four weeks of treatment, a period of stability is reached which lasts for months thereafter (Brown and Laughren, 1981). Prolactin levels tend to be elevated in patients on intramuscular therapy (Chalmers and Bennie, 1978), and while not correlating with the serum levels of the neuroleptics, may be a predictor of the dopamine blockade at the hypothalamopituitary axis. Patients who develop extrapyramidal side effects to these drugs tend to have higher prolactin levels (Kolakowska et al., 1979), and hyperprolactinaemia is often associated with sexual disorders, especially in men (Schwartz et al., 1982).

The most interesting test that has been introduced into psychiatry in recent years is the dexamethasone suppression test (DST). Not only has this a rather specific application to psychiatry, but its very introduction emphasizes the potential value of measurement in clinical psychiatric practice. The trend of the discipline is thus to follow in the direction of progress in medicine, namely the supporting of purely clinical diagnoses by laboratory confirmation. The details of this and some other neuroendocrine tests are reviewed in Chapter 9.

Finally, lumbar puncture is of value in psychiatric practice. Thus, in cases of suspected cerebral syphilis serological investigation is required, and in some cases of undiagnosed dementia the presence of, for example, an oligoclonal immunoglobulin pattern may lead to a diagnosis of multiple sclerosis. In certain situations the radiologist uses the CSF to aid diagnosis, such as the administration of isotopes intrathecally and following their distribution over 48 hours, as was used in the diagnosis of normal pressure hydrocephalus. In this condition abnormally high concentrations of the isotope persist in the ventricles, with little or none being seen in the cortical subarachnoid space. This has now been superseded by CT scanning with isohexol.

BIOCHEMICAL INVESTIGATIONS

Technology

In recent years the ability to measure substances of biological importance in body fluids, from plasma, saliva, CSF and urine has increased considerably. Further, the detection of small quantities with reliable, quick and relatively inexpensive techniques has been important in expanding the use of biological tests in psychiatry. Gas chromatography and high performance liquid chromatography (HPLC) use the separation of compounds on columns and their analysis by sensitive detectors. In the former, the substance to be measured is carried in a gaseous phase into a column in which the separation takes place. Detectors at the end of the column measure and quantify the compounds. A particularly powerful detection method is mass spectroscopy. In this technique the substance to be measured is ionized electrically or chemically, and the application of magnetic and electrical forces separates the fragments in relation to their mass and electrical charge. In HPLC the contents of the separation column are forced in under high pressure, and their subsequent density allows excellent separation of compounds when the sample is injected rapidly through it. Since, unlike gas chromatography, there is no need to create gaseous derivatives, HPLC is cheaper and simpler. When combined with mass spectroscopy, HPLC is capable of quantifying picomolar concentrations.

Radioimmunoassay (RIA) has also been important. In this, a biologically radiolabelled compound is combined with a very specific immunoglobulin molecule—the complex which is then quantified by competitive binding to antibody. After an incubation period when the binding of the labelled and unlabelled substances have equilibrated, the bound and the unbound portions are separated. As the concentration of the unlabelled portion increases, the amount of bound radioactivity decreases and the appropriate quantitative calculations can be made from standardized curves.

Many RIAs are available in kit form and are widely used in the assessment of neurohormones. There are many difficulties, however, with RIA, not the least being the specificity of the antibodies, and often there are discrepancies between the results obtained with biological assays (bioassay—the direct measurement of changes in isolated tissue responsive to the substance, for example a hormone) and the results of RIA.

Another technique is the radioreceptor assay, in which binding to a specially prepared suspension of receptors is calculated. Again the biologically active compound competes with known radio-actively labelled ligands for the receptor, and the bound portion is assessed and compared to a standard. This technique has been especially helpful in the measurement of serum drug levels.

THE EEG

The early publications of Hans Berger, the founder of the EEG, between 1928 and 1935 were almost totally ignored. However, the confirmation of Berger's findings by Adrian and Matthews in 1935 that the electrical rhythms of the brain were detectable through the skull led to the rapid development of EEG machines and their evaluation in clinical practice. Normal and abnormal rhythms came to be described, and their relationship to underlying disease explored. The use of the EEG rapidly found use in the detection of such pathology as a cerebral tumour, and the recording of epileptic seizures led to advancements in the detection and classification of seizure types.

Although it was hoped that the EEG would bring important rewards for psychiatry, summing up the early years' experience, Hill commented: '. . .strictly within this field disappointingly little has emerged' (Hill, 1950, p.319). Over time the role of the EEG in the assessment of patients has been well evaluated, and recent developments, using sophisticated computed and statistical methods, suggest that the full impact of the EEG for psychiatry has yet to be reached.

The EEG signal

The signal finally reflected on the EEG trace represents only an average of the electrical events generated by the dendrites of neurones in the superficial cortical layers. It thus represents the graded sum of the exitatory and inhibitory potentials from many thousands of neurones lying under the recording electrode. Theoretically, if the cells are firing at random, the potentials should average out. The fact that there is a recordable rhythm implies that synchronization has occurred, suggesting the existence of some pacemaker. The thalamus is one structure from which EEG generators derive, although the genesis of the synchrony required for the spike of an epileptic focus is likely to be different from that leading to the generation of the normal alpha rhythm. The existence of multiple origins for synchrony may be postulated, and similar waveforms may not necessarily be derived by the same mechanism.

EEG traces

In the laboratory the patient has electrodes attached to the scalp, and usually eight or sixteen channels are recorded. These are referred to by a standardized notation known as the International 10–20 system. It should be noted that an average electrode spacing is some 5–6 cm, and, since much cortex is buried in the sulci of the brain or is too medial to influence the surface EEG, in a typical examination only some 20 per cent of the cortex is sampled, usually for only a small period of time. Better recordings from such structures as the medial temporal lobes can be obtained by using special electrode placement such as nasopharyngeal or spenoidal leads. The former requires electrodes to be placed through the nares to rest in the nasopharynx under the base of the skull. With sphenoidal electrodes, the tip is placed in the region of the foramen ovale. Activation procedures for enhancing normal and abnormal features of the EEG are usually employed and include hyperventilation, photic stimulation, sleep inducement or sleep deprivation, and the administration of epileptogenic agents such as pentylenetetrazol.

Interpretation of the recordings involves recognition not only of the type of waveform but also its voltage, frequency and polarity. The EEG is, in general, composed of relatively high voltage slow waves of up to 20 hertz (Hz, or cycles per second), and traditionally several different rhythms are recognized. The alpha rhythm has an 8–13 Hz frequency, and tends to appear in the relaxed but awake state. It is most prominent occipitally, and is attenuated or blocked by eye opening. Theta rhythm is 4–7 Hz, and delta is that below 4 Hz. Rhythms faster than 13 Hz are beta, and are more prominent frontally. Many psychotropic agents such as barbiturates or benzodiazepines increase beta. The mu rhythm is a central rhythm of the same frequency as alpha, which does not block with eye opening but does so with movement. It is seen in about one-fifth of young adults.

Age is an important determinant of the normal EEG, especially in early years. At birth theta and delta rhythms dominate, increasing in frequency with maturation, alpha becoming established around 13. The full adult pattern is not reached till the mid-twenties. Paroxysmal activity, including focal spikes or sharp waves, may be seen in nearly 3 per cent of normal children, increasing to nearly 10 per cent if provocative techniques or sleep studies are done (Eeg-Olofsson *et al.*, 1971). Frontal and in particular posterior temporal theta activity is not infrequently recorded in younger people, and its presence is thought to relate to brain maturation. Its detection should not be interpreted as evidence of epilepsy in patients having 'funny turns'.

An individual's EEG is characteristic, and studies of twins reveal important genetic determinants (Hill, 1950). The correlation with intelligence is poor. Level of awareness is crucial to the EEG wave pattern, and marked changes occur with the onset of sleep. Thus in the drowsy state, alpha waves tend to come and go, and as sleep supervenes the rhythms slow. Deeper sleep is characterized by delta activity, while in paradoxical sleep (REM), there is fast desynchronized activity. During the orthodox, slow wave stage, a number of other EEG events may be observed. Sleep spindles are bursts of low-voltage 13–15 Hz activity, and K-complexes, delta waves associated with spindles, may be seen. During a night's sleep, REM activity occurs in four to six periods lasting up to 30 minutes approximately 90 minutes apart. Typically the first REM period starts after about 90 minutes, and the total REM time for the average adult is 20–25 per cent of total sleep time.

EVOKED POTENTIALS

The electrical events generated by the brain following a simple stimulus are small, and in the sea of background activity will not be detected. By the technique of averaging the results of many similar stimuli, the signal to noise ratio is enhanced and the so-called evoked potential recorded. Thus, visual, auditory or somato-sensory stimuli are repetitively presented, and after each event the electrical activity of the brain is recorded. The averaged evoked potential is derived from computer analysis of the data, and is a series of waveforms of negative and positive voltage. The actual form of the event-related potential varies with the sensory stimulus, its modality and the cognitive processes involved in its perception. The first waves represent the arrival of the signals by the specific sensory pathways, the later waveforms reflecting activation over slower, polysynaptic paths. The former seem independent of the psychological state of the individual, while the latter

130

vary with the state of the subject and the meaning and relevance of the stimulus. The latency and amplitude of the early response seem related to the strength of the stimulus such that amplitudes increase and latencies decrease with increasing stimulus intensity. This, however, is not invariable, and in some subjects increased intensity leads to smaller responses (Shagass, 1972). The presentation of a stimulus and the evocation of a response alters a subsequent evoked response for a short period of time. It has been suggested that alteration in the recovery of this change may relate to psychopathology (Shagass, 1972). Changes in the waveforms of evoked potentials are widely used in the diagnosis of various diseases, an obvious example being multiple sclerosis (see Figure 1).

In addition to the shorter 'exogenous' latency responses, a number of the 'endogenous' event-related slow potentials have been described. These include the P300 wave, the contingent negative variation (CNV) and motor potentials such as the Bereitschaftspotential. The P300 wave refers to a positive response component seen some 300–500 ms after the stimulus, said to relate to a process of cognitive appraisal of the stimulus. It has a centroparietal distribution for all sensory modalities, and its latency increases with diminishing discrimination of presented stimuli. It has been suggested that it may be related to the laying down of memory traces (Karis *et al.*, 1984).

The CNV is derived by giving a subject a stimulus, to be followed some brief time later by another which requires some response. The first serves as a warning stimulus, in expectancy of the second (expectancy wave is an alternative name). The wave

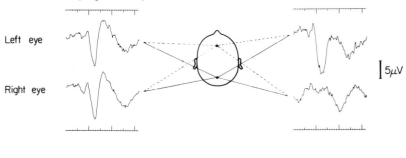

Normal   Optic Neuritis

Figure 1. A visual evoked potential showing a normal pattern, and, for comparison, a similar potential from a patient with optic neuritis. (Kindly supplied by Dr M. Halliday, Institute of Neurology.)

consists of a slow negative shift in potential, especially in the vertex and frontal regions. Originally described by Walter and colleagues in 1964, it relates to such psychological processes as motivation, attention and heightened attention (see Figure 2). It is increased by such factors as certainty that the stimulus will occur and interest in the stimulus. It is diminished by distraction and boredom, and its character may be altered in psychopathology. The CNV should not be confused with the 'readiness potential' or Bereitschaftspotential which is a similar slow negative potential that arises about one second before voluntary movement. It is maximal in the precentral parietal region, and may be broken down into a number of separate components (Shibasaki *et al.*, 1980).

Some other techniques

In recent years other sophisticated variations of EEG recording have come into use, including prolonged monitoring and computerized analysis leading to continuous mapping of brain electrical activity.

There are two main forms of prolonged monitoring, namely videotelemetry and ambulatory monitoring. In the former the patient is filmed by a videocamera, usually in a specially designed laboratory or ward, and the EEG is recorded simultaneously. Both the picture and the EEG trace are sent to an adjoining room where they are displayed on a split screen to be viewed together. The EEG and the patient's behaviour can thus be correlated.

With ambulatory monitoring, the EEG is recorded for a prolonged period of time using a portable cassette recorder strapped to the patient's body. The technique requires the use of special head-mounted amplifiers that diminish muscle and other artifacts. Although with this method there is no accompanying visual image of the patient, the apparatus can be worn at home or in the school without interference to daily activities. A disadvantage of both these investigations is the limited number of channels that can be recorded and the interference that still occurs on the record at crucial times, such as during a seizure.

The use of computerized EEG methods allows profiles of the average amount of activity in various wavebands over time to be derived. The EEG record can be broken down into frequency components which are quantified using electronic filters and integrators, and electrical power determined according to selected frequency bands by using the mathematical technique of Fourier

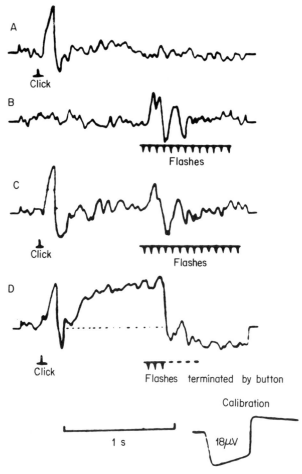

Figure 2. Showing the contingent negative variation CNV. Averages of responses to twelve presentations. A, response in frontovertical region to clicks; B, flicker; C, clicks followed by flicker; D, clicks followed by flicker terminated by the subject pressing a button as instructed. The CNV appears following the conditional response and submerges the negative component of the imperative response. (Reprinted with permission from Walter *et al.*, *Nature*, **203**, pp.380–384. Copyright © 1964 Macmillan Journals Limited.)

analysis. This has been particularly useful in psychopharmacology, for example noting the influence of different classes of drugs on these measurements.

Brain electrical activity mapping (BEAM) is a topographic mapping technique that condenses information from the EEG or evoked potential and presents it as a coloured map. Data are broken down into a matrix of some 4000 elements, and a map is coded depending on the amount of electrical activity at each point. The resulting image can be an average of a series of images from a group of patients, and that data can be compared with that collected from another group. Areas of statistical differences between groups can be displayed as coloured maps, a technique known as significance probability mapping.

Finally, a new technique known as magnetoencephalography (MEG), in which extracranial magnetic fields derive from the brain's electrical potentials, has been introduced. The magnetic fields are not influenced by the scalp as EEG potentials are, and are more localized. It will be possible using MEG to provide information from deeper cortical structures which is at present impossible with the EEG without using depth electrodes.

BRAIN IMAGING TECHNIQUES

CT scans

Both angiography and pneumoencephalography, widely used prior to the introduction of the CT scan, provided only indirect information and did not show brain tissue directly. In contrast, the CT scan provided a computerized reconstruction of the brain image (Figure 3).

A typical scanner is composed of an X-ray source, a detector, a computer for image construction and an image display system. A fine beam of X-rays is generated and projected through the patient's head. The apparatus then rotates through one or more degrees and another projection is made. The process is repeated until all points in a plane, around 180 degrees, have been probed from many directions. During the passages of the X-ray photons through the tissues of the head they will interact with intrinsic electrons, and either be scattered or be captured. In either case they will not reach the detector. The more important event is scattering, which is dependent on tissue density. The final image represents a matrix display, a kind of grid map composed of many adjacent squares. Each square represents the average density of the tissue in the area of the square and a volume of tissue lying underneath it. The small square as seen is called a pixel, and the volume of tissue it represents is the voxel (see Figure 4).

It is obvious that if the voxel is composed of all the same tissue, then the density reflected in the pixel will faithfully reflect the

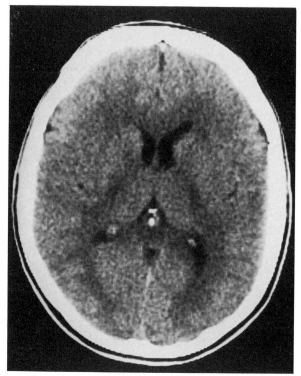

Figure 3. A normal CT scan. The slight asymmetry of the ventricles reflects the patient's head position during scanning.

quality of the represented area. However, if within the voxel there are, in addition to the soft tissue elements, bone, fluid or air, then the average reading will be altered which may lead to a misinterpretation of the presence of pathology in that tissue. This is known as the partial volume effect, and is an important source of error in CT data. The depth of the voxel varies with different machines from 2 to 13 mm. The usual matrix is made up of a 160 × 160 or 320 × 320 matrix. Although original scanners used single beams, later models use multiple collimated beams and detectors and allow reconstruction of the X-ray data to produce sagittal and coronal, as well as axial, views.

The units of density on one of the scales used are referred to as Hounsfield units, named after a pioneer of the CT technique. On this scale zero is the representative of water, air being –500 and brain tissue in the region of +15 to +18. An alternative is the EMI unit, which is half the value of the Hounsfield unit. Some machines

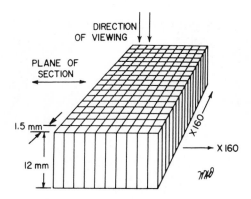

Figure 4. In the interpretation of CT scans it is important to understand that the small square seen from above as a picture element (pixel) actually represents the average radiodensity of the entire underlying volume element (voxel). A small amount of solid bone encroaching into any fraction of this voxel will slightly increase the pixel value and may be misinterpreted as abnormal soft tissue. A small fraction of air could produce a misleading slight lowering of average density. This is known as the partial volume effect. Even a small fraction of solid calcium occupying the voxel (such as found in almost all pineal glands) causes an obvious change in pixel brightness. (Reproduced with permission from Oldendorf, *Quest for an Image of the Brain.* Copyright © 1980 Raven Press, New York.)

allow for direct assessment of densities in the selected region of interest (ROI).

The scan can be contrasted by giving an iodinated contrast medium which, on account of its efficient electron capture, deletes X-rays and increases tissue radiodensity.

A grey scale, ranging from white to black, allows the ultimate visual display, and the scale is set to allow maximum visualization of tissues of interest. This procedure relates to window width and level. The latter refers to setting the scale so that it is centred on the attenuation (X-ray absorption) value of most relevance, and the width refers to the range of other tissue attenuations to be included in the grey scale. Thus, if the window width is set at 20 and it is equally weighted either side of the level, then ten units above and the same below will be included in the grey scale. Values outside of this range will appear either as all white or all black.

The CT scan has dramatically altered neurological practice and has had a major impact on psychiatry. The most important clinically has been the detection of structural lesions in association with psychopathology, for example cerebral tumours or meningiomas (see Figure 5).

It allows the effective early evaluation of patients with dementia by relatively non-invasive techniques (see Chapter 11), and is

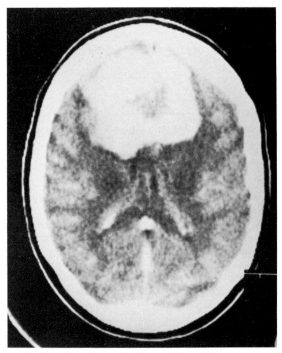

Figure 5. CT showing frontal meningioma. The patient presented with a typical major affective disorder, responsive to antidepressants.

providing us with prognostic and treatment information in such disorders as schizophrenia. It has been important in psychiatric research, notably by reinforcing what had been shown in earlier times with other techniques, namely that patients diagnosed as schizophrenic show abnormalities, especially cortical sulcal widening and ventricular enlargement (see Chapter 8).

Roberts and Lishman (1984) reviewed the results of CT scans taken at one psychiatric hospital in the first year of use of a scanner. Of 323 patients, 29.1 per cent had definitely abnormal scans and 26.3 per cent equivocally abnormal scans. While in the majority of cases the scans confirmed a clinical impression of the presence of a lesion, in 11.7 per cent of cases the scan was influential in determining the clinical practice of the referring physician. Similar data are recorded from other centres (for example Larson *et al.*, 1981), emphasizing the value of the technique in psychiatric practice. In certain selected settings, such as mental retardation or psychogeriatrics, the rate of abnormalities is likely to be even higher, although paradoxically, in some countries, such groups are likely to have poor access to routine scanning facilities.

Magnetic resonance imaging (MRI) scan

The elegant demonstration of the brain's structure by the CT scan is already being superceded by MRI. While more expensive, and as yet not widely available, in a few years MRI is likely almost to replace conventional CT technology.

Although the technique, also referred to as nuclear magnetic resonance (NMR), has been used in spectroscopy for some time, the formation of images derives from the work of Lauterbur (1973), who used the term zeugmatography. The principle involves the examination of the physicochemical environment of proton nuclei in tissue based on the inherent electromagnetic forces that exist in such electrically charged particles.

Briefly, any object that has charge and velocity produces a magnetic field perpendicular to it. A charged nuclear particle spinning in the body's tissues thus produces a magnetic field, although in this case the field is referred to as the angular magnetic moment with a vector perpendicular to the axis of rotation. A charged nuclear particle, spinning about its axis acts like a tiny bar magnet, and, before the application of an external magnetic field, the sum total magnetization of many of them spinning in human tissues is zero, since their direction of movement is random. On application of an external magnetic force the tiny magnets are aligned, just as an ordinary compass needle will align in the Earth's magnetic field. The alignment is parallel (or antiparallel) to the external field. The protons in such a setting actually spin, like a spinning top, around the alignment of the applied field, a process referred to as precession. Protons, which possess their own inherent specific precession, once aligned can now be excited by the momentary application of a radiosignal broadcast at their own specific frequency (the Larmour frequency) from a radiofrequency transmitter. This process may be likened to a tuning fork and a guitar string. Thus, if we have six strings tuned to different frequencies and a tuning fork for one of those frequencies is struck nearby, then only that string will resonate; if we have a series of guitars, then all the strings of that frequency will respond. So it is with protons in human tissue. If now the tuning fork is silenced, the guitars will continue to give off a sound, and this can be picked up by a receiver and measured (see Figure 6).

138

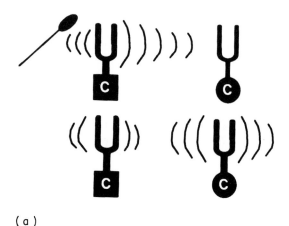

(a)

(b)

Figure 6. (a) Showing the principle of resonance if tuning fork is struck; an adjacent one of the same tone will vibrate and emit sound (upper). This will persist after the first tuning fork is removed (lower). (b) Principles of MRI. (Reproduced with permission from Young, *NMR Imaging: Basic Principles.* Copyright © 1984 Raven Press, New York.)

The procedure of imaging makes use of the fact that waves emitted from the nuclei differ in both frequency and amplitude, the former locating the position of the particular nucleus in the body and the latter reflecting the number of nuclei present at that position. Thus, within the static externally applied magnetic field, energy is imparted to the parallel protons, exciting them to a higher energy level by radiofrequency waves of exactly the right frequency, and after the signal is finished electromagnetic energy of the same frequency will be given off, detected by a receiver coil. After the application of the radiofrequency pulse, the magnetization returns exponentially to its pre-excitement level, a process referred to as relaxation. This may be defined by two time constants, referred to as T_1 and T_2, of which T_1 is always greater than T_2.

The T_1, or spin-lattice, relaxation time, representing relaxation along the longitudinal axis, is the time taken for the protons to recover their previously aligned position in the static field after excitation in this axis by a 180 degree pulse. In practice, due to the configuration of most scanners, a so-called inversion recovery image is used to give a T_1 weighted image.

The T_2 relaxation time, representing relaxation in the transverse plane (hence transverse relaxation time), is the exponential time constant which results from decay of coherence, due to the interaction of the spinning nuclei. It relates to energy exchange between protons, and is also referred to as the spin–spin relaxation time. T_2 is thus a measure of the length of time the tissue maintains its temporary transverse magnetization, perpendicular to the external magnetic field following a 90 degree pulse. The spin echo is proportional to the proton density and T_2, and is frequently used for T_2 measurement.

Thus, each tissue has a specific T_1 and T_2 value, and they essentially reflect the physicochemical environment of the proton nuclei. The T_1 relates to the interactions of protons with surrounding nuclei, the T_2 depending on interactions of protons with each other. In the brain, the proton behaviour measured relates to the hydrogen nucleus, most commonly of CNS water. Thus the spinning atomic nucleus will behave like the spinning top only if it has an odd atomic mass or number, an atom with an even number being non-magnetic. While NMR spectroscopy can image ^1H, ^{13}C, ^{15}N, ^{19}F, ^{23}Na and ^{31}P, imaging is largely at present confined to hydrogen nuclei.

In practice, the requirements for clinical brain imaging are a large superconducting bore magnet, a radiofrequency transmitter coil that may also act as a receiver, a computer and a display system. With present techniques the patient lies in the magnet for approximatly an hour, and many slices are imaged. The actual imaging technique involves a series of choices for sequencing related to the direction and timing of the radiofrequency pulses delivered, the data being spatially encoded to provide information on proton density, T_1 and T_2 times. Since it is an electronic process, reconstruction can be done in any direction, and is usually slice encoding. Inversion recovery and spin echo techniques are the most widely employed. By exploiting differences between the relaxation times of different tissues, heightened contrast between them is achieved, and hence better images. The use of contrast media such as gadolinium DTPA is becoming available to further aid tissue differentiation. These cross the blood–brain barrier in small quantities and alter the relaxation time of tissues, inversion recovery images being particularly sensitive.

The static magnet activates all protons, and gradient magnets activate specific cuts. The derived images have a low spatial resolution, in some machines being as low as 0.8 mm square. Most pathological conditions increase the length of T_1 and T_2, free water having even higher values. Since on T_1 images increasing the time darkens the image, and on T_2 images it lightens the image, on T_1 images, CSF and pathological areas are relatively darkened, and vice versa on T_2 images. Both T_1 and T_2 are shorter in white matter than in grey, but the signal from bone is very weak and it is not well visualized on images. This has an enormous advantage for imaging in neuropsychiatry since the bony structures of the cranial vault, which on CT imaging so often obscure the structures of interest such as the temporal lobes, are not present (see Figure 7). A disadvantage is that calcified lesions are not well visualized (see Figure 8). A summary of the advantages and disadvantages of MRI are shown in Table 1, and further examples of scans in Figures 9 and 10.

Table 1   Advantages and disadvantages of MRI

Advantages	Disadvantages
No radiation	Noise discomfort
Minimal risk[a]	Claustrophobic
Good grey/white discrimination	Limited discrimination
Less degradation of image with movement	between pathologies
	Length of scan time
No bone artifacts	Artifacts from
Clear strutural images	ferromagnetic material
Ability to visualize several planes	(e.g. tooth filling)
Potential for functional imaging	

[a]Only patients with cardiac pacemakers, intracranial magnetic clips or in the first trimester of pregnancy should not be scanned.

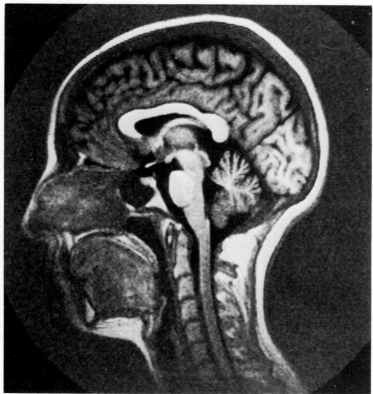

Figure 7. A normal MRI scan. Note the absence of bone artifacts, and the clear delineation of anatomical structures. (Kindly supplied by Dr D. Miller, Institute of Neurology.)

There is the potential to use quantitative information from the scans, especially actual T_1 and T_2 measurements for studying structural changes, and, with higher strength magnets, to image other atoms such as ^{31}P.

Cerebral blood flow (CBF) and metabolism

The techniques described above for brain imaging provide essentially anatomical data, and to the present time have given information about structural changes in the brain. In contrast, CBF and metabolism reflect on the function of the brain. It is

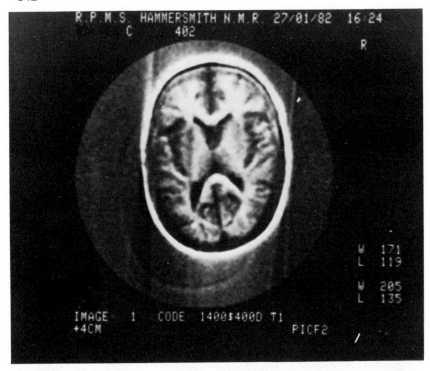

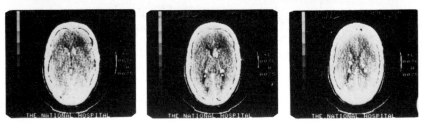

Figure 8. MRI of a patient with tuberose sclerosis and, beneath, corresponding CT scan. Note the poor calcification of tubers on the MRI image.

important to emphasize that the resulting images are based on complicated mathematical modelling, itself based on suppositions about the biochemical activity of the brain in non-diseased states, and that the resolution of current machines is far less than that for MRI. Although assessment of whole brain CBF has been available for many years, it was the development of regional analysis in the 1960s and the combination of these techniques with computed imaging to provide PET that has revolutionized our knowledge in this area.

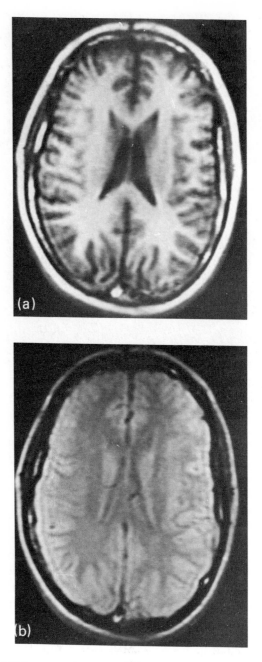

Figure 9. (a) MRI contrasting inversion recovery with (b) spin echo sequences. (Kindly supplied by Dr D. Miller, Institute of Neurology.)

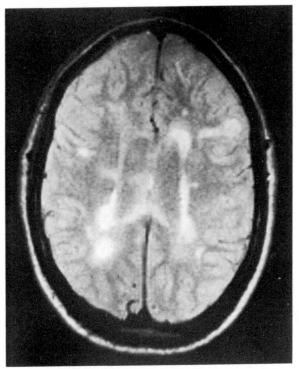

Figure 10. MRI in multiple sclerosis with spin echo sequence. Note in particular the periventricular sites of demyelination. (Kindly supplied by Dr D. Miller, Institute of Neurology.)

The use of radioactive isotopes to aid in diagnosis initially involved the administration of gamma ray emitting compounds such as technetium 99 to outline blood–brain barrier defects and enhance the visualization of, for example, cerebral tumours. The first successful measurement of CBF was with the nitrous oxide technique, introduced by Kety and Schmidt (1948). This required sampling of blood entering and leaving the brain with the inhalation of the gas. Since the latter was non-metabolizable but freely diffusable, if the arteriovenous (A-V) difference after steady state was achieved was known, blood flow could be determined. In the technique, blood samples were taken from an artery and the internal jugular vein, and it was thus highly invasive. In addition, originally, only whole brain CBF was calculated. The principle behind these techniques was that the amount of substance carried to the brain per unit time by the arterial blood equals the amount leaving it by the venous blood, plus the amount accumulated in addition to that metabolized, the latter, with the nitrous oxide, being zero. Since after a time equilibrium between the brain tissue and venous blood is reached, the CBF could be calculated based on an equation containing the observed tracer concentrations in arterial and venous blood.

A variant of the method employed 85-krypton and a longer period of blood sampling. The second-generation methods, rapidly developed, relied on the rates that similar isotopes were cleared from the brain, traced by recording the decline in radio-activity over the scalp with scintillation counters. The isotopes were given either by inhalation or intracarotid injection, and included 85-krypton and 133-xenon. The number of detectors available has increased, and it is now possible to image regional CBF (rCBF) from many areas on both sides of the brain. In practice, tracer is given, and the 'clearance curve' of its arrival and elimination from the region is plotted. By comparison to theoretical values obtained from a physiological model, the CBF is derived. The initial slope index (ISI) is an early flow index frequently used. Tracer is monitored for approximately 10 minutes after administration and calculations of both grey and white matter flow are derived. The spatial resolution of the technique is limited, and interference from the contralateral hemisphere reduces the sensitivity, especially for detecting asymmetries. Early artifacts, such as the problem of contamination of blood from extracerebral sources, have been overcome, but haemoglobin values, due to the affinity of xenon for haemoglobin, and the arterial CO_2 tension have to be taken into account. CO_2 is a potent vasodilator of cerebral vessels, and hyperventilation, for example due to anxiety, may lower the $PaCO_2$ and the CBF.

In normal healthy adults, the mean CBF is around 50 ml/100 g of brain tissue per minute, the values for grey and white matter being approximately 80 and 20 ml/100 g per minute respectively. Normally a tendency to greater values frontally is found, and a slow decrease with advancing age (Frackowiak *et al.*, 1980).

Advantages of the CBF techniques, especially xenon inhalation, include: being a non-invasive procedure, it is quick to perform; the ability to repeat images after a short time interval; and, especially compared to PET, its inexpensiveness. Its limitations are the low spatial resolution (2–4 cm), inability to provide three-dimensional imaging and its failure to give information on deep cerebral structures.

PET

As noted, the main source of cerebral energy is glucose, but provided that there is coupling between oxygen consumption and ATP production, energy metabolism can be deduced from measuring oxygen use. Although under normal conditions there is coupling between the CBF and the cerebral metabolic rate of oxygen use ($CMRO_2$), and thus assessment of CBF may provide information regarding metabolism, in pathological states or with hypercapnia or hyperventilation the relationship is lost. Measurement of $CMRO_2$ using the technique of Kety and Schmidt was possible, but, with the autoradiographic work of Sokoloff *et al.* (1977) and the technology of computed tomography, the development of PET has allowed for the assessment of both CBF and metabolism, in vivo, on a regional basis.

In PET radioactive isotopes of biological substances are created by a cyclotron, which fires protons at a nucleus of, for example, carbon. The latter gains protons and becomes unstable, being an 'antiparticle' to a negatively charged electron. When in tissue, it combines immediately with an electron, the two particles converting their mass into radiation energy. They subsequently annihilate. The latter gives rise to the release of two coincident gamma rays of equal energy which travel at 180 degrees to each other (see Figure 11).

The presence of these rays is picked up by the detectors of the scanner, positioned such that they only record coincident events, these being separated from other non-simultaneously released gamma rays. Thus the decay event is known to have taken place on a line connecting the two detectors. Detection cameras are placed in a ring around the patient's head, the exact structure being dependent on the system used. Computerized reconstruction of the image is performed using technology similar to that of CT scanning. However, it is essential to recognize a fundamental difference between the two techniques, namely that in CT, rays from an external source are passed through the patient's brain, while in PET, rays are emitted from the brain, detected and quantified. Further, the image of PET is indeed an image, and one of tissue tracer distributions. It is not an anatomical map as provided by MRI and CT.

The spatial resolutions of the machines vary, but typically are between 7 and 15 mm. For technical reasons related to the finite range of the decay of positrons, the maximum resolution is in the

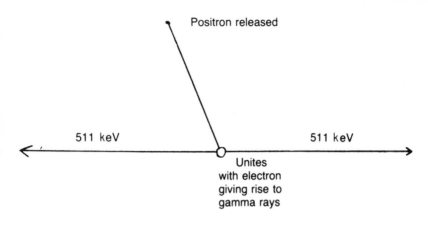

(a)

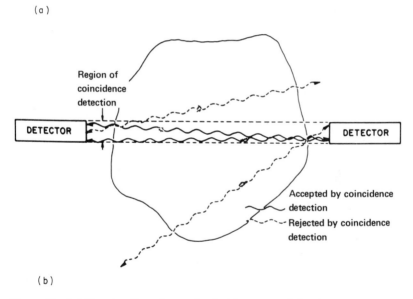

(b)

Figure 11. (a) Showing the release of coincidence rays following positron anni-hilation. (b) Showing the detection of coincidence rays by the scanner.

region of 2–3 mm. In order to obtain accurate readings from a structure, it should have a size twice that of the resolution of the machine.

The main biologically interesting positron emitters created include carbon-11, nitrogen-13, flourine-18 and oxygen-15. In practice, since all but flourine-18 have short half-lives, the patient has to be in close proximity to the cyclotron for the investigations to be carried out. With flourine labelled isotopes, with a half-life of 110 minutes, the substance can be transported to the patient over considerable distances.

Depending on the isotope used, PET provides information on several parameters including cerebral blood volume, CBF, cerebral metabolism and, more recently, with the successful labelling of transmitter ligands, neuroreceptor function.

At the present time there are two main systems for imaging metabolism, that based on oxygen and that on glucose or deoxyglucose. In the oxygen-15 technique, the patient continuously inhales trace amounts of oxygen-15 labelled carbon dioxide (CO_2) and oxygen. The CO_2 is rapidly converted in the lungs to $H_2^{15}O$, and is distributed throughout the arterial tree, about 20 per cent reaching the brain. There it equilibrates rapidly with tissue water. Since this is removed continuously by the venous system, at steady state the concentration of radioactivity measured will reflect both the delivery to and the decay from the tissue. Thus, at steady state, it is possible, using mathematically derived formulae with various corrections, to calculate the blood flow.

Similarly, the ^{15}O is delivered to the brain attached to haemoglobin, and there is used to fuel the Krebs cycle for the production of ATP, the radioactive oxygen appearing in water as a result of the metabolism. Again, with sophisticated mathematics and correction for sources of error (Lammertsma *et al.*, 1981), it is possible to define the oxygen extraction fraction (OEF)—the fraction of available oxygen extracted from the blood—and from this and the CBF, the $CMRO_2$ is calculated.

The fluorodeoxyglucose (FDG) method relies on the ingenious yet simple principle developed by Sokolof *et al.* (1977). Thus, glucose, when administered, is taken up into tissue and rapidly metabolized to CO_2 and H_2O and cleared from the brain. However, deoxyglucose is taken up and phosphorylated to deoxyglucose-6-phosphate, but this is not metabolized further as there are no available enzymes for its further degradation. In addition there is no functional dephosphorylase, so it can not reenter the precursor pool. As a consequence it gets trapped in the tissue, and its presence is directly measured and quantified since the radioactive deoxyglucose emits positrons which lead to the production of coincidence annihilation gamma rays detected by the scanner. In contrast to the short half-life of ^{15}O (123 s), that of FDG is in the region of 110 minutes; hence its use entails a longer study and requires careful control and monitoring of the patient's state during the uptake period. The metabolic handling of this analogue of glucose has then to be equated with that of glucose, if the derived measurements are to be used to reflect neuronal metabolism. The relationship has been found constant under many conditions, mathematically referred to as the lumped constant, but the latter has been derived essentially from animal models and may break down in certain pathological states leading to erroneous calculations.

Innovations in PET technology are progressing rapidly. Some of the newer machines, referred to as time-of-flight, attempt discrimination of the time of arrival of the paired gamma rays to actually localize the disintegration spatially. More relevant has been the ability to label other biologically active substances such as transmitters and their precursors, amino acids and psychoactive drugs. At present, one active area is the labelling of dopamine receptors. Ideally, in order to be visualized, the radiotracer use for receptor study should have a high affinity for the receptor, high specificity and readily cross the blood–brain barrier. For dopamine receptors, N-methylspiperone may be used, which, when labelled with carbon-11, flourine-18 or bromine-76 or -77, attaches preferentially to dopamine receptors (D2), and in frontal cortex to 5-HT receptors. A ratio between binding at the caudate nucleus and the cerebellum (relatively free of dopamine receptors) is one calculation obtained. Carbon and flourine labelled L-dopa is now available to detect the precursor pool for dopamine, and in animals the cholinergic receptor has been visualized. ^{11}C labelled buprenorphine to assess opiate receptor binding, radioactively labelled benzodiazepines such as flunitrazepam and diazepam, or antagonists such as RO 15-1788, and labelled ketanserin for 5-HT$_2$ receptors can also be used.

Interpretation of the data accumulated with PET is subject to a multitude of errors, which at the present time are probably responsible for the confusion in some of the data, especially with regard to psychiatric illness. Some of these are listed in Table 2.

In spite of these, much data has been collected in patients and volunteers, brain function being studied in a variety of physiological states. Thus, using either the earlier blood flow techniques or later PET, it has been possible to confirm a number of previously held theories regarding brain–behaviour correlates. Most investigators have demonstrated a so-called hyperfrontality, with blood flow and metabolism tending to be greater in the frontal when

Table 2 Potential artifacts in the interpretation of PET data (from De Lisi and Buchsbaum, 1986)

Compound as tracer
1. Half-life and breakdown rate of label
2. Purity of the compound
3. Differences between oxygen and glucose
4. Differences between labels, e.g. $^{18}F/^{11}C$

Experimental conditions
1. Variation in anxiety and emotional state of subject
2. Psychiatric state of patient
3. Task performed during the uptake period
4. Variation in sensory inputs, e.g. eyes open/closed
5. Prolonged uptake period with inconstant physiologic changes
6. Variation in blood sampling procedures
7. Failure to control for age and sex

Instrumentation
1. Limited resolution
2. Non-uniform resolution
3. Scatter and partial volume effects
4. Inadequate number of planes sampled
5. Need to standardize adequately to phantoms
6. Variation in head size and shape
7. Head movement
8. Change in distribution of tracer compound during the scan procedure from first to last slice

Data analysis
1. Inaccuracy of models to describe biochemical kinetics
2. No appropriate model for some substances
3. Kinetic constants used derive from animals
4. Differences in the kinetics between white and grey matter
5. Difficulties in matching some slices among individuals
6. Undersampling of anatomical structures
7. Overinterpretation of assumed anatomical details
8. Computerized methods do not account for anatomical differences among individuals
9. Accounting for cortical folding
10. Lack of serial determinations of data in the same individual over time to know normal variation

---

compared with the occipital areas. With visual stimulation, uptake in the occipital areas increases, progressively with greater complexity of the visual stimuli. With auditory information, regardless of the stimulus, increased values are detected in both auditory cortices and the frontal cortex. With verbal stimulation activation of the left frontal cortex accompanies the temporal lobe stimulation, the left-sided laterality being present regardless of the ear stimulated. The asymmetries closely parallel the known anatomical differencies of Heschl's gyrus and the planum temporale. Interestingly, using chords of complex harmonic composition leads to a greater increase of the right temporal cortex, except in musically sophisticated subjects who show a relative left posterior hypermetabolism. This suggests that the activation in response to stimuli is varied, not only by the stimulus, but also by the cognitive stategy of the subject (Phelps and Mazziotta, 1983).

An increase in activity is seen with speech, but not however maximally in the classical speech areas of Broca and Wernicke, but in a Z-shaped distribution affecting the prefrontal areas and some of the temporal lobes on both sides of the brain. Frontal activation is also seen with planning of tasks and thinking. Even thinking of words internally, without actually speaking, will activate frontal areas. On performance of a motor task with one hand there is an expected increase in the contralateral motor area of the cortex. However, when someone is asked to plan a motor act by rehearsing it in his mind, then the increase is seen in the supplementary motor area and the prefrontal cortex. In other words, purely intrinsic mental activity leads to focal areas of brain activation. These findings emphasize the importance of the frontal areas for the performance of language, thinking and planning. While the findings have been more prominent in CBF studies, they have also been seen with metabolic studies using PET.

SPECT

One of the main difficulties of the conventional CBF studies with xenon has been the restriction of the images to the cortical surface. CT techniques have been applied to the methodology using a rotating gamma camera with radiochemicals such as 123-iodoamphetamine used as tracers. This is present in brain long enough to allow CT imaging, and tomographic slices of brain can be reconstructed. While the resolution of the technique is less than that of PET, it is considerably less expensive and becoming of value in neuropsychiatric studies.

CHAPTER 6

Disorders of the limbic system

The anatomy and physiology of the limbic system have been described. It has been pointed out that the discovery of the limbic system and the development of an understanding of its links with behaviour have been of fundamental importance to biological psychiatry. In this chapter it is intended to discuss some of the conditions that primarily affect the function of the limbic system. However, it is not implied that other conditions do not affect these brain areas, and indeed, as will be shown in later chapters, it is suggested that many conditions that lead to psychopathology in some fashion involve the limbic system. What distinguishes the conditions described in this chapter is that they destroy limbic tissue, and the limbic system bears the brunt of the disease process.

By isolating this group of conditions it is not intended to imply that the limbic system somehow operates in isolation from the rest of the brain. Thus, critics of the limbic system concept note that brain research is increasingly emphasizing holistic models of brain function, and, especially with our increasing knowledge of brain anatomy and chemistry, it becomes difficult to separate one functionally different region of the brain from another (Brodal, 1969). This view is correct, but dissection of brain syndromes on the basis of sites of known abnormalities has been influential in the neurosciences, and the principle is appropriate for understanding the development of psychopathology. This is not to return to the old localizationist views, with the implication that functions are localized exclusively in discrete brain areas. It is an attempt to analyse the role of different anatomical systems in relation to behaviour as a whole, with the full knowledge that any destruction of brain leads to both the effects of that lesion in that area and the continued, but now different, action of the rest of the brain.

In clinical neurology, the essence of the clinical examination since its introduction has been to delineate clinical signs which reflect disturbances in one or other part of the nervous system. Symmetrical inequality, whether of reflexes, tone or sensation, is given prime place, since in clinical practice, at least prior to the

introduction of CT scanning, one important aspect was the identification of structural lesions which would lead one side of the body
to perform inappropriately. A distinguishing feature of neurology
in contrast to psychiatry stems from the success of the former in
developing methods of detection of such localizations from clinical
examination.

Two of the most important events that have led to the restructur-
ing of our views have already been discussed. The first was encephalitis lethargica; the second the introduction of the EEG into
clinical practice. Thus, the psychopathology seen following the
encephalitis was so striking that its significance was and is impossible to ignore. The EEG reinforced the idea that some areas of the
limbic system were susceptible to specific pathology, and these
regions, notably the medial temporal areas, were the very areas
which were being linked to emotion and behaviour in animal
investigations. The suggestion of Gibbs (1951) that patients with
temporal lobe epilepsy were more prone to psychiatric illness than
patients with other forms of epilepsy emphasized the significance
of the limbic structures for psychiatry. In this chapter some limbic
system disorders are reviewed, while the psychopathology of epilepsy is discussed in Chapter 10. In view of the close links to the
frontal cortex, frontal lobe syndromes are included here.

TEMPORAL LOBE DISORDERS

Encephalitis

In various parts of the world encephalitis is endemic, and the CNS
seems a specific target organ for some neurotropic viruses such as
that of St Louis encephalitis. Further, conditions such as measles
and the acquired immune deficiency syndrome (AIDS) may lead
to encephalitis, although here the viruses affect many body organs
as well as the brain. Among the viruses are some that appear to
preferentially invade certain CNS structures, including the rabies
virus, herpes simplex virus and that which causes encephalitis
lethargica. All three seem to have some predilection for the limbic
system.

In general, the prodromal symptoms of encephalitis are non-
specific, with a fever, headache and drowsiness. In severe cases
this progresses to stupor and coma, and convulsions may be seen.
At this acute stage, CSF changes occur such as an increase in

protein and cells, mainly mononuclear in type. Identification of the virus type by detection of a rising viral antibody titre in serum is sometimes possible. Antiviral drugs such as acyclovir, which inhibits DNA synthesis, may be given in the acute stages, with variable success.

Herpes simplex encephalitis, responsible for what previously was referred to as acute necrotizing encephalitis, is the commonest cause of fatal encephalitis in patients. Following a non-specific prodromal period, there is often the relatively sudden onset of a change of affect, and evidence of focal CNS involvement. Seizures are common. Aphasia and progressive paraparesis, and the presentation of an acute organic brain syndrome with confusion, disorientation and drowsiness are seen. The initial behaviour disturbance may be quite bizarre, the patient doing things seemingly quite out of character, and hallucinations may be reported. The EEG is abnormal, sometimes showing characteristic repetitive slow wave discharges from one or other temporal region.

The disease is due to HSV-1 virus, either as a de novo infection or due to activation of a previously acquired but dormant virus (Longson, 1985). The virus leads to marked necrosis of infected brain areas, but the brunt of the pathology is on the frontal and temporal lobes. Brain biopsy reveals HSV in the neuronal tissue. The mortality rate is high, around 70–80 per cent, in spite of the availability of newer antiviral agents. Among the survivors the subsequent psychopathology is severe. This may become manifest during recovery (Greenwood et al., 1983) and continue thereafter. Notable are an amnesic syndrome (see below; Rose and Symonds, 1960), hypermetamorphosis (overattention to external stimuli), a tendency to explore objects orally, agnosias, eating and drinking indiscriminantly and inappropriate sexual displays. Irritability, easy distractability, aggressive outbursts, emotional blunting, periods of apathy and depression and episodes of restlessness and overactivity are seen in most patients. Some survivors of herpes simplex encephalitis exhibit parts of the Kluver–Bucy syndrome. Hierons et al. (1978) provided both clinical and pathological data on ten patients who survived from 3 to 39 years. The most affected areas of the brain were the anterior part of the temporal lobe, the uncus and the amygdaloid nucleus, the hippocampus and the dentate fascia, the insula and the parahippocampal, posterior orbital and cingulate gyri. This relative selection can sometimes be

156

identified on CT scan (see Figure 1), even more subtle pathology being seen with MRI (see Figure 2).

The reasons for the limbic location of the virus are not clear, but several explanations have been given. These include the progression of the virus from the trigeminal ganglia where it is dormant, travelling along the trigeminal nerve to the dura mater in the anterior and middle fossae; via the olfactory pathways following intranasal innoculation; and via anterograde spread from the trigeminal ganglion to the brainstem and trigeminal nuclei, hence to the locus coeruleus and raphe nuclei and ascending to limbic structures (Damascio and van Hoesen, 1985).

Management of these patients can be extremely complicated. The indiscriminate behaviour and aggressive outbursts, while being helped by major tranquillizers, are often severe enough to require institutionalization, and the amnesias and agnosias make rehabilitation difficult. The seizures are poorly controlled by conventional anticonvulsants.

The possibility that mild forms of herpes encephalitis occur, which, while generally having a good prognosis, may, if latent, be involved in the development of psychiatric illness, has been suggested (Klapper *et al.*, 1984). Lycke *et al.* (1974) found a significantly higher than expected prevalence of several viral antibodies

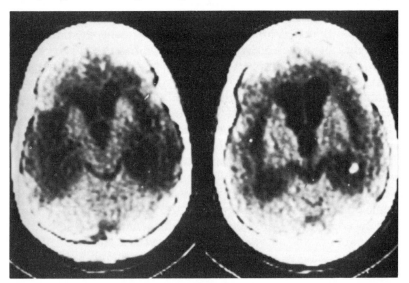

Figure 1. Showing the CT scan of a patient following herpes simplex encephalitis. Note the extensive destruction of the limbic system and related structures.

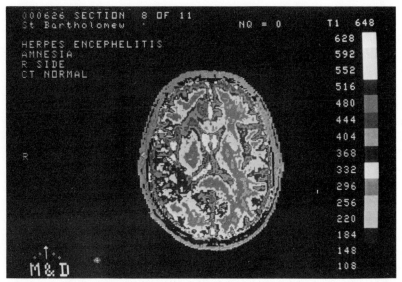

Figure 2. MRI of a patient after herpes simplex encephalitis. The CT was normal. Note increased T_1 values in the right temporal lobe.

in psychiatric patients, notably for HSV, measles and varicella-zoster viruses. Patients classified as depressed and demented had the strongest association. Cleobury et al. (1971) reported an increase in HSV-1 neutralizing antibody in aggressive psychopaths, while Halonen et al. (1974) confirmed that HSV-1 titres were higher than in controls for patients with schizophrenia, psychotic depression and 'other psychiatric diseases' which included personality disorders. In the latter study, neither measles nor rubella antibody titres were elevated.

The possibility that the viral infection may damage limbic structures during development and thus lead to personality changes or psychiatric illness is postulated by several of the authors. Glaser and Pincus (1969), following case descriptions of five cases of subacute encephalitis, all presenting with disturbed behaviour at some point in their illness and in appearance similar to depressive or schizophrenic illness, suggested the term 'limbic encephalitis' for the clinical picture of a subacute or chronic encephalitis, which commonly involves the limbic system. This especially damages the medial portions of the temporal lobes, and they implicated herpes simplex, measles or rabies viruses. They speculated that possible neurotransmitter differences or metabolic requirements of the susceptible structures lead to the selective damage.

Subacute sclerosing pan encephalitis (SSPE) is a disorder usually seen in childhood or adolescence presenting as a progressive dementia with behaviour disturbances and sometimes hallucinations, associated with myoclonic jerking, seizures and a characteristic EEG pattern. Pathologically, viral inclusions are seen, and these may particularly affect the temporal lobes and subcortical nuclei. Florid psychiatric presentations resembling schizophrenia have been described (Koehler and Jakumeit, 1976), as have subacute forms presenting with unusual behaviour, paranoid delusions and hallucinations (Himmelhoch *et al.*, 1970).

In rabies, virus is transmitted to the brain along the peripheral nerves following infection from the bite of an infected animal, usually a dog. The classic pathological sign is the presence of Negri bodies, which contain viral antigen, especially in the pyramidal cells of the hippocampus. Patients experience profound anxiety, and irrational, hyperactive behaviour is seen. Hydrophobia is said to be a distinguishing feature of the clinical state.

Other pathologies

Of the other conditions affecting the temporal lobes, of importance are those which lead to epilepsy, and the frequent association of temporal lobe epilepsy (TLE) with a variety of psychopathologies is discussed in Chapter 10. In particular, personality changes, aggression and psychotic disorders, the latter often taking on a schizophreniform pattern, have been most investigated. Tumours, referred to as hamartomas, cerebrovascular accidents (CVA) and the effects of head injury may all lead to temporal lobe damage and provoke psychopathology. Head injury is discussed below under frontal lobe syndromes.

Neoplasms, of which gliomas are the commonest, affect all brain regions, but the suggestion that psychopathology is more commonly associated with limbic tumours emerges from several sources. This has been well reviewed by both Davison and Bagley (1969) and Lishman (1978).

There is an increased incidence of cerebral tumours in populations of psychiatric hospital patients, many of whom are only diagnosed at post-mortem. Based on a literature review, Davison and Bagley concluded that the association of a diagnosis of schizophrenia and cerebral tumour exceeded chance. No particular pathological type seems involved, although correlations to the site have been reported. Tables 1 and 2 are taken from Davison and Bagley (1969, p.129) and Lishman (1978, p.269) respectively.

It can be seen that there is a significant association between temporal lobe tumours and psychosis, and that, since in some series patients with epilepsy were not included, this is not attributable to the epilepsy. Malamud (1975), in a series of 245 cases of intracranial tumour, reported that 155 presented various mental symptoms, of which 18 (11.5 per cent) were diagnosed as 'purely functional disorders'. In all these cases, the limbic system was involved, notably the amygdaloid–hippocampal region, the cingulate region and the area of the third ventricle. In over 60 per cent the diagnosis was schizophrenia.

In addition to psychosis, aggression, apathy, amnesia, irritability and depression are all noted with temporal lobe tumours, and there is some evidence that pathology of the dominant hemisphere is more likely to present with affective changes.

Hamartomas, areas of abnormal tissue of developmental origin, include such pathologies as angiomas. The latter are composed of dilated blood vessels that are fed by cerebral arteries and drain into one or more cerebral veins that may present anywhere in the brain.

Table 1 Localization of cerebral tumours in 77 psychotic cases from the literature compared with two unselected series. Statistical significance of differences calculated by χ^2 method. Values of p refer to difference between psychotic group and each of the two unselected series

Site of cerebral tumour	% of 600 cases of Walther-Büel, 1951 (276)	% of 530 cases of Keschner, Bender and Strauss, 1938 (233)	% of 77 psychotic cases	
Frontal	29.0	24.7	19.5	
Temporal	13.0	16.2	35.1	$p<0.001$
Parietal	10.0	10.6	—	
Occiptal	5.3	2.0	1.3	
Cerebellum	10.3	14.0	5.2	$p<0.01$
Cerebellopontine angle	8.3	6.8	1.3	
Hypophysis and suprasellar	9.3	6.8	19.5	$p<0.01$
Third ventricle	—	3.0	9.1	
Brainstem	4.7	3.6	3.9	
Midbrain and basal ganglia	—	2.6	1.3	
Pineal	—	2.0	3.9	
Supratentorial	76.7	75.7	89.6	$p<0.01$
Infratentorial	23.3	24.3	10.4	

Table 2   Incidence of mental symptoms with cerebral tumours

Location of tumour	From Keschner et al. (1938) (excluding paroxysmal disturbances)			From Hécaen and Ajuriaguerra (1956a) (including paroxysmal disturbances)		
	Number of cases	% with mental symptoms	% with mental symptoms 'early'	Number of cases	% with mental symptoms	% with mental symptoms 'early'
All tumours	530	78	15	439	52	18
All supratentorial	401	87	18	354	56	19
All infratentorial	129	47	5	85	40	12
Frontal	68	85	25	80	68	20
Temporal	56	93	29	75	68	28
Parietal	32	81	19	75	52	16
Occipital	11	82	9	25	52	32

Although no specific studies of their psychopathological correlates have appeared, their presence in the temporal lobes is quite common, and may be associated with psychotic episodes. In some patients this is schizophreniform, and, although often associated with epilepsy, this is not invariable. Dementia, in the setting of recurrent haemorrhages, is one outcome.

In a series of patients that had temporal lobectomy for temporal lobe epilepsy, and in whom pathology was determined, Taylor (1975) observed an association between those with 'alien tissue', including small tumours, hamartomas and areas of focal dysplasia, and the development of a schizophrenia-like psychosis.

Since the middle and posterior cerebral arteries supply regions of the temporal lobe it is interesting that occasionally psychosis occurs as a manifestation of cerebrovascular accidents (Davison and Bagley, 1969). However, specific implication of the temporal lobes has not been demonstrated, with the exception of an amnestic syndrome following posterior cerebral artery infarctions.

Finally, Corsellis et al. (1968) reported on cases of limbic encephalitis associated with systemic carcinoma. The features were convulsive episodes, followed by amnesia, with disturbances of affect, usually depression and anxiety and sometimes hallucinations. At post-mortem the amygdaloid nucleus, the hippocampus, the fornix and the mamillary bodies were most affected, and the pathological picture was similar to the cases of HSV encephalitis.

Amnestic syndromes

One of the best defined of the temporal lobe syndromes is that of amnesia. Since the description of Korsakoff's psychosis in the last century, the amnestic syndrome associated with alcoholic encephalopathies has been well documented. This memory disorder comprises an inability to recall information acquired before the illness (retrograde amnesia) and an inability to acquire new information, referred to as anterograde amnesia. Clinically such patients are able to repeat the digit span normally, thus having an intact short-term memory, and in pure cases other cognitive abilities are unimpaired. Other symptoms reported in Korsakoff's psychosis include mood disturbances, especially apathy and an air of detachment, lack of insight and initiative, and lack of spontaneity. Confabulation may occur, but not in all cases.

While there are still disagreements as to the precise anatomical lesions that underlie this state, it seems that the mammillary bodies are particularly involved, although some implicate the dorsal medial nucleus of the thalamus (Victor *et al.*, 1971). A deficiency of vitamin B_1 is thought to be responsible in alcoholics. In patients with destructive lesions of the hippocampal–limbic circuits, similar amnestic deficits have been seen. Included among the pathologies are temporal lobectomy (in which one hemisphere was removed, and a damaged contralateral one led to an effective bilateral loss of temporal lobe function), occlusion of the posterior cerebral arteries, subarachnoid haemorrhage, following cerebral anoxia, head trauma and meningitis.

There is argument as to whether the pattern of amnesia is the same with the different pathologies and also as to which elements of the temporal lobes need be damaged for the amnesia to occur. Nonetheless, the evidence indicates that integrity of the limbic system links between medial temporal and diencephalic structures are essential for the laying down of memory traces and retrieval and that a variety of causes may result in an amnestic state.

FRONTAL LOBE SYNDROMES

Although there are now many extensive documentations of the frontal lobe syndromes (Blumer and Benson, 1975; Fuster, 1980; Stuss and Benson, 1984), it is remarkable how frontal lobe pathology often goes unnoticed and how the relevance of frontal lobe syndromes in man for understanding behaviour has been neglected.

Early clinical reports, such as that of the American Phineas Gage who, after his frontal lobes were shattered by a metal bar in an accident, underwent marked personality change (Harlow, 1868), emphasized the role of the frontal cortex in behaviour. The observations of Jacobsen (1935) on lesions in primates, the careful reports of the consequences of head injuries in the Second World War and those on patients examined after leucotomy, all led to the delineation of specific deficits of behaviour associated with lesions to this area of the brain.

Various pathologies lead to frontal damage, including trauma, tumours, cerebrovascular accidents, infections and some degenerative diseases. Of the latter, Pick's disease seems to have a particular predilection for the frontal and temporal lobes. Anterior cerebral artery rupture is most likely to lead to frontal lobe damage, although the middle cerebral artery does supply the lateral parts of the orbital gyri and the inferior and middle frontal gyri.

One of the specific behavioural deficits seen after frontal lobe damage is related to attention, patients showing distractibility and poor attention. They present with poor memory, the latter sometimes being referred to as 'forgetting to remember'. The thinking of frontal patients tends to be concrete, and they may show perseveration and stereotypy of their responses. The perseveration, with inability to switch from one line of thinking to another, leads to difficulties with arithmetical calculations such as serial sevens or carry-over subtractions.

An aphasia is seen, but this is different from both Wernicke's and Broca's aphasia. Luria (1973) referred to it as 'adynamic aphasia'. The patients have well-preserved motor speech and no anomia; repetition, the hallmark of a perisylvian aphasia, is intact. However, they show difficulty in propositionizing, and active speech is severely disturbed. He suggested that this was due to a disturbance in the predictive function of speech, that which takes part in structuring sentences. The syndrome is similar to that form of aphasia referred to as transcortical motor aphasia.

Other features of frontal lobe syndromes include reduced activity, particularly a diminution of spontaneous activity, lack of drive, inability to plan ahead and lack of concern. Sometimes associated with this are bouts of restless, aimless uncoordinated behaviour. The affect is often disturbed, with apathy, emotional blunting, and the patient showing an indifference to the world around him. Clinically this picture can resemble a major affective disorder with psychomotor retardation.

In contrast, on other occasions, euphoria and disinhibition are described. The euphoria is not that of a manic condition, however, having an empty quality to it. The disinhibition can lead to markedly abnormal behaviour, sometimes associated with outbursts of irritability and aggression (see Figure 3).

So-called Witzlesucht has been described, in which patients show an inappropriate facetiousness and a tendency to pun.

Some authors have distinguished between lesions of the lateral frontal cortex, most closely linked to the motor structures of the brain, which lead to disturbances of movement and action with perseveration and inertia, and lesions of the orbital areas, interlinked with the limbic and reticular systems, which lead to disinhibition and changes of affective life. The terms pseudodepressed and pseudopsychopathic have been used to describe these two types respectively (Blumer and Benson, 1975). A third syndrome, the medial frontal syndrome, is also acknowledged, marked by akinesia, and associated with mutism, gait disturbances and incontinence. The features of these differing clinical pictures have been listed by Cummings (1985) and are shown in Table 3. However, in most patients the picture is one of a mixture of the syndromes.

In some patients, paroxysmal behaviour disorders are recorded. These tend to be short lived, and include episodes of confusion and perhaps hallucinations. These are also thought to reflect transient disturbances of the frontolimbic connections. Finally, following massive frontal lobe lesions, the so-called apathetico–akinetico–

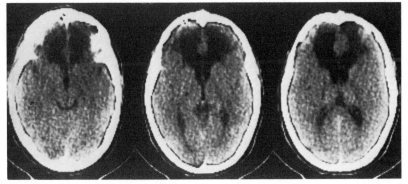

Figure 3. CT scan of a patient with extensive frontal lobe damage after head injury. The only clinical manifestation was a solitary episode of theft from his wife.

Table 3   Clinical characteristics of the three principal frontal lobe syndromes (from Cummings, 1985, p.58)

Orbitofrontal syndrome (disinhibited)
    Disinhibited, impulsive behaviour ('pseudopsychopathic')
    Inappropriate jocular affect, euphoria
    Emotional lability
    Poor judgement and insight
    Distractibility

Frontal convexity syndrome (apathetic)
    Apathetic
        (occasional brief angry or aggressive outbursts common)
    Indifference
    Psychomotor retardation
    Motor perseveration and impersistence
    Loss of set
    Stimulus boundedness
    Discrepant motor and verbal behaviour
    Motor programming deficits
        Three-step hand sequence
        Alternating programmes
        Reciprocal programmes
        Rhythm tapping
        Multiple loops
    Poor word-list generation
    Poor abstraction and categorization
    Segmented approach to visuospatial analysis

Medial frontal syndrome (akinetic)
    Paucity of spontaneous movement and gesture
    Sparse verbal output (repetition may be preserved)
    Lower extremity weakness and loss of sensation
    Incontinence

---

abulic syndrome may occur, in which patients lie around passively unaroused, unable to complete tasks or listen to commands.

    Further clinical signs associated with frontal lobe damage include sensory inattention in the contralateral sensory field, abnormalities of visual searching, echophenomena such as echolalia and echopraxia, confabulation, hyperphagia and various changes in cognitive function. Recently, the term utilization behaviour has been used for an exaggerated tendency to grope objects and use them (L'Hermitte, 1983).

Detection of frontal lobe damage can be difficult, especially if only traditional methods of testing are carried out. Indeed, this point cannot be overemphasized, since it reflects one of the main differences between neurological syndromes, that affect only elements of a patient's behaviour, such as a paralysis following destruction of the contralateral motor cortex by a tumour or CVA, and limbic system disorders. In these the whole of a patient's motoric and psychic life are influenced and the behaviour disturbance itself reflects the pathology. Thus, the standard neurological examination will be normal, as may the results of psychological tests such as the Wechsler adult intelligence test (WAIT). Special techniques are required to examine frontal lobe function, and care required finding out how the patient now behaves and how this compares with his premorbid performance.

The orbitofrontal lesions may be associated with anosmia, and the more lesions extend posteriorly, the more neurological signs such as aphasia (with dominant lesions), paralyses, grasp reflexes and oculomotor abnormalities become apparent. Of the various tasks that can be used clinically to help detect frontal pathology, those given in Table 4 are suggested. However, not all patients with frontal damage show abnormalities on testing, and not all tests are exclusively found abnormal in frontal lobe pathology.

Cognitive tasks include the word fluency test, in which a patient is asked to generate as many words as possible beginning with a single letter in one minute (the normal being around 15). Proverb or metaphor interpretation can be remarkably concrete. Problem solving, for example carry-over additions or subtractions, can be tested by a simple question (see Table 4); serial sevens is difficult to perform.

Laboratory-based tasks of abstract reasoning include the Wisconsin card sorting and other sorting tasks. The essential nature of these is to arrange a variety of objects into groups depending on one common abstract property, for example colour. In the Wisconsin card sorting task, patients are given a pack of cards with symbols on them which differ in form, colour and number. Four stimulus cards are available, and the patient has to place each response card in front of one of the four stimulus cards.

Table 4   Some useful tests of frontal lobe function

Word fluency
Abstract thinking (If I have eighteen books and two bookshelves, and I want twice as many books on one shelf as the other, how many books on each shelf?)
Proverb and metaphor interpretation
Wisconsin card sorting task
Other sorting tasks
Block design
Maze test
Hand position test (three-step hand sequence)
Copying tasks (multiple loops)
Rhythm tapping tasks

The tester tells the patient if he is right or wrong, and the patient has to use that information to place the next card in front of the next stimulus card. The sorting is done arbitrarily into colour, form or number, and the patient's task is to shift the set from one type of stimulus response to another based on the information provided. Frontal patients cannot overcome previously established responses, and show a high frequency of perseverative errors. These deficits are more likely with lateral lesions of the dominant hemisphere.

Patients with frontal lobe lesions also do badly on maze-learning tasks (especially the Porteus maze which requires advanced planning of the path to be followed) and block design. They show perseveration of motor tasks and difficulty carrying out sequences of motor actions. Skilled movements are no longer performed smoothly, and previously automated actions such as handwriting or playing a musical instrument are impaired. Tests such as asking the patient to follow a succession of hand positions (with the hand first placed flat, then on the side and then as a fist on a flat surface) or being asked to tap aloud a complex rhythm (for example two loud and three soft beats) are impaired. Perseveration (especially prominant with deeper lesions in which the modulating function of the premotor cortex on the motor structures of the basal ganglia are lost; Luria, 1973) may be tested by asking the patient to draw, for example, a circle or copy a complex diagram with recurring shapes in it which alternate with one another. The patient may continue to draw circle upon circle, not stopping after one revolution, or miss the pattern of recurring shapes (see Figure 4).

In many of these tasks there is a discrepancy between the patient's knowing what to do and being able to verbalize the instructions, and the patient's failure of the motor act.

It should be emphasized that some of the tasks, for example the word fluency task, are more likely to be affected by dominant side lesions, and the inhibition of motoric tasks relates to the dorsolateral syndrome.

The neuroanatomical bases for the frontal lobe syndromes have been explained as follows (Luria, 1973; Stuss and Benson, 1984). The lateral areas are most closely linked to the motor structures of the anterior part of the brain, thus leading to the motor inertias and perseverations seen with these lesions. They are more pronounced after dominant hemisphere lesions, when the speech-related disorders become manifest. More posterior lesions seem to link to difficulties with the organization of movement, anterior ones resulting in difficulties of motor planning and a dissociation between behaviour and language. Elementary motor perseveration probably requires lesions that are deep enough to involve the basal ganglia. Disturbances of attention are related to disruption of the brainstem–thalamic–frontal system, and the basal (orbital) syndromes are due to disruption of the frontal–limbic links. Loss of inhibitory function over the parietal lobes, with release of their activity, increases the subject's dependence on external visual and tactile information, leading to echophenomena and utilization behaviour.

Teuber (1964) suggested that the frontal lobes 'anticipate' sensory stimuli that result from behaviour, thus preparing the brain for events about to occur. The expected results are compared to actual experience and regulation of activity results. More recently, Fuster (1980) has proposed that the prefrontal cortex plays a role in the temporal structuring of behaviour, synthesizing cognitive and motor acts into purposive sequences.

A number of findings are relevant to understanding these frontal syndromes. These include (a) the frontal location of the CNV; (b) the profuse afferents to the frontal cortex from limbic structures, notably the amygdala and related subcortical structures to the orbitofrontal cortex; (c) the sensory and motor information, deriving from virtually all cortical regions outside the primary sensory areas projecting to the dorsolateral frontal cortex—there are reciprocal efferents, allowing modulation and monitoring of

168

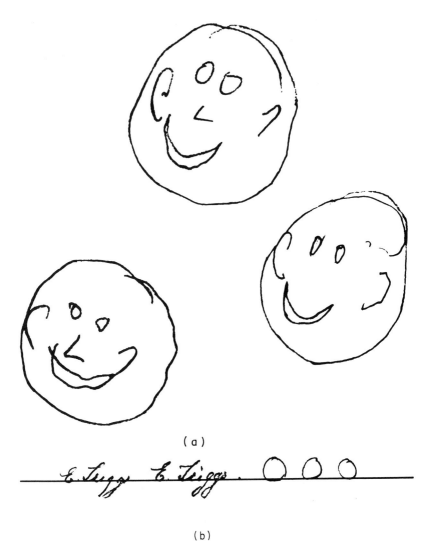

(a)

(b)

Figure 4. (a) The patient was asked to draw a face, but repeated the act as shown. Frontal lobe damage was shown both on CT and MRI scans. (b) The patient was asked to write her name. This was immediately repeated. On being asked to draw a circle, the patient repeats the act.

diffuse cortical activity and its integration with limbic information relating to biological needs and motivation; (d) the specific projection from the mediodorsal thalamic nucleus relating both to memory and limbic afferents; and (e) the descending motor outputs to the striatum. Thus, lesions of the lateral convexity disrupt sensory–emotional–motor links, leading to inappropriate monitoring of the environmental relevance of events and failure of motoric programming. In contrast the limbic disruptions of the orbital cortex lead to disconnection of the frontal regulatory systems from information of emotional relevance leading to the disinhibition and impulsivity.

Disorders implicating frontal lobe function

As noted, frontal lobe syndromes may be seen following a variety of insults, some of them destroying relatively selectively frontal lobe tissue. However, the frontal lobes appear involved in a variety of other disorders, and in some of them frontal lobe symptoms are detected. The evidence for frontal lobe involvement in depressive illness and schizophrenia is reviewed in later chapters. Of the dementias, Pick's disease and normal pressure hydrocephalus specifically affect this area (see Chapter 11), and of the tumours, frontal meningiomas, especially if slowly growing, may be missed and lead to florid psychopathology (see Chapter 5, Figure 5). These tumours, arising from the arachnoid villi and attached to the dura, commonly arise along the superior saggital sinus, in the suprasellar region and from the spenoidal ridge. They may locally invade bone, allowing them to be detected on skull X-ray, but are rarely malignant.

Intoxicants such as alcohol may preferentially damage frontal areas, sometimes apparent on CT scans of alcoholics. Demyelinating conditions such as multiple sclerosis, with multiple periventricular lesions, may also lead to frontal lobe problems.

Syndromes of abnormal awareness have also been related to frontal pathology (Stuss and Benson, 1984). These include the Capgras syndrome, in which patients acknowledge a person as looking like a relative or friend but maintain they are someone else in disguise, and reduplicative paramnesia, where patients who know, for example, the name of the hospital they are in will place it out of context such as in their own town.

Head injury

In many instances of trauma, it is the head which receives the injury, often with fracture of the skull and death. However, especially with improved intensive care techniques, survival from often severe injury is common, yet the morbidity may be profound. The sequelae of the injury will depend to some extent on which areas of the brain are damaged, although prediction based on simple neurological principles will fail in many cases. Thus, neuronal damage frequently occurs in areas of brain subserving functions outside those of the primary motor and sensory areas of the brain. Many years ago, Denny-Brown and Russell (1941) showed that even minor head injuries altered brainstem activity, while others reported, in animal experiments, loss of neurones in brainstem areas, the extent of the loss relating to the severity of concussion (Groat and Simmons, 1950). Human data likewise reveal cell loss after trivial injuries (Oppenheimer, 1968).

The mechanism of subtle brain damage following head injury was explored in monkeys by Pudenz and Sheldon (1946). They took photographs of the movement of the brain following a blow to the head, using a special transparent material that replaced the animals' calvaria. They found that brain movement lagged behind movement of the skull, such glide being greatest in the parietal and occipital lobes. However, the relative lack of movement in the frontal and temporal lobes, held rigid by the bony anterior fossae, led to strains in the cerebral tissue, laceration and damage. Thus, the anterior temporal and the frontal lobes are highly susceptible to damage from head injury, and so-called contracoup lesions are commonest at these sites.

The implications of this, in the light of the above, are clear. Often such patients show normal neurological function with standard tests, and traditional psychometry and CT scan may be normal. However, the behavioural and emotional sequelae are often severe, and reflect limbic system disruption, often due to frontal and temporal lobe damage. Thus, follow-up studies of head-injured patients show that psychopathology is frequently present, and with more severe injury, personality changes and psychoses are reported. These are commoner in patients with left-sided injuries, frontal lesions being more often associated with personality change and temporal ones with psychoses (Hillbom, 1960; Lishman, 1978). The presence of limbic lesions is one explanation for continuing psychopathology in head-injured patients, several years after the insult, and the lack of association between one index of severity, the post-traumatic amnesia, and personality change (Brooks and McKinlay, 1983). Further, it explains the development of post-traumatic neurosis in some patients with head injury and the failure of traditional neurological screening methods to help understand such problems (Trimble, 1981b).

Cingulate lesions

Being contiguous with the frontal cortex anteriorly, and forming a crucial part in some limbic circuits, it may be anticipated that cingulate pathology leads to behavioural changes. Curiously there are few reports in the literature that specifically concern this gyrus and its nuclei. Electrical stimulation leads to complex sustained environmentally relevant motor acts and vocalizations (Talairach *et al.*, 1973; Wieser, 1983), and responses such as anxiety, tension, hallucinations and negativism (Laitinen, 1979). Further, neuro-surgical lesioning of the cingulum is used in the relief of some conditions, notably obsessive compulsive neurosis (see p.401). Serious behavioural abnormalities, including bulimia, increased sexual activity, aggression and schizophreniform-like states have been reported with cingulate tumours (Malamud, 1975; Angelini *et al.*, 1980).

OTHER LIMBIC SYSTEM LESIONS

A variety of subcortical structures which are linked to the limbic system are involved in disease processes including the basal ganglia, the thalamus and areas of the limbic midbrain such as the VTA.

Lesions in the area of the ventral striatum include tumours which are reported to lead to rage attacks and increased irritability (Valenstein and Heilman, 1979). Disorders of the basal ganglia, for example Parkinson's disease and Huntington's chorea, are commonly associated with psychopathology (see Trimble, 1981a), notably depression in the former and personality changes and psychoses in the latter. Thalamic lesions are linked to dementia (Smythe and Stern, 1938) and the amnesia of alcoholism. Indeed, a variety of diencephalic tumours, notably hypothalamic, pituitary, suprasellar and third ventricular may provoke psychopathology, usually with a marked amnestic component, fluctuating levels of consciousness, hypersomnia and confabulation. When the hypothalamus is compromised, endocrine disorders may develop, with sexual dysfunction, appetite changes and polyuria and polydipsia. Davison and Bagley (1969) noted that tumours in the suprasellar region and hypophysis are overrepresented in patients with tumours that develop psychosis, and Lishman (1978) refers to transient manic behaviour, psychotic depression, personality changes and some features reminiscent of frontal lobe pathology with apathy, disinhibition, indifference and denial with pathology at this site.

Lesions of the VTA and interrelated limbic nuclei may be related to marked behaviour disturbances in man. Notable among the pathologies involved is encephalitis lethargica. This condition, arising in epidemic proportions from the influenza epidemics following the First World War, is of the encephalitides, the most frequently associated with schizophreniform states (Davison and Bagley, 1969). These tended to emerge as long-term sequelae, notably associated with neurological deficits and Parkinsonian features. The clinical picture may exactly resemble schizophrenia, paranoid-hallucinatory states predominating. The family histories do not reveal an excess of genetic loading for schizophrenia, and premorbid schizoid personalities are said to be rare (Davison and Bagley, 1969).

The main pathology in the condition is microscopic foci of inflammation, mainly in the grey matter of the midbrain and the basal ganglia. Von Economo (1931) noted that it was the region of the aqueduct, the tegmental region, and the posterior wall, floor and the basal parts of the lateral walls of the third ventricle that were mainly affected. The next most important sites were the hypothalamic region, the thalamus, the lenticular nuclei and the substantia nigra.

Such disorders are not confined to the history books, and similar cases are still seen sporadically (Hunter and Jones, 1966). The suggestion that a similar encephalitis may be responsible for some cases of schizophrenia is an active area of current investigation (see Chapter 8).

Case reports of upper brainstem lesions leading to psychiatric disturbances are found in the literature associated with tumours, cerebrovascular accidents and intoxications (Trimble and Cummings, 1981). These are often associated with disorders of eye movement. This reflects the close proximity of the nuclei that regulate eye movement to those that, when disrupted, may provoke psychopathology. Cummings (1985) suggested that these lesions alter the function of the main monoamine pathways to the limbic forebrain, in keeping with the animal literature which relates VTA lesions to a hyperactive, hypoemotional, disinhibited behaviour pattern, the extent of which correlates with dopamine denervation (Glowinski et al., 1984).

CONCLUSIONS

The psychopathological pictures described in this chapter are varied, and much of the data is based on clinical impression. In some cases, for example in relation to cerebral tumours, it is often difficult to know if the disturbances of the mental state relate more to non-specific factors such as cerebral oedema than to the siting of the lesions in certain structures. Nonetheless, certain facts emerge. Thus, disorders of the limbic system frequently present with psychiatric symptoms, and in some cases this resembles very closely the presentation of well-recognized psychiatric disorders such as schizophrenia. Limbic pathology presents as a behavioural syndrome, in the sense that the patient's behaviour is altered in its entirety, rather than as some isolated area of altered function as seen after a lesion to the primary sensory or motor cortex. The essential feature of limbic system disturbances is that they do not lead to traditional neurological localizing signs, and with exceptions, for example the eye movement disturbances of VTA lesions or the often more subtle extrapyramidal or other motor signs and release reflexes with basal ganglia and frontal lobe syndromes, the disturbances of behaviour are the predominant aspects of the presentation.

The behavioural similarity of patients with such lesions to psychiatric states is such that many patients reported in the literature were initially not diagnosed as having the underlying neurological disorder, and were often poorly investigated.

The extent to which differing clinical pictures are encountered with differing sites of the lesions is not clear, although psychotic states seem commoner after temporal lobe (especially dominant side lesions) and mesodiencephalic disturbance, while apathy and emotional blunting reflect more on frontal, especially lateral frontal, damage. Amnesic disturbances relate to temporo-thalamic disorganization.

The relationship of the type of pathology to the type of behaviour change is also unclear, but generally acute lesions seem to result in psychopathology as part of an organic brain syndrome with clouding of consciousness, while chronic pathologies such as encephalitis and epilepsy lead to symptoms in the setting of clear consciousness. A caveat is that mesencephalic lesions lead to marked fluctuations of consciousness.

CHAPTER 7

Personality disorders and the neuroses

In this, and the following chapters on the affective disorders and the psychoses, the biological underpinnings of psychopathology will be reviewed. Following an introduction, genetics, somatic, metabolic and biochemical findings, neurochemical and neuropathological information, and then the literature on neurological illness, including the abnormalities from special investigations, are referred to. Biological treatments are discussed in Chapter 12.

INTRODUCTION

The personality disorders and the neuroses are taken together on account of their close relationship clinically, and the historical associations that unite them. The classification of the personality disorders in Chapter 2 and the accompanying theoretical discussion emphasizes several points. First, attention was drawn to the fundamental distinction of Jaspers between personality development and a process. Secondly, the two main ways of defining personality were noted, namely the ideal and the statistical. The classification given bears more on the former, and emphasizes the framework of the DSM III. The latter has attempted to abandon the term neurosis, and familiar terms such as reactive or neurotic depression are not seen. A form of depression less severe than major affective disorder is referred to as dysthymic disorder, often associated with prolonged and persistant lowness of mood beginning early in life. This is associated with chronic psychosocial stresses and 'personality disorder. . .merges imperceptibly into this condition' (American Psychiatric Association, 1980, p.221). Patients with personality disorders, especially those referred to as avoidant or dependent personalities, display lifelong anxiety with bouts of panic and exacerbation under stress.

Thus, in these typologies there is not always a clear separation between personality style and certain categories of illness that used to be referred to as neurotic. If the alternative, quantitative approach to personality disorders is taken, as adopted by

Schneider (1959), separation between individuals takes on even less clear boundaries, personality disorder relating to a statistical deviation from the norm. Schneider's model blurs the distinction between the neuroses and personality disorders, defining personality disorders as conditions through which either individuals themselves or society suffer. Some other models of psychopathology confuse boundaries even further. For example, the Meyerian reaction types, which minimized endogenous variables at the expense of 'reactions' to environmental events, drew no clear distinctions between personality idiomorphs, neurosis and psychosis. Freudian psychoanalysis also failed in this regard, the pathogenesis of all forms of psychopathology being similar in that they represent deviant childhood developments with libidinous fixations and later regressions.

In contrast, Jaspers' model emphasizes clear distinctions between personality and illness, not only phenomenologically, but also developmentally. Illness is a new feature, skewing the development of personality, leading to phenomena that could not be understood in terms of development. The changes in personality brought about by illness were qualitative, and 'the observer has a vivid feeling of the gulf which has torn mutual understanding apart. . .' (Jaspers, 1963, p.574). However, even Jaspers did not clearly separate the neuroses from personality disorders. He thus states: 'The psychic deviations which do not wholly involve the individual himself are called neuroses, and those which seize upon the individual as a whole are called psychoses. . .the neuroses embrace the wide field of personality disorder. . .' (p.575).

Thus, behaviour in both a neurosis and a person with a personality disorder was seen to derive from understandable, normal psychic life, differing in degree only from normal behaviour. As Slater and Roth (1969) pointed out, this was an extremely useful clinical distinction, enabling clearer delineation of such illnesses as schizophrenia, and their distinction from the excessive reactions of various personalities. Further, it led to success in distinguishing various primary mood disorders from secondary mood changes, the endogenous from other forms. This breakdown into primary and secondary is not employed in the DSM III, but is used by some. Secondary depression is that which occurs in the presence of preexisting psychiatric disorders or chronic medical illnesses (Feighner *et al.*, 1972; Goodwin and Guze, 1984), amongst which are to be included personality disorders.

Thus, concepts of personality and neurosis seem to have been intertwined by several groups of authors, often writing from different perspectives. The blurred boundary has had many consequences. For one, terminology became a labyrinth of confusion. Neurotic depression and its distinction from endogenous depression became an area of intense research, the outcome of which is not clear to this day. Variants of terms such as depressive reaction, psychogenic reaction, depressive personality and others added confusion, and people with abnormal personalities were wrongly classified as having psychiatric illnesses.

This last point is more fundamental than is often appreciated, and itself has consequences. First, if the illness represents the outcome of a process, then it may be possible to identify that process biologically. Hence the search for biological markers in psychiatry. In some cases these markers will be identifiable as abnormal tissue pathogens, for example as in an encephalitis. In others, the neurochemical constituents alone may be at variance, and detection of the change rests in identifying change from the normal expected range. If patients with personality disorders are confused in a group with those having an illness, then the sought abnormality will be diluted and not found. This problem frequently arises with research into depressive illness, where patients with personality disorders are wrongly categorized as having a major affective disorder. A similar problem arises in drug trials, where heterogeneous populations masquerade for homogeneous ones, and real differences between active drugs and placebos may be minimized. Attempts such as the DSM III to more rigidly define categories and provide exclusions as well as inclusions are helpful, but are still quite imperfect.

A second consequence relates to the image of psychiatry with non-medical people. Patients with personality disorders often develop depressive symptoms in the setting of social stress, and may be thought, by the uninitiated, to have what psychiatrists refer to as major affective disorder. As many such people respond, albeit temporarily, to manipulation of their social environment, it is assumed that all psychopathology can likewise be remedied. This thinking, combined with lay confidence in non-biological therapies that characterized psychiatry a generation ago, has led to marked distractions in the attempts to understand the biological bases of psychopathology.

If personality structure and the neuroses are intertwined as suggested, and patients with personality disorders are susceptible to the development of secondary psychopathology, it might be expected that there would be many studies of the relationship between personality and psychiatric illness. In reality there is little concrete information, and much is clinical lore. For example, it is said that cyclothymic personalities are more prone to depressive illness, and an anxious personality is likewise prone to anxiety states and panic attacks. Similarly, the obsessional is at risk for obsessive compulsive disorder and the hysterical personality to hysteria. This line of thinking leads on to consideration of personality traits and their relationship to states. Traits are persistent underlying attitudes, while states are temporary manifestations, and will take two forms. Trait exaggeration is one form, in which a flowering of the premorbid personality is seen. The other is symptoms that arise de novo. Thus, traits and states do not always go hand in hand; the development of obsessive compulsive disorder or hysteria is not necessarily dependent on the premorbid personality as predicted by some theories. Further, the evidence that personality types are aetiologically linked to major psychiatric illness is not available. As Schneider (1959) observed:

> Reactions to external events are on the whole non-specific for the personality type. They have a universal quality, since all of us are at some time sad, or anxious, about something. However, the smaller the stimulus that liberates the feeling of sadness or anxiety and the more abnormal the reaction in its degree, appearance, and duration and the more abnormal the ensuing conduct, the more weight we can place on the personality factor (p.44).

With regards to depressive symptoms, some authors described so-called depressive personalities (Schneider's (1959) depressive psychopaths) as people continually pessimistic, with constant anxiety about themselves and their world. This style, however, is not found in the DSM III. Cyclothymic disorder, appearing with affective disorders, replaces both this and cyclothymic personality disorder, emphasizing the illness rather than the personality. There is some literature supporting the link between cyclothymic personality and manic depressive illness, notably the finding of an excess of cyclothymic personalities among the relatives of manic depressive patients (Slater, 1936; Kallmann, 1954), and evidence of cyclothymic behaviour in between illness episodes in manic depressive patients (Winokur and Tanna, 1969).

The strongest associations between personality traits and neurosis are encountered between compulsive personality disorder and obsessive compulsive disorder. In Kringlen's (1965) study, over 70 per cent of patients with the neurosis had such a personality style. Another postulated relationship is between the symptoms of conversion hysteria and the hysterical personality. However, clinical estimates note that only 18–21 per cent of patients with conversion symptoms conform to this style (Merskey and Trimble, 1979), supported in studies of similar populations using standardized rating scales to assess personality (Wilson-Barnett and Trimble, 1985).

In summary, the links between personality styles and neurotic illnesses are not so clear. In some clinical settings, notably the anxiety and affective neuroses, disentangling the constitutional elements in the clinical picture is difficult, especially with limited patient contact. It is often only with time that the personality vulnerabilities of patients become exposed, and the nature of the psychopathology becomes clearer.

GENETICS OF NEUROSES

There is considerable evidence that genetic factors are of importance in personality disorders and some of the neuroses, well reviewed by Slater and Roth (1969) and more recently by McGuffin (1984b). Animal studies have permitted the selective breeding of anxiety-prone rats (Broadhurst, 1975). These show greater corticosterone, ACTH and prolactin responses to stress, and lower ^{3}H-diazepam binding in various cortical structures and the hippocampus than non-anxious counterparts (Gentsch et al., 1981).

In humans, the familial prevalence of anxiety neurosis is high, over 50 per cent of first-degree relatives suffering from the same disorder (Noyes et al., 1978). The incidence of neurosis and clinical ratings of personality similarities are greater in monozygous (MZ) twins in comparison to dizygous pairs, even in MZ twin pairs reared apart from an early age. In the study of Shields (1962), MZ twins reared apart were more alike than those raised together, leading to the suggestion that the common environment of the twins is less relevant for this aspect of personality development than genetic factors. Shields (1954) showed that MZ twin schoolchildren resembled one another with regards to the pattern of their neurosis, the mean concordance rate taken from several studies of neurotic identical twins being given as 61 per cent by Tienari (1963). In the latter's own study of 21 identical twin pairs classified as neurosis cases, only five had a normal co-twin, 13 pairs having a co-twin with either neurotic personality, a neurosis or an immature personality. With regards to the clinical picture, the tendency towards concordance was clearest with phobic and obsessional cases (91 per cent). These data are supported by the later study of Cary and Gottesman (1981) showing seven out of eight MZ and only five of thirteen DZ twins to be concordant for phobias. A similar but even greater discrepancy between MZ and DZ twins was found for the obsessional neuroses. In contrast, no genetic contribution has been reported for the presentation of hysteria, in the sense of conversion symptomatology (Slater and Roth, 1969).

There is, in addition, considerable evidence that genetic factors contribute to sociopathy. Concordance between MZ twins with regards to criminality has been reported by several groups (Lange, 1929; Christiansen, 1974), supported by adoption studies which show higher rates of offences in adopted children in cases where the natural father is known to the police (Hutchings and Mednick, 1975).

One problem of many of these clinical studies is the vague classification of the neuroses, and in many instances the diagnoses were purely given on a retrospective analysis, case notes being relied on for the historical data. Further information comes from studies using rating scales of psychopathology to quantify symptomatology. Gottesman (1962) gave the Minnesota multiphasic personality inventory (MMPI) to twins and derived an hereditability index for the scales. The highest values were for Si (social introversion) and Pd (psychopathic deviation), while only low values were reported for Hy (hysteria). Likewise there is evidence for genetic factors in the personality dimensions extraversion–introversion using the EPI, recent estimates of hereditability values being 50 per cent (Flǿderus-Myrhed et al., 1980). Studies using phobia questionnaires reveal MZ twins to be more alike than DZ twins with regards to the pattern of their fears (Torgersen, 1979), and using the Leyton obsessional inventory, Murray et al. (1981) suggest heritabilities of 0.44 and 0.47 for obsessional traits and states respectively.

Some further evidence for a contribution of genetic factors to personality development derives from patients with chromosomal abnormalities. The contention that patients with trisomy 21 (mongolism) or a translocation variant are friendly and jovial is hard to evaluate, especially in the presence of subnormality. More data have been accumulated in patients with Y chromosome abnormalities, notably XYY males. Such individuals tend to be taller than normals, are overrepresented in prison populations and show poor impulse control and aggressivity. Neither height nor socioeconomic class explain such observations (Dorus, 1980). Other studies, of patients with variability in length of the Y chromosome, although supportive of an association with excessive criminality and aggression, are not conclusive (Dorus, 1980). XYY males show an excess of neurological problems, including EEG abnormalities, mild to moderate ventricular enlargement on pneumoencephalography, a tendency to clumsiness, incoordination and hyperactivity, and occasionally epilepsy (Hakola and Iivanainen, 1978).

In comparison, disorders of the X chromosome present different behavioural profiles. Klinefelter's syndrome (XXY) is linked with hyposexuality, sexual deviancy, lack of self-assertiveness and immaturity. Puberty is often delayed and developmental language defects are common (Money, 1975; Walzer et al., 1978). In contrast, lack of one X chromosome in Turner's syndrome (XO) leads to a specific vulnerability for visuoconstructive cognitive deficits, and patients are reported to be phlegmatic, showing an inertia of emotional arousal (Money, 1975). While most of these assessments have been clinical, they do suggest that different chromosomal aberrations lead to differing personality profiles.

It may be concluded, as it was by Slater and Roth (1969), that 'heredity factors play an important role in the development of personality' (p.68). Slater further defined the 'neurotic constitution', emphasizing the link between liability to neurotic breakdown and personality, noting its quantitative variability. The severity of a traumatic event required to provoke breakdown varied inversely with the constitutional deviation. The symptoms of the breakdown were related to the personality of the patient, and the more susceptible the constitution, the more the past history of the patient revealed other features of neuroticism. Genetic factors of a multifactorial kind were postulated as contributing to the predisposition.

SOMATIC VARIABLES

The older literature has much reference to body build and personality characteristics, much of which seems now of little relevance. Psychophysical variables associated with anxiety have been investigated, notably monitoring autonomic activity (Lader,

1969). Lower skin conductance, more spontaneous fluctuations, increased sweating, and diminished habituation of autonomic indices to stimulation, monitoring such variables as blood pressure, the EMG and forearm blood flow, have been reported. Patients with conversion hysteria have high levels of arousal and very poor habituation, in spite of displaying minimal overt anxiety (Lader, 1969). The galvanic skin response is the sudden increase in skin conductance that can be observed with appropriate stimuli, and, since it can be abolished by atropine, it is thought to be dependent on the activity of sweat glands. Its habituation is delayed in those with anxiety states, the habituation being negatively correlated with ratings of anxiety (Lader, 1969).

There has been interest in an association between panic disorder and mitral valve prolapse. The latter may present with symptoms similar to anxiety, although the emphasis is on palpitations and chest pain. Early reports suggested that a high percentage of patients diagnosed as panic disorder had this condition (Kantor *et al.*, 1980), although later series, using more stringent cardiological criteria, did not confirm this (for example Shear *et al.*, 1984). Whether the occurrence of the two conditions when seen together is coincidence, or reflects some underlying autonomic dysfunction associated with both, is not clear.

METABOLIC AND BIOCHEMICAL FINDINGS

In contrast to the affective disorders and the psychoses, there is a dearth of information regarding metabolic and biochemical links with the personality disorders or the neuroses. The data derive from an era when peripheral mechanisms were thought to be predominant in causing anxiety, a hangover from the old James–Lange hypothesis. This postulated that bodily changes directly follow the perception of an exciting stimulus and that the feelings of these same changes, as they occurred, represented the emotion. The autonomic nervous system, and in particular adrenaline, became a focus of interest. Anxious patients have an increased output of catecholamines in their urine, and adrenaline infusions provoke somatic symptoms of anxiety or exacerbate anxiety in anxious patients (Breggin, 1964). Further, noradrenaline stimulates the production of lactic acid and free fatty acids, both of which are raised in anxiety states. Isoprenaline, a beta receptor agonist, when infused provokes tachycardia more readily in the anxious (Frolich *et al.*, 1969).

The lactic acid link has been taken further following the suggestions of Pitts and McClure (1967) that lactate was responsible for the anxiety. In their studies they gave anxious patients and normals intravenous sodium lactate, and nearly all the former (93 per cent) developed severe anxiety, starting within a few minutes of the infusion. This was not seen to the same extent in the normals (20 per cent), or following glucose–saline infusions. Since lactate combined with calcium chloride was much less effective in provoking anxiety they suggested that the lactate complexed calcium, lowered it, and thus interfered with neurotransmission.

These observations have been replicated by several groups, the main clinical conclusion being that lactate provokes anxiety, and more specifically panic in susceptible patients. In a recent study testing the validity of the DSM III classification of anxiety disorders, lactate infusions provoked panic in 7 per cent of patients with social phobias, 44 per cent of agoraphobics and 50 per cent of panic disorder patients (Liebowitz et al., 1985). Possible mechanisms of this effect have recently been reviewed by Levin et al. (1984) and are given in Table 1.

The lactate induction of panic is widely used in anxiety research. In their own studies, Klein and colleagues (Liebowitz et al., 1985) infuse 0.5 M racemic sodium lactate over a 20 minute period. They report that the induced panic is not accompanied by hypocalcaemia, alkalosis or elevated plasma catecholamines. They argue that it is a centrally driven phenomenon, possibly via alteration of the $NAD^+/NADH$ ratio with accumulation of this reduced product, or through a rise in cerebral CO_2 secondary to lactate

Table 1 **Some possible mechanisms of lactate-induced panic attacks** (from Levin et al., 1984, p.83)

1. Lowering of ionized calcium
2. Metabolic alkalosis
3. Beta adrenergic hypersensitivity
4. Peripheral catecholamine release
5. Central noradrenergic stimulation
6. Hyperventilation
7. Endogenous opiod dysregulation
8. Altered NAD^+ to NADH ratio
9. Non-specific stress

infusion, since panic can also be provoked by inhalation of CO_2. Thus, following infusion, the lactate is converted to pyruvate in the liver, generating bicarbonate which dissociates to CO_2 and water, both of which readily diffuse into the CNS.

One of the peripheral markers that has been studied in personality disorders is platelet MAO activity. The enzyme MAOB is present in human platelets, and its activity, and that of central MAO, is thought to be under genetic control although the mechanism of the inheritance is not clear. Levels are relatively stable over time, with a tendency to increase with advancing age.

It has been suggested that reduced platelet MAO may represent a marker of genetic vulnerability for psychopathology (Murphy *et al.*, 1974). In non-patient studies, there is an association between platelet MAOB activity and personality variables. Murphy *et al.* (1977) noted an inverse relationship with higher MMPI scores, and higher ratings on a sensation seeking scale in males only. Plasma amine oxidase activity held a similar relationship, while another enzyme, dopamine beta hydroxylase, showed no correlations to personality scales. Volunteers with the lowest MAO activity showed elevation of most of the MMPI subscales, showing profiles similar to patients with psychiatric illness and low MAO activity. Comparable data are reported by others (Schooler *et al.*, 1978; Fowler *et al.*, 1980), emphasizing the association in particular between low MAO activity in platelets and sensation seeking, the correlations, for example, to extraversion on the EPI being much weaker (Oreland *et al.*, 1984).

Other studies indicate that children with low platelet MAO activity are more active at birth and are more likely to display neurotic traits in early childhood and that adults with low platelet MAO are more likely to be impulsive, monotony avoiders and aggressive. Buchsbaum *et al.* (1976) noted those with low platelet MAO to have more psychiatric contacts, to attempt suicide more frequently, to have a higher familial incidence of psychopathology, a greater number of convictions and to use illicit drugs more than those with high MAO activity.

In contrast to these data, there are reports that platelet MAO is increased in patients with panic disorder (Gorman *et al.*, 1985).

In animals, a correlation between low MAO activity and brain serotonin and its metabolites is reported, notably in a strain of mouse with high anxiety, irritability and aggression (Oreland *et al.*, 1984), and in primates, low MAO platelet activity relates to exploratory sensation-seeking activity. Biochemically, the relationship to serotonin activity in the brain, confirmed in human autopsy material (Adolfsson *et al.*, 1978), suggests that, while in no way being a specific marker for any personality type, platelet MAO activity, especially MAOB, may indicate vulnerabilities to certain personality attributes and psychiatric illness. In one recent follow-up study of low MAO subjects, Coursey *et al.* (1982) reported that they had more psychopathology and job instability than high MAO counterparts, and Perris *et al.* (1984) noted that low MAO subjects reported less life events prior to the development of depressive disorders than others.

Several groups have noted increased urinary or plasma catecholamines in anxious subjects. The difficulty with the plasma assessments from earlier studies was the insensitivity of the assay procedures, and thus more studies have been done on urine. Excretion of both adrenaline and noradrenaline are noted in anxiety-provoking situations, increased adrenaline relating to threatening or uncertain situations and noradrenaline to states of challenge, including those leading to anger or aggression (Schildkraut and Kety, 1967). Mathew *et al.* (1980a) have reported that both noradrenaline and adrenaline are increased in patients with generalized anxiety disorder compared with controls, decreasing after a course of biofeedback.

To date, there are few hormonal investigations of patients with either personality disorders or the neuroses. The absence of thyroid hormone at crucial stages of early life is known to markedly alter development. The clinical picture of thyrotoxicosis has long been recognized to simulate anxiety neurosis, and assessment of thyroid function is still required in the evaluation of anxiety states. In view of the overlap, the reports of blunted TSH responses to TRH in panic disorder patients are of interest (Roy-Byrne *et al.*, 1985a). Basal levels of TSH seem only slighty diminished and routine thyroid function tests are within normal limits.

There is one report of a blunted growth hormone response to intravenous clonidine in obsessive compulsive disorder patients, who also displayed higher MHPG and noradrenaline plasma levels than controls (Siever *et al.*, 1983). The similarity of the clonidine response to that seen in affective disorders (see p.262) suggests a biological affinity between the two, the authors suggesting an association with increased presynaptic and decreased postsynaptic noradrenergic responsiveness.

Generally patients with anxiety neurosis or panic disorder show normal cortisol suppression with the DST (Roy-Byrne et al., 1985b), and suppression does not relate to anxiety symptoms in depressed patients (Saleem, 1984). Similarly, patients with obsessive compulsive disorder show normal DST suppression (Lieberman et al., 1985). In contrast, there are reports of some patients with the borderline personality having abnormal patterns of DST, although this is most likely related to underlying mood disorder.

NEUROCHEMICAL INVESTIGATIONS

Anxiety disorders

The two main areas of neurochemical investigation relating to the neuroses are the association of anxiety with abnormal adrenergic activity and the link with benzodiazepine receptors.

The interest in adrenergic mechanisms relates to the early observations that drugs such as the beta stimulants provoked many of the peripheral effects of anxiety and the finding that these were blocked by specific beta receptor antagonists. In particular, drugs such as propranolol diminish the heart rate, inhibit palpitations, decrease tremor and inhibit the release of free fatty acids. In addition, the beta blockers have a long and respectable clinical use in anxiety. One hypothesis to emerge is that in anxiety there is an increased sensitivity of adrenergic, specifically beta receptors. Some suggest this is a peripheral phenomenon supporting the James-Lange hypothesis, but this is not supported by several findings. First, in general, catecholamine related compounds used to stimulate and block the anxiety symptoms cross the blood–brain barrier, and may thus be exerting their effects centrally. Secondly, the available evidence with regards to panic disorder does not show increased responsiveness. Thus, Gorman et al. (1983) have shown that propranolol pretreatment fails to prevent lactate-induced panic attacks, and Nesse et al. (1984) report that panic patients actually decrease their heart rate after an infusion of the beta stimulant isoproteranol. Thirdly, panic disorder responds better to imipramine than propranolol (Kathol et al., 1981). Fourthly, many of the infusion investigations were not carried out under double-blind conditions, and it is uncertain to what extent the infusions themselves acted as a non-specific stressor.

In contrast, alternative theories emphasize the primacy of central mechanisms in anxiety and panic, sometimes seen as a rival to the peripheral theory. The origins of this revert to Cannon (1927). He acknowledged the work of others who previously had shown that decorticate animals could still experience anxiety. His own investigations showed that emotions could be generated by stimulation of CNS structures, and the experience of anxiety was not dependent on peripheral changes. For this theory, the somatic manifestations experienced in anxiety are an effect, not the cause, and it follows that the biochemical changes such as those of the catecholamines were also secondary. As noted in Chapter 4, there is some evidence from animal data to support the theories of Gray (1982), which gives a central role to the septohippocampal regions in anxiety. His theory also involves the monoamine system, regulating activity in the hippocampus.

Central monoamine activity in anxiety-panic disorder has been studied, with particular reference to noradrenaline and the locus coeruleus, which when stimulated provokes anxiety in animals. Drugs that increase locus coeruleus firing, and thus release of noradrenaline, such as yohimbine, provoke anxiety in man (Helmberg and Gershon, 1961), while the alpha-2 agonist clonidine, which reduces locus coeruleus activity, is anxiolytic, albeit modestly (Hoehn-Saric, 1982; Uhde et al., 1985). Similar down-regulation of activity is seen with tricyclic antidepressants, also effective in some anxiety patients (Nyback et al., 1975), propranolol and benzodiazepines.

A possible estimate of central catecholaminergic activity is measurement of the MHPG in urine and plasma. Ko et al. (1983) reported that plasma levels of this metabolite correlated highly with rated anxiety in patients with the phobic anxiety syndrome, and both clonidine and imipramine inhibited a panic-induced MHPG increase. In a more extensive investigation of alpha-2 receptor function in anxiety, Charney et al. (1984a) gave yohimbine to healthy subjects and drug-free patients with agoraphobia or panic attacks. In the patients the rise of plasma MHPG levels correlated with patient rated anxiety, nervousness and the frequency of reported panic attacks. This was interpreted as evidence for impaired presynaptic noradrenergic regulation in their patients. This is supported by the observation of diminished yohimbine platelet binding in panic disorder patients (Cameron et al., 1984).

Another putative neurotransmitter of interest in anxiety is the purinergic system. Thus caffeine is anxiogenic, even provoking anxiety in normal controls at high levels (Uhde et al., 1985).

Caffeine is an inhibitor of adenosine, itself a potent neuromodulator which has anticonvulsant effects, and antagonists are proconvulsant.

Understanding of the benzodiazepine receptor has been of importance. As noted, there are hints of an association between central benzodiazepine receptor binding and anxious traits in animals, and in patients, the benzodiazepines are most successful in the treatment of anxiety disorders. The discovery of the benzodiazepine receptor, at first in animals (Braestrup and Nielsen, 1982), but now demonstrated in human brain using PET (Mazière et al., 1986), was a landmark in our understanding of the neuroses, and is of great significance for biological psychiatry. Thus, the possibility of discovering abnormalities of brain structure and function in patients with major psychopathology has been a continuous endeavour, but the neuroses and personality disorders have been somewhat excluded. Indeed, the concept of biological therapies for neuroses has been criticized, and medications such as the benzodiazepines have been discouraged. The concept of endogenous anxiety has been ignored, and the essentially biological nature of the neuroses sacrificed on the Cartesian shrine.

It has to be of interest therefore that benzodiazepine receptors exist in profusion in the human brain; that in animal models, anxiety levels can be related to such receptors; and that in man, benzodiazepines are anxiolytic. Further, benzodiazepine receptors are found in high concentration in such structures as the temporal, frontal and visual cortices, and the cerebellum (Mazière et al., 1986), and their antagonists provoke anxiety in animals and man. These antagonists displace radioactively labelled benzodiazepines from their binding sites, and reverse their behavioural and physiological effects. Two commonly used compounds are beta-carboline-3-carboxylate (beta-CCE) and Ro 15-1788, which appear anxiogenic when given alone. A derivative of beta-CCE has been given to man, and shown to provoke severe anxiety (Dorrow et al., 1983). These data raise the possibility that an 'endogenous anxiolytic' exists within the brain, and Sandler (1983) has proposed the name 'tribulin' for this. Although not chemically specified, it has a molecular weight less than 500, and its output is increased by stress in animal models. Tribulin is both an inhibitor of benzodiazepine receptors and an endogenous MAOI, which increases in output following benzodiazepine withdrawal.

Aggression

As noted in Chapter 4, animal studies fail to provide a clear picture of the neurotransmitter changes associated with aggression, although 5-HT, GABA, catecholamines and choline were most likely to be involved. Brown *et al.* (1979) studied the CSF metabolites of males with a history of aggressive, violent or impulsive behaviour, and found significantly lower 5-HIAA levels, aggression scores showing a significant negative correlation with the metabolite level. A less significant and positive relationship to the MHPG levels was also recorded. A further interesting finding was that those with a history of a suicide attempt had a lower 5-HIAA and a higher MHPG than those with no such attempts. In a separate study, patients with the borderline personality were investigated, and significant negative correlations were recorded between CSF 5-HIAA and psychopathic deviate scores of the MMPI and a history of aggression (Brown *et al.*, 1982). Again an association of low metabolite levels to suicide attempts was noted.

Similar data have been reported by others. For example, Linnoila and colleagues, in a study of incarcerated murderers, reported low 5-HIAA levels compared with normal controls (Linnoila and Martin, 1983), and Lidberg *et al.* (1985) noted the same both in men convicted of criminal homicide and a group who attempted suicide. In addition, there are several reports of patients with affective disorder and schizophrenia who attempt suicide, especially by violent means, showing low 5-HIAA levels, discussed further in Chapter 9.

In such populations, those with low CSF 5-HIAA are rated significantly higher on the Rorschach test for aggression. Impulsivity is one feature shown by many of these patients, suggesting an association with the personality attributes noted with low MAO levels reported above. A further link between the studies is that alcoholism itself is associated with low platelet MAO levels (Oreland *et al.*, 1984) and abstinent alcoholics also have low 5-HIAA CSF levels (Ballenger *et al.*, 1979; Linnoila and Martin, 1983); impulsive aggression in such subjects is related to the low 5-HIAA.

These data are compatible with some of the animal data, and emphasize the relationship of 5-HT and its metabolites to certain aspects of human behaviour. The genetic evidence and the links to MAO activity suggest that some personality variables, notably impulsivity, sensation seeking, aggressiveness and proneness to alcoholism, may have biochemical correlates, notably with the serotonergic system and its regulation through MAO.

Another finding related to aggression is higher levels of phenylacetic acid in the plasma of aggressive psychopaths (Sandler, 1978). This is the major metabolite of phenylethylamine, the enzyme involved being MAOB. Phenylethylamine is closely related to amphetamine. One interpretation suggests that there is an excess of endogenous phenylethylamine production and, rather as amphetamine can improve impulse control and aggression in children with attention deficit disorders, that this represents a compensatory reaction of the body to curb aggressive tendencies.

Obsessive compulsive disorder

Patients with obsessive compulsive disorder seem to respond preferentially to the tricyclic drug clomipramine, reputed to be more selective for inhibition of 5-HT uptake. This is seen in patients who do not have an accompanying affective disorder (Thoren et al., 1980a) and the response is better in patients with higher pretreatment levels of CSF 5-HIAA and HVA (Thoren et al., 1980b) and in those whose 5-HIAA level falls the most with clomipramine treatment. In a more recent study, Insell et al. (1985) confirmed the rather specific response of this disorder to clomipramine, which may be enhanced by addition of the serotonin precursor L-tryptophan (Rasmussen, 1984), and reported higher CSF 5-HIAA levels in obsessionals. These high levels stand in contrast to the low values reported for patients with impulsive, aggressive conditions. Interestingly, zimelidine, an apparently selective inhibitor of 5-HT uptake, was ineffective in ameliorating the obsessional symptoms, in contrast to some reports of benefits with such selective compounds as fluoxetine.

NEUROPHYSIOLOGICAL AND NEUROLOGICAL DATA

The close similarity of EEG patterns in identical twins was established long ago (Lennox and Lennox, 1960), as was the frequency of abnormalities in patients referred to as aggressive or psychopathic (Hill, 1952). In particular, bilateral theta activity in temporal and central regions was reported. These data were reinforced by Williams (1969), whose studies revealed a far higher incidence of abnormal EEGs in aggressive psychopaths than in individuals selected for stability, such as flying personnel, and by

Stafford-Clarke and Taylor (1949), who found over 70 per cent of motiveless murderers to have abnormalities. Monroe (1970), reporting on 70 psychiatric patients, noted, with activation, that those who demonstrated high amplitude paroxysmal slow waves were more likely to be seriously aggressive to themselves or others. Patients diagnosed as suffering from episodic dyscontrol frequently have EEG abnormalities, again the majority being temporal lobe in origin (Bach et al., 1971).

These data are supplemented by observations that psychiatric patients with no history of epilepsy but a temporal lobe focus on the EEG are more likely to be aggressive (Treffert, 1964; Tucker et al., 1965) and the depth electrode studies, which indicate that feelings of dyscontrol and rage are primarily associated with discharges in the amygdala and hippocampus, in both epileptic and non-epileptic patients (Heath, 1982).

In a more systematic study of the behavioural correlates of rhythmic midtemporal discharge, an abnormality frequently associated with psychopathology (see p.267), Hughes and Hermann (1984) noted a relationship between the frequency of such discharges and abnormal MMPI profiles. Further, patients with borderline personality disorder have a high frequency (46 per cent) of EEG abnormalities, including non-focal spike or sharp wave activity and, on occasions, posterior temporal spike-wave discharges (Cowdry et al., 1986).

These data suggest links between cerebral dysrhythmia and certain personality features, and the emphasis is on impulsive aggressive behaviour. The association is in particular with posterior, often bilateral, temporal paroxysmal discharges. The aetiology of the dysrhythmias is unclear, but may reflect maturational factors, possibly genetically determined, earlier brain damage or a functional disturbance of brainstem–limbic system structures.

Evoked potential studies have also been carried out, although attempts to correlate changes to personality variables have not been reliably reproduced (Shagass, 1972). The CNV has been shown to be of higher amplitude in two studies of psychopathic patients (Howard et al., 1984), although the meaning of this is unclear.

Substantial evidence that personality and the brain are closely entwined stems from observations of patients with various neurological conditions, or who have suffered trauma to selected regions of the brain. Generally, any brain lesion may disrupt personality, and some authors refer to an 'organic personality change' (Lishman, 1978). This includes irritability and restlessness, lassitude, poor concentration, loss of initiative and excessive emotionality. There may be poor tolerance for change, withdrawal, insecurity and anxiety. With more severe damage, extremes of this picture are seen, with social disorganization, loss of interest in the self, explosive irritability, shallowness of affect and a blunting of emotional responses. In such situations, an exacerbation of preexisting personality traits is seen, for example aggressive people exhibiting outbursts of anger, and perhaps violence, with minimal provocation. While many of these features are non-specific, their recognition is important. Slater (1943), in his work on the neurotic constitution, noted how cerebral injury predisposed to neurosis, suggesting that in such cases the clinical picture would emerge with less of a premorbid predisposition. Stengel (1949) made the point that 'often a neurotic syndrome forms round a nucleus of symptoms due to structural damage, especially when the latter is slight', making the clinical point that 'it is difficult and unprofitable to attempt to demarcate the neurotic superstructure from what is called its organic basis'.

Patients, often following even trivial head injuries, may develop a variety of symptoms, sometimes referred to as post-traumatic neurosis. The DSM III post-traumatic stress disorder covers some of the clinical features, but is quite restrictive in its definition. There is always debate about the pathogenesis of these syndromes, especially if there is a compensation issue outstanding (Trimble, 1981b), but in head injury cases subtle neuronal damage, especially when the constitutional liability is slight, may be important and must always be considered.

The most substantial evidence that the brain is intimately involved in the structure of the personality comes from the observations on patients with frontal lobe damage. This is discussed in more detail in Chapter 6, where the main elements of the frontal lobe syndrome have been presented. These include reduced activity, lack of drive, loss of appropriate affect with indifference and blunting, inability to plan appropriately, impulsivity with irritability and aggression, and marked impairment of relationships with others. One recognized form of this has been termed 'pseudopsychopathic', reflecting the similarity of the behaviour to that form of personality disorder.

In contrast, changes of personality related to temporal lobe pathology are different. The issue of personality disorders in relation to epilepsy are discussed in Chapter 10 where the arguments in favour of a 'temporal lobe syndrome' and the relation to aggression are rehearsed. This has been most strongly advocated by Geschwind and his group from Boston. The increased association between personality disorders and epilepsy crystallized more clearly following the introduction of the EEG, which led to a fuller understanding and identification of temporal lobe epilepsy. It was suggested that patients with such an origin of their seizures were more likely to show personality changes. Such clinical information seemed in keeping with the growing literature on the role of the temporal lobes in animal behaviour, in particular the description of the Kluver–Bucy syndrome. Alterations of aggressive potential, sexual behaviour, affective tone, appetites for food and sex, and motoric life are described in association with other limbic system conditions where the burden of the pathology is in the temporal lobes, in keeping with the data on epilepsy.

Waxman and Geschwind (1975) defined the interictal behaviour syndrome of temporal lobe epilepsy, emphasizing alterations in sexual behaviour, hyperreligiosity and hypergraphia, a tendency towards extensive and often compulsive writing. They suggested that in some patients the syndrome appeared before any seizures, and when present, even in the absence of further evidence, might suggest dysfunction at this specific anatomical site. They contrasted this picture both with the frontal lobe syndrome and with the Kluver–Bucy syndrome, having some characteristics almost opposite to the latter. The religiosity may be seen as sudden religious conversions or as a growing interest in mystical and religious themes, often with behaviour quite out of keeping with the patient's normal behaviour. There may be compulsive church attendances, or repetitive bible reading, or obsessive attachment to an unorthodox group. Alternatively, there may be an interest in the cosmic and supernatural, or the conviction that the person has some special significance in the world, some messianic mission.

Meticulous attention to detail is another feature, with viscosity or stickiness pertaining to an idea which is continually worked over. There may be circumstantiality of speech, with prolonged and tortuous explanations being given, often for trivial events. This to some extent may be reflected in the hypergraphia, with detailed and meticulous accounts of events being recorded, often with a moral or religious theme.

The disturbed sexuality is usually referred to as hyposexuality, with indifference to sex and minimal sexual contacts. In other patients it may manifest as plasticity of responses, with somewhat unusual proclivities developing.

It is emphasized that the constellation of symptoms and signs that make up the syndrome are not necessarily maladaptive, and often patients display remarkable talents and are productive and valuable members of their societies. Waxman and Geschwind suggested that ongoing interictal abnormal electrical activity in the limbic system may be responsible for the behaviour changes, a theme taken up by Bear and Fedio (1977). In their own studies of patients with temporal lobe epilepsy, using a behavioural rating scale constructed from literature descriptions of abnormalities recorded in association with the condition, they reported such factors as humourlessness, circumstantiality, philosophical and religious interest, and obsessionalism to be features of the syndrome. Many items correlated with the length of seizure history. Their interpretation of the findings was that the epileptic focus somehow led to enhanced associations between affect and stimuli, a so-called 'functional hyperconnection' (p.465) between neocortical and limbic structures, possibly inhibiting events that normally prevent fortuitous sensory and affective connections. This can be seen as the opposite of the Kluver–Bucy syndrome. In the latter the limbic dysfunction leads to failure to attribute stimuli their appropriate emotional significance with hypermetamorphosis, emotional blunting, diminished fear and aggression, and inappropriate sexual behaviour (limbic agnosia).

The above data implicate the limbic system and related structures in determining personality, and show how it is possible to influence personality by altering its function or structure. There is also evidence that some of the neuroses are clearly linked to limbic activity, particularly anxiety and panic disorder.

The Kluver–Bucy syndrome, with diminished anxiety as a central feature, has already been described. It might be anticipated that stimulation of medial temporal structures leads to anxiety. Such is indeed the case. Heath (1982) correlated changes in various brain sites with emotions using intracerebral EEG recordings, and noted, in some patients, how the affect fear related to subcortical discharges. This has been replicated by several other groups, including Gloor et al. (1982) and Wieser (1983). The former recorded from, and stimulated, electrodes implanted in neocortical and allocortical sites in patients awaiting neurosurgery. Of 35 patients, 50 per cent exhibited some kind of experiental phenomenon with recorded activity, fear being the commonest. The responses required limbic system discharges and could not be evoked by purely cortical discharges. The amygdala was particularly involved, a structure also identified in the studies of Wieser. He stimulated various brain regions, again using implanted electrodes, and reported fear on activation of the amygdala and periamygdaloid area.

The evidence from patients with epilepsy points in a similar direction. Williams (1956) recorded the ictal emotional experiences of 100 patients with epilepsy, and noted fear in 61. It was seen mainly with an anterior or midtemporal location of the seizure origin. Cases of partial status epilepticus, with an origin in the temporal lobes and fear as a clinical manifestation, are described (Henriksen, 1973), and clinically on occasions it can be very difficult to distinguish a panic attack from an epileptic aura of fear.

Of interest with regards to cerebral function in panic disorder are the data using PET. Reiman et al. (1984), using radioactively labelled oxygen, measured CBF in patients satisfying DSM III and Feighner criteria for the condition. Their data were compared with controls, and a subgroup with lactate-induced panic were also identified. When the left–right ratio of the CBF for the patients was analysed, it was significantly lower in the region corresponding to the parahippocampal gyrus, in the lactate-sensitive group. Further, after completion of the study, the authors analysed a further 20 neurologically normal volunteers, and found one with a similar abnormal ratio in the same region. The subject was challenged with lactate and developed panic attacks. The siting of this abnormality, detected in vivo in a group of biologically susceptible patients, homogeneous for their response to lactate, is in keeping with the importance of the limbic system in this condition, and with some of the theories of anxiety derived from animal studies, such as those of Gray (1982) which specifically implicated the septohippocampal system.

The association between CNS abnormalities and hysteria is often reported. Whitlock (1967) noted that 62.5 per cent of patients with conversion symptoms had coexisting organic disorder, compared with only 5 per cent of controls. Merskey and Buhrich (1975) reported that 61 of 89 such patients had organic disease, epilepsy being the commonest condition, and Slater and

Glithero (1965), in a follow-up study, reported that a high frequency of organic pathology emerged over time in patients diagnosed with hysteria.

Examination of the laterality of the symptoms of hysteria reveals an excess of left-sided complaints, especially the anaesthetic areas. These, reported over 100 years ago by authors such as Briquet (1859) and Charcot, are 'positive' neurological signs of hysteria (Trimble, 1986). Briquet noted that anaesthesia occurred in 93 cases of 400, and that in 70 it was on the left side. Similar observations have been made by several others (see Trimble, 1986c), especially for female patients. Flor-Henry (1983) has speculated that this reflects underlying cerebral organization. He points out that there is evidence of unequal decussation in the pyramidal tract, more fibres of the left crossing to the right than vice versa, with more ipsilateral projections to the right side. Further, left hemisphere lesions tend to provoke bilateral motor abnormalities and right-sided ones unilateral contralateral effects, and sensory representations are discrete in the dominant hemisphere and diffuse in the non-dominant hemisphere. Thus, the chances of bilateral or unilateral left-sided changes following disruption of the right side were greater.

Galin *et al.* (1977), in contrast, proposed an explanation based on the particular properties of the non-dominant hemisphere for processing unconscious information. In keeping with the laterality observations and the possible link of non-dominant hemisphere dysfunction to conversion symptoms is the observation that patients with brain lesions on that side tend to show 'la belle indifference' (Gainotti, 1969); the known association of neglect and denial of illness (anosognosia) to damage of the right parietal and possibly frontal areas; and the association between conversion symptoms and depression (Wilson-Barnett and Trimble, 1985), the latter itself being linked with non-dominant hemisphere dysfunction (see Chapter 9).

The connections of the inferior parietal lobule, dorsolateral frontal cortex, cingulate gyrus, thalamus and RAS are known anatomically, and lesions at such sites may lead to inattention and neglect in animal models or in patients with cerebral lesions. This has led to the postulate of an arousal system based on these anatomical structures. The posterior parietal area is a polymodal association cortex, receiving massive amounts of sensory information from sensory areas of brain, and is intimately connected with the frontal association areas, themselves linked to thalamus.

The latter is the main receptive area for ascending sensory information via the lemniscal and related pathways, and hence this neuroanatomical circuitry regulates, with associated limbic connections, the quality and quantity of sensory information we receive. Inattention and loss of the ability for selective attention, a feature of many psychopathologial states, may be dependent on such neural systems.

Patients with Briquet's hysteria have been examined as a separate subgroup of hysteria patients and shown to respond abnormally on neuropsychological tasks, suggesting bifrontal and non-dominant hemisphere dysfunction (Flor-Henry, 1983). However, the latter, according to Flor-Henry, is a reflection of an associated affective disorder bias of female sex overrepresentation and the conversion symptomatology. He further argues that this syndrome of stable hysteria in the female has its counterpart in psychopathy in the male, and is fundamentally a dominant hemisphere dysfunction reflecting imprecise verbal communication, affective incongruity and conversion symptoms.

The neurological associations of obsessive compulsive disorder are apparent from the literature, although not well recognized. Thus, clinically this syndrome would seem the 'most neurological' of the neuroses, and in many patients the quality of the thoughts and compulsions are of psychotic intensity. The syndrome seems rather arbitrarily labelled a neurosis, with the supposed assumption that in doing so its pathogenesis was understood in psychodynamic terms.

Tuke (1894) was one of the earliest writers to recognize the cerebral underpinnings of the condition, quoting with approval the ideas of Laycock and Jackson. Since then the evidence for the neurological associations of obsessive compulsive disorder stems from such disorders as encephalitis lethargica, Parkinson's disease, the Gilles de la Tourette syndrome and the remarkable response of some patients to selective neurosurgical lesions. The encephalitis pandemics of the early part of this century led to the rich variety of neuropsychiatric symptomatology descibed by von Economo (1931). These included obsessive and compulsive behaviours (Neal, 1942). Many patients had postencephalitic Parkinson's disease, and in some the compulsive behaviour was 'awakened' by L-dopa therapy (Sacks, 1973). The association between Parkinson's disease and obsessive compulsive traits has been frequently mentioned, either in terms of rigid, moralistic and inhibited premorbid personality profiles or the development of obsessive compulsive symptoms in association with the motor manifestations of the disease (Todes and Lees, 1985). Obsessional slowness, the extreme time required by some patients to carry out acts, may be likened to failure of executive motor planning, similar to that which must underlie Parkinson's disease.

The Gilles de la Tourette syndrome is characterized by multiple tics, including vocal tics, which usually manifest before the age of fifteen (Trimble, 1981a). Although they wax and wane with time, the condition once established seems lifelong. Some of its manifestations are responsive to drugs that block dopamine receptors such as haloperidol, pimozide and sulpiride. The richness of the condition, however, extends far beyond the tics, and the motor symptoms include a great variety of complicated movements, many of which have a compulsive quality. Further, some 30–50 per cent of patients have obsessive compulsive phenomena, equivalent in severity to obsessive compulsive disorder as defined by the DSM III (Trimble and Robertson, 1986). These symptoms are closely interlinked with some of the central features of the syndrome such as coprolalia and echophenomena, suggesting close biological links between the motoric and psychological phenomena.

The evidence that psychosurgery is influential in the relief of obsessive compulsive phenomena has been reviewed by Flor-Henry (1983), and points to anterior cingulate lesions as being the most important target area. The observations of Talairach et al. (1973), in which patients' brains were stimulated electrically, showed that excitation of the cingulate area provoked forced integrated motor behaviour, similar in nature to compulsive movements. Such observations, combined with the known anatomical connections of the cingulate gyrus to the frontal cortex, and the role of the latter in the regulation of sensory motor integration and motor planning (Stuss and Benson, 1984), imply a potential neuroanatomical circuit involved in obsessive compulsive disorder.

Other evidence for a neurological involvement comes from observations of increased birth abnormalities (Capstick and Seldrup, 1977), especially in patients with more bizarre rituals, and case reports of the condition developing after a head injury (Hillbom, 1960; McKeon et al., 1984). There is a long history of an association between epilepsy and forms of obsessional thinking, sometimes reflected in hypergraphia, associated mainly with temporal lobe epilepsy (see Chapter 10), and EEG studies of obsessive compulsive patients reveal significant abnormalities in 6–60 per cent (Flor-Henry, 1983). Evoked potential investigations show shorter latencies and reduced amplitude of the N200 component of the visual evoked response (Ciesielski *et al.*, 1981) to patterned stimulation, similar to that seen in psychotic patients. Shagass *et al.* (1984) reported high amplitude somatosensory N60 waves in the disorder, again found in schizophrenic patients, and a lower amplitude P90. These data were taken to support notions of excessive arousal in these patients, but, in addition, implicate and support a suggestion of Flor-Henry that there is a deficit of left frontal inhibition, leading to an inability to inhibit verbal ideational representations and their motor counterparts.

Insel *et al.* (1982) reported that patients with obsessive compulsive disorder have abnormal sleep patterns and shortened REM latencies, similar to patients with affective disorder, reinforcing the clinical and biochemical links between the two.

There are also reports of abnormal psychological test profiles in these patients, reflecting cerebral impairment (Insel *et al.*, 1983), in particular frontal lobe involvement (Flor-Henry, 1983; Behar *et al.*, 1984), and one report of CT scan abnormalities with increased ventricular–brain ratios. A recent PET study has shown significantly increased metabolism in the left orbital gyrus and bilaterality in the caudate nuclei in obsessive compulsive disorder patients compared with controls (Baxter *et al.*, 1987).

CHAPTER 8

Schizophrenia

INTRODUCTION

Over time, many of the illnesses termed by Cullen as neuroses have melted away into more clearly defined neurological conditions with a recognizable structural basis. So it is with Kraepelin's concept of dementia praecox. Although for him it represented a disease, whose origins may often be found in early life, its pathogenesis and physiological accompaniments largely eluded him. Bleuler, recognizing the heterogeneity of the condition, used the term 'disease group'. . . 'about analogous with the group of the organic dementias' (Bleuler, 1924, p.373), while Slater and Roth (1960) refer to schizophrenia as a term 'for a group of mental illnesses characterized by specific psychological symptoms' (p.237). Gradually over time some aetiological factors have become clarified.

Schizophrenia therefore should be considered not as a disease, but, like epilepsy, as a syndrome, recognized by a collection of signs and symptoms, which has diverse pathogeneses. It is suggested that the symptoms represent the outcome of abnormal cerebral functioning, itself provoked by disease processes, some of which we readily recognize. However, it is important to understand that, as with the neuroses, as time passes, and as the cerebral basis of schizophrenic symptoms becomes clearer, then the clinical diagnostic category gets whittled down, and preferred pathological diagnoses are given. This is one process whereby medicine advances, and the principle is as important in psychiatry as in other areas of medicine. Thus, Parkinson's disease, dementia and epilepsy are no longer thought of as clearly defined entities with a common cerebral pathology, but as recognizable conditions on clinical grounds, perhaps with common underlying functional change that helps explain the symptom pattern, but with several pathological antecedants.

The concept that schizophrenia is a single disease entity has led to much confusion in psychiatry, even leading some authors to the fanciful conclusion that it does not exist (Szasz, 1976). However, as noted in Chapter 2, there are clearly laid-down operational criteria for the condition, and, as will be noted in this chapter, we indeed have a considerable, but often unacknowledged, amount of information in regard to its pathological associations. There will be arguments over the precise definitions, if only because they are operational and clinical, but this is common with many conditions. How to define epilepsy is an elusive problem (see Chapter 10), and whether or not the subcortical dementia of affective disorder should rightly be included with the dementias is a contemporary issue about which there is much debate (Cummings and Benson, 1983). The point of clarifying definitions for research and communication between scientists is to sharpen up the possibilities of discovery and to aid understanding; hence the widespread use of such systems as the ICD 9 and the DSM III. However, these are not immutable, and indeed allow for change and upgrading in line with medical knowledge. So it will be with schizophrenia, as our concepts change with time to incorporate new findings.

GENETICS

The contribution of genetics to schizophrenia has been long recognized, but often curiously neglected in some pathogenic explanations of the disorder. It has been reviewed in detail by Slater (Slater and Roth, 1960), and more recently by McGuffin (1984b). In brief, the twin studies show impressive differences in rates of concordance between monozygous and dizygous pairs, and the adoption data indicate that there is a greater incidence of schizophrenia and schizophrenic spectrum disorders in those who, adopted to normal parents, have a biological parent with the condition.

A table summarizing the more recent data indicating concordance rates from 35 to 58 per cent in monozygous and from 6 to 26 per cent in the dizygous pairs is shown in Table 1.

While there were several criticisms of the early data, for example the method of ascertainment of the zygosity and in the clinical diagnostic criteria for the schizophrenia, later studies have attempted to overcome these. Some authors (Gottesman and Shields, 1972; Kendler and Robinette, 1983) noted that the more severe the illness the more likely the concordance in monozygous pairs, and Kallmann (1946), whose own series noted a 91.5 per cent concordance for monozygous twins living together, reported a rising familial incidence of the condition as subjects approach a

Table 1   Recent twin studies in schizophrenia

Study	Concordance	
	Monozygous (%)	Dizygous (%)
Kringlen (1967)	45	15
Pollin *et al.* (1969)	43	9
Tienari (1971)	35	13
Fischer (1973)	56	26
Gottesman and Shields (1972)	58	12
Kendler and Robinette (1983)	40	6
Mean	46.1	13.5

genetic relationship with index cases. Thus, compared to a percentage expectation of 0.9 per cent for the general population, the equivalent figure for half-sibs was 7.1 per cent, for parents was 9.2 per cent, for full-sibs 14.2 per cent, for children 16.4 per cent, for dizygous co-twins 14.5 per cent and for children of two schizophrenic parents 39.2 per cent. After a review of the data, Slater concluded 'the evidence is very strong that the genetical constitution of an individual contributes a large part of his total potentiality of becoming schizophrenic' (Slater and Roth, 1969, p.246). McGuffin (1984) calculated that the heritability of the condition was 0.66, genetic factors thus accounting for two-thirds of the variance in vulnerability to the disorder. A similar figure (68 per cent) has been given by Kendler (1983), who notes that this is similar to that for diabetes and hypertension, and rather in excess of that for epilepsy, peptic ulcer and coronary artery disease.

There is some suggestion that schizophrenic probands resemble their affected relatives with regards to subtype, although there is much overlap, and twin and adoption studies which may clarify this issue have not been conducted. Leonhard (1980) has suggested, on the basis of family studies, that periodic catatonia has a high genetic loading, and Perris (1974) noted the same for cycloid psychosis. Winokur (1977) reported that paranoia may also be genetically separate.

McGuffin *et al.* (1984) examined the heritabilities of a twin population using six different sets of operational criteria for schizophrenia. Those of Feighner and the RDC criteria gave the highest heritability, while the Schneiderian criteria had a heritability value of zero. Dworkin and Lenzenweger (1984) examined the case histories of MZ twins, in whom at least one had schizophrenia, and assessed concordance for positive and negative symptoms. Their results suggested that negative symptoms may have the greater genetic component.

With regards to interpretation, the contention that environmental factors are so important, in that the environment of monozygous twins is said to be more alike than that of dizygous pairs, has been discounted by the adoption studies. Heston (1966) showed that the adopted children of schizophrenic mothers, removed from them shortly after birth, had a higher incidence of the illness than the adopted children of non-schizophrenic mothers. These findings have been replicated and extended by a series of studies on Danish patients, including investigation of the relatives of adopted children who later became schizophrenic (Kety, 1983). These studies have not only shown the higher incidence of schizophrenia among the biological relatives, but also an overrepresentation of the schizophrenia spectrum of disorders. Further, there was an overrepresentation of schizophrenia or schizophrenia spectrum disorders in the biological relatives of adopted schizophrenic patients, significantly greater than among the relatives of non-schizophrenic adopted controls. In addition, in investigations of paternal half-siblings of schizophrenic probands, the incidence of schizophrenia was higher than in control cases, ruling out intra-uterine contributions to the congenital effects.

Replication studies (Kendler *et al.*, 1981), particularly improving the criteria for schizophrenia spectrum disorders, have been conducted. The prevalence of schizotypal personality disorder was significantly higher in the biological relatives of schizophrenic adoptees than controls, but this was not the case for delusional disorder of the non-schizophrenic type or anxiety disorder.

These adoption studies, particularly the careful analysis of the Danish patients, have confirmed the genetic contribution to schizophrenia, and identified the concept of the schizophrenia spectrum more clearly.

With regards to the mode of inheritance, several authors favour polygenic as opposed to monogenic transmission (Kendler, 1983), mathematical models failing to provide evidence for the latter. To date, no genetic markers linking to schizophrenia have been described, although molecular genetic studies are now under way. However, the identification of such a marker will only be successful if there is a major gene effect (either a single or a small number) or if there is a subgroup with such a component. HLA markers have been claimed, but results of various studies are variable. McGuffin *et al.* (1981), after review of the available literature, noted that the most persistent genetic marker to date was HLA A9 with paranoid schizophrenia, and the more consistent associations (found by more than one group) relate to HLA A9 and B5.

SOMATIC VARIABLES

Some earlier investigators emphasized a relationship of bodily constitution to psychopathology, noting the aesthenic typology to be schizothymic and to possess a predisposition to develop schizophrenia (Kretchmer, 1936). Such findings have little relevance today, especially since so many patients are receiving neuroleptic medications that may dramatically alter the bodily habitus.

Of recent interest has been the reporting of abnormalities of muscle endplates in schizophrenic patients. Using muscle biopsies stained for motor neurones and terminals, Crayton and Meltzer (1976) reported the size and dispersion of terminal bulbs to be abnormal in psychotic patients, with larger and more variable endplate arbourization, and low density of endplate neural structures. Although similar findings were seen in some manic depressive patients and no association was noted with type or length of illness, the authors felt the findings may indicate regenerative processes of previously denervated fibres, reflecting perhaps altered CNS physiology. These data are in keeping with other evidence of disturbed muscle pathology in psychotic patients. A number of authors have noted an increase in serum creatine phosphokinase in acute psychoses. This does not simply reflect on the use of intramuscular injections or methods of restraint since elevations are found in a proportion of first-degree relatives and there is some correlation with the alpha-motor neurone abnormalities noted on biopsy. Further, mean creatine kinase levels during a hospital admission are also elevated (Meltzer *et al.*, 1980).

METABOLIC AND BIOCHEMICAL FINDINGS

One early finding that has been replicated was that of abnormal nitrogen balance in patients with periodic catatonia (Gjessing,

1947). Thus, phases of stupor and excitement were associated with nitrogen retention, with later compensatory increased excretion. In such patients it was claimed that alteration of nitrogen input, by reducing protein intake, altered the course of the illness.

The concept that endogenous neurotoxins exist, derived from the abnormal metabolism of various chemicals, was encouraged by the observations of psychoses resembling schizophrenia that could be provoked by the ingestion of various psychotropic drugs such as LSD, mescaline and amphetamine. Attempts were made to identify abnormal compounds in the blood and urine of schizophrenics, some authors reporting success, although much of the early data was not replicated. Heath *et al.* (1957) reported an abnormal enzyme, similar to caeruloplasmin in schizophrenic plasma, which they called taraxein. When injected into volunteers this led to an acute psychosis. The view of these authors was that such an abnormal toxin provoked behavioural changes by influencing specific neuronal structures, notably the septal region of the brain. They also postulated autoimmune mechanisms, brain dysfunction being consequent on brain tissue destruction by autoantibodies.

From these ideas arose the transmethylation hypothesis (Smythies, 1976). Thus, several hallucinogenic compounds were seen to be closely related chemically to the endogenous catecholamines and indolamines, notably being methylated derivates. It was suggested that abnormal transmethylation of these compounds might produce hallucinogenic methylated monoamines related to the pathogenesis of at least some forms of schizophrenia. Administration of methyl donors such as methionine to schizophrenics gave variable results, but, especially when combined with a monoamine oxidase inhibitor, led to the exacerbation of symptoms in some 40 per cent of patients. These studies did not, however, distinguish between an acute organic brain syndrome and true exacerbation of schizophrenic symptoms (Wyatt *et al.*, 1971).

Further support for the transmethylation hypothesis has come from attempts to isolate the endogenous psychotoxin, notably methylated derivates of serotonin such as dimethyltryptamine (DMT), 5-methoxydimethyltryptamine and bufotenin. DMT is present in the body and CSF, but the evidence that it is raised in patients with schizophrenia is equivocal. More recent data suggest it may be elevated in psychotic rather than only schizophrenic patients at the time of an acute illness episode (Oon *et al.*, 1975). Since in animal models stress alone increases DMT levels, these data may reflect a non-specific effect, and do not support a substantial role for DMT in schizophrenia.

Smythies has also put forward a second transmethylation hypothesis, which is referred to as the 'one carbon cycle' hypothesis (Smythies, 1983). The essence of this is that methylation is an essential part of brain function and that, if disrupted, then neuronal activity will be interfered with. It is thus not any product of the methylation which is important but the methylation itself. The process of methylation involves especially methionine, S-adenosylmethionine (SAM) and folic acid. These relationships are shown in Figure 1.

In the brain, a methyl group is contributed to homocysteine from methyltetrahydrofolic acid to create methionine, in a reaction which requires the presence of both B_{12} and SAM. Methionine

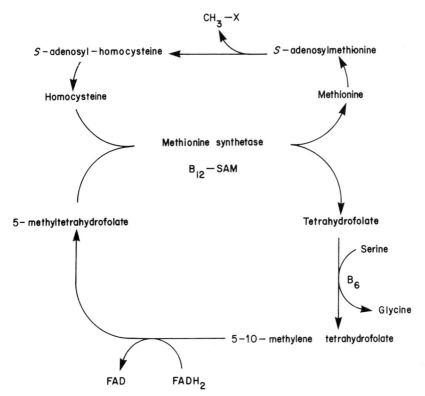

Figure 1. Showing the relationships between the folate cycle, SAM and transmethylation. (From Reynolds and Stramentinoli, 1983.)

only provides methyl groups after conversion to SAM. Thus, it is converted to SAM, the physiological methyl donor, in a series of reactions that involve folate coenzymes. It is clear that trans-methylation reactions influence monoamine synthesis, and in addition are involved in membrane reactions and gene expression. Further, there has been a long history of clinical observations suggesting that folic acid deficiency may be associated with psycho-pathology. While much of this relates to affective disorder (Reynolds and Stramentinoli, 1983), there are case reports of schizophrenia-like psychoses appearing in patients with folic acid deficiency, showing improvement following folate therapy.

A related theme is the possibility that 5-HT is involved in schizophrenia. Thus, methionine may inhibit the uptake of tryp-tophan into the brain by competitive blockade (Smythies, 1976) and schizophrenia may in part reflect defective tryptophan metab-olism. The results of supplementary trytophan loading in patients has provided only equivocal results, and to date the role of indol-amines in the psychoses remains to be clarified.

Platelet MAO activity in schizophrenia has been studied by many authors. In general, the values are low, although, as similar data are noted in some other psychiatric conditions, it is not specific for schizophrenia. The subject has been reviewed by sev-eral authors (De Lisi et al., 1982; Siever and Coursey, 1985), and attempts have been made to link specific clinical variables with the low activity. Patients with paranoid symptoms probably have the lower levels, and in studies of normals, an inverse correlation between the paranoia score on the MMPI and MAO levels has been noted. Several authors link low values to hallucinations and delusions, others with poor outcome. Baron et al. (1980) identified students that had abnormally high or low levels of MAO, and found that 70 per cent of those with low levels and none with high levels had a diagnosis of borderline schizophrenia. This same group also reported that schizophrenic patients with a high genetic load have reduced levels in contrast to those with non-familial schizophrenia, and relatives with low MAO are more often affected with schizophrenia spectrum disorders than the high MAO relatives (Baron et al., 1984).

Reveley et al. (1983) examined MAO in MZ twins discordant for schizophrenia, normal MZ and DZ twins and controls. The MZ pair with a schizophrenic co-twin had significantly lower values than the healthy MZ twins and the other controls, the MZ schizo-phrenics having only slightly lower values than their healthy co-twins.

Although some authors have failed to find low MAO in schizo-phrenic patients, and further show that neuroleptic treatment may itself lower MAO (Owen *et al.*, 1981), the consistency of the data and the findings in twins, relatives and volunteers suggest some association, genetically determined, between MAO and vul-nerabilities to these behaviour patterns, and are in agreement with the adoption studies that both schizophrenia and related spectrum disorders need to be considered together.

Low platelet MAO has been implicated in both the trans-methylation and the dopamine (see below) hypotheses of schizo-phrenia in the sense that reduced MAO activity may reflect an impaired capacity to degrade monoamines or their abnormal metabolites, thus increasing the load of these substances in the brain.

The dopamine hypothesis

In recent years the predominant biochemical hypothesis of schizo-phrenia has been the dopamine hypothesis, and a considerable amount of research work has been carried out investigating dopamine and its metabolites in patients. The hypothesis emerged in the wake of the introduction of the phenothiazines in the 1960s; the recognition of the similarity of a psychosis induced by amphetamine to schizophrenia, and that in small doses they can activate symptoms in patients; and the discovery that the principal mode of action of the phenothiazines is to block dopamine recep-tors. The ability of neuroleptic drugs to block dopamine receptors correlated better than other biochemical effects with their efficacy in the control of psychotic symptoms (Snyder *et al.*, 1974). The dopamine hypothesis which emerged thus suggested that schizo-phrenia was the result of overactivity of dopamine neurotransmis-sion in the CNS and that neuroleptics acted by reducing this. However, the evidence was largely circumstantial, and over time modifications have had to be made.

In animal models, behavioural disturbances provoked by dopamine agonists given systemically or by injection into the limbic forebrain were reversed by neuroleptic drugs (Anden, 1975), and the ability of these compounds to inhibit dopamine-sensitive adenylcyclase stimulation is proportional to their clinical potency, with notable exceptions, namely the butyrophenones. However, the recognition of different classes of dopamine receptors and the fact that only D1 activity is linked to adenylcyclase activity has helped explain this apparent discrepancy.

Generally the evidence that neuroleptics act at dopamine receptors in the limbic system is strong (Scatton and Zivkovic, 1984). Electrophysiologically their iontophoretic application antagonizes the depression of cellular activity induced by the application of dopamine agonists, and binding studies show that a variety of neuroleptics specifically bind to dopamine sites within the limbic system. Further, they increase the metabolism and turnover of dopamine, an effect related to the feedback activation of neurones following the postsynaptic receptor blockade.

Early on it was noted that some neuroleptic drugs were less frequently associated with extrapyramidal side effects. The latter were thought to occur with the blockade of dopamine receptors in the striatum, and the reason why some drugs, notably thioridazine, clozapine and sulpiride, did not do this required explanation. Some evidence pointed to differential effects at limbic and non-limbic sites (ventral and dorsal striatum respectively), either due to anticholinergic properties (strong with thioridazine and clozapine, anticholinergic effects being greater in non-limbic striatal areas) or due to preferential action on different receptor subpopulations at the two sites (Scatton and Zivkovic, 1984—see also Chapter 12), drugs such as sulpiride acting mainly at the limbic receptors. It seems that the effects of neuroleptic drugs on psychotic symptoms relate to changes of dopamine turnover in the limbic forebrain at least, while the development of extrapyramidal symptoms is related to the corpus striatum (Crow et al., 1979a). Further, the antipsychotic effect most likely relates to blockade of D2 dopamine receptors.

An effective demonstration of the antipsychotic effect of dopamine antagonism has been provided by Crow et al. (1979a). Patients with acute schizophrenia took part in a double-blind trial of treatment with flupenthixol, comparing the alpha isomer, which blocks the dopamine receptor, to the beta isomer, which does not. The former had a significant effect compared to placebo, although this was confined to only certain symptoms, referred to by the authors as 'positive'. Thus, using the Krawiecka scale, the improvements were seen on scores for delusions, hallucinations and speech incoherence, but not on poverty of speech or affective flattening.

One problem for the dopamine theory relates to the time course of the clinical effect. Thus, prolactin, which is elevated by blocking dopamine receptors (the prolactin inhibitory factor probably being dopamine), rises much faster than the noted clinical improvements, which do not become manifest for two or three weeks after commencing treatment. In contrast, the extrapyramidal effects often arise within 48 hours. This paradox has some explanation in terms of adaptive effects to the acute blockade in dopamine systems. Thus, CSF studies indicate that the initial rise of dopamine turnover diminishes after time (van Praag, 1977b), as does the plasma level of HVA (Pickar et al., 1984), and similar tolerance of the biochemical effects has been observed in animals. However, it seems that the tolerance relates more to dopamine receptors in the caudate areas, less in the limbic forebrain and not at all in the frontal cortex (Scatton and Zivkovic, 1984). The latter finding may relate to the lack of autoreceptors in frontal areas.

Another line of evidence has been to observe the effects of drugs known to increase dopamine activity on the symptoms of schizophrenia. Paradoxically, administration of the dopamine agonists L-dopa and apomorphine seems to improve symptoms in some patients (Buchanan et al., 1975; Tamminga et al., 1977). In some reports the effect is on such symptoms as apathy, isolation and blunted affect (Gerlach and Luhdorf, 1975); in others it is on hallucinations and delusions (Tamminga et al., 1977). However, several carefully conducted trials have failed to replicate these findings (Ferrier et al., 1984b; Syvalahti et al., 1986). It is suggested that any observed effect is due to inhibition of dopamine release by interaction with presynaptic receptors.

More direct evidence of abnormal dopamine activity in schizophrenia has been hard to demonstrate. If dopamine is overactive in the CNS, then low basal levels of prolactin may be expected, but studies generally have been negative. In contrast, provocation tests using apomorphine and measurements of either growth hormone (raised by dopamine agonists) or prolactin have been more successful. Growth hormone responses have been reported to be greater in patients with first-rank symptoms (Whalley et al., 1984), with delusions, hallucinations and thought disorder (Meltzer et al., 1984), and to be both increased (Meltzer et al., 1984) and blunted in association with negative symptoms and in chronic schizophrenia (Ferrier et al., 1986). Prolactin baseline levels and apomorphine-induced prolactin suppression have been shown to correlate inversely with the presence of positive symptoms

(Johnstone *et al.*, 1977; Ferrier *et al.*, 1984b), especially in patients with normal ventricular size on CT scans (Kleinman *et al.*, 1982b). Although the interpretation of such findings may be easily blurred by the effects of medication on hormonal release, these studies were on drug-free patients, and the results tend to support the hypothesis that at least some symptoms in schizophrenia are related to dopaminergic mechanisms, notably hallucinations, delusions and thought disorder, similar to the ones shown to respond preferentially to dopamine antagonist drugs.

Other estimates of dopamine activity have related to peripheral markers. Plasma dopamine has been reported to be elevated in some studies (Bondy *et al.*, 1984). Measurement of dopamine beta-hydrolase, the enzyme that converts dopamine to noradrenaline, has provided inconsistent results (Castellani *et al.*, 1982). Other markers have included the reporting of reduced platelet cyclic-AMP production (Kafka *et al.*, 1979) and elevated spiperone binding to lymphocytes apparently unrelated to treatment (Bondy *et al.*, 1984). Further evidence that links dopamine to schizophrenia, notably from CSF and post-mortem studies, are discussed below (see Table 2).

Table 2   Main arguments in favour of and against the dopamine hypothesis

---

In favour:
1. Amphetamine-induced psychosis produces a schizophrenia-like illness.
2. Amphetamine exacerbates schizophrenia.
3. Drugs that block dopamine receptors are antipsychotic in relationship to their blocking potential.
4. Post-mortem and endocrine studies.
5. Animal models of dopamine agonism resemble psychosis, and are reversed by dopamine blocking agents.

Against:
1. Time course between administration of a dopamine blocker and clinical response.
2. Dopamine agonists have an inconsistent effect on psychosis.
3. Direct evidence of increased dopamine activity is poor.

Noradrenergic hypothesis

An alternative to the dopamine hypothesis is the noradrenergic hypothesis, suggested by Stein and Wise (1971). This was based on the idea that the central noradrenergic pathways, then shown to be related to a central reward system, might degenerate and lead to at least some of the symptoms of schizophrenia. Generally the data are less favourable to this hypothesis, although several studies indicate a role of noradrenergic mechanisms in some symptoms of schizophrenia. This has recently been reviewed in detail (Kleinman *et al.*, 1985). No noradrenergic abnormalities have been reported in urine of schizophrenic patients, although there is one report of increased levels in the plasma of drug-free patients (Ackenheil *et al.*, 1979). Neither plasma nor urine MHPG or VMA levels have been consistently abnormal in schizophrenia, most studies showing no difference from controls. CSF and neurochemical data are discussed below. Attempts to assess the functions of alpha-2 adrenergic receptors have been done either by direct measurement of platelet binding or by changes of metabolites after challenge with clonidine. Alpha-2 receptors have been reported as increased in platelets in only a minority of subjects, probably schizoaffective (Kafka *et al.*, 1980), while others have noted decreased binding in a group with negative symptoms and poor response to treatment (Rosen *et al.*, 1985), with subsensitivity of MHPG release to a clonidine challenge (Sternberg *et al.*, 1982).

Other studies

Early investigations of endocrine function in schizophrenia yielded inconsistent results and were aimed in particular at examination of the thyroid and adrenal glands. Schizophrenia-like psychoses have been described in association with several endocrinopathies including hypo- and hyperthyroidism and hypoparathyroidism (Lishman, 1978). The prolactin and growth hormone data, utilized more as a method of challenging hypothalamic–pituitary function as opposed to implicating the hormonal changes themselves as pathogenic, have been discussed. Few other studies of endocrine function in schizophrenia have been recently carried out, although there are reports of lower LH and FSH levels in chronic schizophrenia, with an inverse relationship to positive symptoms. There seems to be loss of normal episodic secretion of LH, possibly reflecting disturbed hypothalamic or limbic system function (Ferrier *et al.*, 1982). Further evidence for this is the finding of blunted

FSH and prolactin responses to thyrotropin releasing hormone in similar patients (Ferrier *et al.*, 1983).

In contrast to affective disorders, the number of schizophrenic patients showing abnormal dexamethasone suppression is low, unless there is coexistent depression (Munro *et al.*, 1984).

Finally, following the discovery of enkephalins, attempts have been made to examine peptide function in schizophrenia, largely by giving peptides to patients and estimating clinical changes. Table 3 lists some of the substances tried, and to date, with the possible exception of the data with des-tyr-gamma endorphin in acute onset patients, the results have been disappointing. In addition, the opiate antagonist naloxone fails to provoke constant changes.

NEUROCHEMICAL INVESTIGATIONS

In order to explore further the dopamine and related neurochemical hypotheses in schizophrenia, many neurochemical investigations have been conducted. The CSF data will be discussed first, followed by neurochemical pathological data.

CSF

The main metabolite assessed in CSF to test the dopamine hypothesis is HVA, although it is suggested that the main source of this is nigrostriatal dopamine and not mesolimbic and mesocortical dopamine. Nonetheless, the anatomical proximity and the overlap between these systems suggests that at least some of it reflects limbic system dopamine function. In general, either the baseline CSF values have been sampled or the accumulation of metabolite

Table 3   Some peptides used in schizophrenia

Peptide	Author
CCK	Lostra *et al.* (1984)
	Albus *et al.* (1984)
Des-tyrosine gamma-endorphin	van Praag *et al.* (1982)
Des-enkephalin gamma-endorphin	van Praag *et al.* (1982)
Beta-endorphin	Berger *et al.* (1980)
Thyroid releasing hormone	Prange *et al.* (1979)

after probenecid administration. The latter technique inhibits the exit of HVA and related compounds from the CSF, diminishing the gradient that exists between ventricular and spinal CSF values. Theoretically this should provide a more accurate determination of metabolite turnover and concentration, but it, too, has methodological difficulties. Not the least is that the results are related to the CSF probenecid levels.

One of the early baseline studies of HVA was that of Rimon *et al*. (1971), who reported normal values, except that patients with paranoid symptoms had elevated levels. Generally, however, the baseline data have failed to show differences between schizophrenics and controls, although Sedval and Wode-Helgodt (1980) reported that high HVA levels were associated with a family history of schizophrenia. The probenecid studies likewise have tended to be negative with singular exceptions. There are two reports of decreased accumulation in patients with Schneiderian first-rank symptoms (Bowers, 1973; Post *et al*., 1975) and a suggestion that those with low values have poorer prognosis (Bowers, 1974). These data are compatible with increased dopamine receptor sensitivity, which subsequently decreased dopamine turnover. Some support for this comes from a recent study in which the relationship between apomorphine-induced growth hormone release and CSF–HVA levels have been assessed in drug-free schizophrenic patients. An inverse relationship was found, those patients with low HVA having a higher release of hormone (Zemlan *et al*., 1985). Thus low HVA was associated with higher dopamine receptor activity, and in addition with first-rank symptoms and thought disorder.

Both CSF levels of DOPAC and dopamine itself are reported as normal in schizophrenia (Berger *et al*., 1980; Gattaz *et al*., 1983b), as are prolactin levels (Rimon *et al*., 1981).

With regards to the noradrenergic hypothesis, MHPG levels are consistently reported as normal (Kleinman *et al*., 1985), although there are reports of increased levels of noradrenaline (Gomes *et al*., 1980; Lake *et al*., 1980), especially in paranoid subtypes.

A variety of other substances have been measured in the CSF of schizophrenic patients, some of the more important ones being shown in Table 4.

Brain neurochemistry

Again, most studies in this area relate to testing the dopamine hypothesis. Studies on post-mortem brains are difficult to interpret. Not only are they derived from patients that have usually

Table 4   Some CSF studies in schizophrenia

Compound	Result	Reference
Dopamine beta-hydrolase	Normal	Lerner *et al.* (1978)
5-HIAA	Normal	Post *et al.* (1975) Gomes *et al.* (1980) Roy *et al.* (1985a)
Cyclic-AMP	Decreased Increased	Biedermann *et al.* (1977) Gomes *et al.* (1980)
Cyclic-GMP	Decreased	Gattaz *et al.* (1983a)
GABA	Normal ($\downarrow$ young females)	van Kammen *et al.* (1982)
Angiotensin-converting enzyme	Decreased	Beckmann *et al.* (1984)
Neurotensin	Decreased (subgroup only)	Widerlov *et al.* (1982)
Copper	Decreased	Tyrer *et al.* (1979)

been on medication, or have used a large dose of psychotropic drugs to kill themselves, but also there are rapid post-mortem biochemical changes that occur. Several groups have set up centres designed specifically for collection of brains and appropriate storage after death, control specimens being treated in the same manner. It seems likely that peptides and receptors are much more stable than monoamines and their metabolites. Generally the areas of brain examined have been those with a high level of the neurotransmitter under investigation, and mainly concentrated on limbic system and related structures.

The majority of studies (at least eight are published) show normal values for both dopamine concentrations and HVA, notably in the caudate nucleus, putamen and nucleus accumbens. However, Bird *et al.* (1979) reported increased concentrations of dopamine in the nucleus accumbens and the anterior perforated substance. In an extended study on over 50 schizophrenic brains, with controls, Mackay *et al.* (1982) confirmed the significant elevations, especially in patients with early onset of illness. Owen *et al.* (1978) reported increases in dopamine in the caudate nucleus, but not in the putamen or nucleus accumbens, and a significant decrease in HVA in the caudate. Farley *et al.* (1977) reported increases in dopamine only in the septal region of chronic paranoid patients.

Reynolds (1983), in a study now replicated twice, has attempted to assess laterality effects in relation to neurochemistry in schizophrenia. Comparing patient brains to controls, dopamine was increased in the amygdala of the schizophrenics, selective for the left side.

Dopamine receptor binding, with such compounds as haloperidol, spiperone, flupenthixol and apomorphine, has also been investigated. Here most of the studies (there are at least six) show increased binding in some areas, although the interpretation of this has led to much debate. A summary of the data is given in Table 5.

The reported increases are in receptor density and the studies of Crow and colleagues (Cross *et al.*, 1981a) with flupenthixol identify the receptor involved as the D2 receptor. With regards to the effects of neuroleptic drugs, Lee and Seeman (1980) had a subgroup free of long-term treatment with neuroleptics, and this population also showed elevated binding. Likewise, Owen *et al.* (1978) observed increased binding in patients who never had neuroleptics or who had no exposure a year prior to death. In contrast, Mackay *et al.* (1982) did not detect binding changes in a small number of patients without neuroleptics for a month prior to death, and Reynolds (1983) noted higher binding in the putamen

Table 5   Studies of dopamine binding

Author	Number	Result
Owen *et al.* (1978)	19	Increase in NA,P,C
Lee and Seeman (1980)	50	Increase in NA,P,C
Reisine *et al.* (1980)	11	Increase in C,P
Reynolds *et al.* (1981)	16	No change (P only examined)
Mackay *et al.* (1982)	48	Increase in NA,C

NA = nucleus accumbens
P   = putamen
C   = caudate nucleus

in patients treated with neuroleptics. Further, Clow *et al.* (1979) suggest that these very same changes can be observed in rat brains given long-term neuroleptics, especially increased receptor density.

A cautious interpretation of these findings is that they do not support a hypothesis of increased dopamine turnover in schizophrenia, with the possible exception of the amygdala studies, but are in keeping with an alternative hypothesis, that of increased postsynaptic receptor function.

Noradrenaline and its metabolites have also been examined. Decreased levels of noradrenaline have been reported in the putamen (Crow *et al.*, 1979b), others have reported no differences (Bird *et al.*, 1979; Winblad *et al.*, 1979) and others selective increases (Farley *et al.*, 1977). MHPG is reported to be elevated in the hypothalamus and nucleus accumbens by one group (Kleinman *et al.*, 1982a). Dopamine beta-hydrolase and monoamine oxidase appear normal.

Recently the results of investigation of peptide activity in brain has been of interest. Levels of angiotensin-converting enzyme were reduced in the substantia nigra and globus pallidus (Arregui *et al.*, 1980). Opiod and naloxone binding is probably normal (Owen *et al.*, 1985). Ferrier *et al.* (1984a), in an extensive study of peptide distribution in limbic structures in schizophrenic and control brains, reported that CCK was reduced in temporal cortex, especially in the hippocampus and amygdala of patients with negative symptoms (type 2 of Crow); somatostatin was likewise decreased in hippocampus in the same group, while VIP was increased in the amygdala of those with positive symptoms (type 1 of Crow). No changes were seen for neurotensin, while substance P was increased in the hippocampus.

Several other compounds have been assessed in various brain regions, and many of these are summarized in Table 6.

Neuropathological data

A related area of research has been neuropathological studies of schizophrenic brains. Although many studies over the years have been carried out, all of them detecting changes in some brains examined, such data are often criticized on account of the lack of consistency of the findings. However, similar criticisms would apply to pathological studies of such disorders as dementia or

Table 6   Some post-mortem biochemical findings

Chemical	Result	Author
GABA	Probably normal	Cross *et al.* (1979)
Glutamic acid decarboxylase	Normal	Bird *et al.* (1979)
5-HT	Increased:	
	Putamen	Crow *et al.* (1979a)
	Lower:	
	Hypothalamus	Winblad *et al.* (1979)
	Medulla oblongata	
	Hippocampus	
	Frontal cortex	Bennett *et al.* (1979)
Tryptophan	Normal	Crow *et al.* (1979b)
Cathechol-*o*-methyl transferase	Normal	Crow *et al.* (1979b)
Tyrosine hydrolase	Normal	Crow *et al.* (1979b)
Choline acetyl transferase	Normal	Bird *et al.* (1979)

epilepsy if it were supposed that they represented the outcome of only a single process.

Early investigators included Alzheimer, Kraepelin and later Papez. As an example of an older study, Bouman (1929) reported that in dementia praecox, parenchymatous degeneration could be seen, characterized by degeneration and sclerosis of the cortex in the absence of glial reaction, affecting predominantly frontal, temporal and prerolandic regions. Von Meduna was impressed by the apparent opposites of the pathology of schizophrenia, with loss of neurones and no glial reaction, and epilepsy, with slight loss of neurones and massive glial reactions. Such 'antagonisms' were one of the lines of thought that led to attempts to treat schizophrenia with convulsions. Several authors noted changes in the region of the third ventricle. In essence these findings have stood the test of time.

Nieto and Escobar (1972) showed gliosis in the periventricular and midbrain areas using glial stains. Hypothalamus, thalamus, septal area, periaqueductal grey and hippocampus were especially affected. Stevens (1982), also using glial stains, in patients hospitalized prior to the use of neuroleptic medication, reported gliosis, maximal in periventricular, periaqueductal and basal forebrain regions. Nuclei involved included thalamus, hypothalamus, septal, bed nucleus of the stria terminalis, substantia innominata, nucleus accumbens and amygdala. Neurone loss or infarction was seen in the globus pallidus, and several cases showed disruption of the fibre bundles traversing the periventricular region such as the fornix and stria terminalis. She interpreted these data as compatible with the evidence of third and lateral ventricular enlargement in schizophrenia (see below), pathology affecting predominantly limbic structures, in particular the substantia innominata, a major outflow of the limbic system where the ratio of input to output cells is huge.

Bogerts *et al.* (1985) studied the brains from the Vogt collection, serial sections of young schizophrenic brains free from ECT, insulin or neuroleptic treatment, complete with good clinical notes. They reported reduced volume in five areas: greatest was the parahippocampal gyrus, others being the hippocampus, amygdala, globus pallidus and periventricular region. The inferior horn of the lateral ventricle also showed enlargement. Bogerts *et al.* (1983) have also reported a reduction in size of the lateral part of the substantia nigra in schizophrenic brains. In comparing their findings in schizophrenia with patients with Huntington's chorea and Parkinson's disease, the hippocampal changes were the most striking.

Stevens (1986) has reported on a clinicopathological correlation of Bogerts' data, and noted that pallidum changes were related to negativism and catalepsy, while thought disorder was more associated with pathology in the parahippocampal gyrus and enlargement of the inferior horn of the lateral ventricle. Hallucinations and paranoia were seen with amygdala and hippocampal pathology.

Further data in relation to hippocampal pathology has been reported by Kovelman and Scheibel (1984). They reported pyramidal cell disorganization in two separate groups of brains from schizophrenic patients, suggestive of disruption at an early stage of CNS development.

The temporal lobe changes reported by both Bogerts and Scheibel were in the left hemisphere, but in their studies this was the only one examined. Crow and colleagues (Brown *et al.*, 1986), in a comparison of brains from patients meeting strict criteria for affective disorder and schizophrenia, noted that the latter had larger temporal horns of the lateral ventricle and thinner parahippocampal gyri. The greater differences were noted in the left hemisphere.

Some of these reports suggested that gliosis was a typical patho-logical reaction in schizophrenic brains. Roberts *et al.* (1985), using material from both Bogerts' and Crow's collections, stained specifically for gliosis using immunocytochemical techniques, and assessed gliosis by densitrometry. Their results were negative, suggesting that at least astrocytes are not involved (the stain, GFAP, being selective for astrocytes and not all glia cells), perhaps supporting the early findings and suggestions of Kovelman and Scheibel that the changes represent developmental anomalies.

Some other recent neuropathological findings reported include decreased Purkinje cell density in the vermis and cerebellar hemi-spheres of treated patients (Jeste *et al.*, 1985), increased thickness of the corpus callosum (Bigelow *et al.*, 1983) and diminished neuronal density in some layers of frontal, cingulate and motor cortex (Benes, 1986).

NEUROPHYSIOLOGICAL AND NEUROLOGICAL DATA

EEG

Soon after the introduction of the electroencephalogram, reports of abnormalities in schizophrenia appeared. Hill (1950) reviewed these as follows: EEGs suggestive of epilepsy were most often seen in catatonia, although generalized non-paroxysmal dysrhythmias and other paroxysmal phenomena were also found. Since then, there have been many reports of EEG abnormalities in schizo-phrenic patients. In a comparison with patients suffering from affective disorder, Abrahams and Taylor (1979) noted that the proportion of EEG abnormalities was twice as great in the schizo-phrenics, who had more temporal abnormalities. Slow wave asym-metries, slow bursts, spikes or sharp waves were the recorded changes, and they tended to be more frequent on the left side. In patients with temporal lobe EEG changes this laterality was associ-ated with formal thought disorder and emotional blunting, but not first-rank symptoms. Although patients were on medications, this did not correlate with the EEG findings.

Hays (1977) divided schizophrenic patients into two groups, those with and those without a family history of psychosis. Abnor-mal EEGs were found in 64 per cent of the latter and 43 per cent of the former; in particular a frontal and temporal asymmetry was seen in those without family histories, the variant being more prominent on the left side.

Investigations of patients using electrodes implanted within the brain have clearly demonstrated abnormalities in schizophrenics, again notably within the limbic system. In a series of studies, Heath (1982) investigated 63 patients with psychosis, 38 being diagnosed as schizophrenic. Spiking was seen in the septal region. This is defined by Heath as an area bordered dorsally by the base of the anterior horn of the lateral ventricle and the head of the caudate nucleus, and ventrally by the free surface of the gyrus rectus of the frontal lobe. It includes septal nuclei, nucleus accumbens, olfactory tubercle and the diagonal band, as well as parts of the gyrus rectus. It has extensive frontal and temporal connections. The abnormalities occurred when, and only when, the patients were actively psychotic. In many cases changes were not observed on surface recordings, and neither were similar findings noted in chronic pain control patients. Violence and aggression were associated with hippocampal and amygdala discharges. Some patients showed activation in sensory relay nuclei in association with hallucinations (for example medial geniculate recordings), and often cerebellar discharges. Similar findings, especially with regards to the septal region, have been reported by others (Rickles, 1969).

Examination of the spectral power of EEG frequencies in schizophrenia reveals more fast beta activity, more theta and delta, and less alpha than normals (Itil, 1975). Psychotic children and those with a high risk for schizophrenia show a similar pattern of changes. Generally these patterns are 'normalized' by antipsychotic medication.

Fenton et al. (1980) noted the changes to be maximal over temporal derivations in acute schizophrenic patients, while chronic patients showed more diffuse slow wave power, notably theta and delta, diffusely or maximally frontoparietally (Kemali et al., 1981).

Stevens and Livermore (1982) used telemetred EEG recordings during psychotic behaviour of schizophrenic patients. They identified so-called 'ramp patterns', characterized by a monotonic decline in power from lowest to highest frequencies, which can be seen in epileptic patients during subcortical spike activity. These were seen only in recordings from schizophrenic patients in their sample, and not in controls. Patients with catatonic episodes showed them in the right temporal region, while 50 per cent of paranoid patients with auditory hallucinations had left-sided ramps, with increased slow activity. Psychotic events recorded clinically were associated with suppression of left temporal alpha frequencies.

Evoked potential studies in schizophrenia are numerous, and the results complicated to interpret. Several reviews are available (Shagass, 1972; Flor-Henry, 1983). Generally, evoked potentials show greater variability and amplitudes are decreased; a subgroup of patients show a 'reducing' pattern of decreasing amplitude with increasing stimulus intensity. Flor-Henry (1983) summarized a review by stating 'the evoked potential characteristics in schizophrenia consistently implicate the left hemisphere, and particularly the left temporal region' (p.215). The CNV also tends to be reduced, maximally over frontal areas.

There are three studies using BEAM in schizophrenia. Morihisa *et al.* (1983) examined patients with and without medication, and reported increased bilateral delta activity frontally and increased posterior beta frequencies, most marked in the left posterior quadrant. Interestingly, Morstyn *et al.* (1983) reported diminished P300 amplitudes in this same region in medicated, but acutely psychotic, patients, a combination of findings suggestive of irritability and hypofunction, similar to that noted in patients with epileptic foci (Morihisa *et al.*, 1983). Guenther and Breitling (1985), again in medicated patients, examined schizophrenics using a variety of motor activation tasks. They noted increased bifrontal delta and theta power, and widespread left hemisphere dysfunction during the tasks.

Radiological studies

There are over 30 studies of pneumoencephalography (PEG) and over 40 using CT scanning in the published literature, several reviews being readily available (Weinberger *et al.*, 1983; Nasrallah and Coffman, 1985; Crow and Johnstone, 1986a). Many of the PEG studies were uncontrolled, with poor characterization of the patient populations. Nevertheless, patients with schizophrenia were shown to display abnormalities, mainly ventricular dilatation, findings which have since been confirmed with well-controlled CT studies. One widely quoted investigation is that of Huber (1957), who reported that nearly 70 per cent of schizophrenic patients had ventricles above the normal size, noting in addition involvement of the third ventricle. Those with poor social adjustment had more abnormal indices. Another is the investigation of Haug (1962), whose blind evaluation comparing over a hundred schizophrenic patients to psychiatric non-psychotic controls showed the former to have more ventricular enlargement and cortical atrophy, the abnormalities correlating with the degree of clinical deterioration.

The first of the CT studies was that of Johnstone *et al.* (1976). They reported ventricular enlargement in seventeen chronic patients, age and premorbid occupation matched with the controls, the enlargement correlating with symptoms such as flattening of affect, poverty of speech and cognitive impairment. Weinberger *et al.* (1979) also reported ventricular enlargement or cortical atrophy in a larger sample of patients, all under 50 years old. This did not correlate with length of hospitalization or duration of illness. Changes affected some two-thirds of patients.

These ventricular abnormalities have now been shown to occur in early onset cases (Turner *et al.*, 1986) and in teenage patients with schizophrenia or schizophrenia spectrum disorder (Schulz *et al.*, 1983).

Patients with evidence suggestive of cerebral atrophy have been shown to have a poorer premorbid adjustment (Weinberger and Wyatt, 1980); to show a poorer response to therapy (Weinberger and Wyatt, 1980; Luchins *et al.*, 1984); to display more minor neurological signs; have abnormal EEGs and show more deviant smooth eye pursuit tracking (Weinberger *et al.*, 1983; Pandurangi *et al.*, 1986). The early findings of a correlation of atrophy, ventricular or sulcal to more negative symptoms and cognitive decline has been replicated in many studies (Crow and Johnstone, 1986a). Further, such patients are more likely to display involuntary movements, are more at risk for a suicide attempt (Levy *et al.*, 1984) and are less often reported to display hallucinations or delusions as a prominent feature of their psychopathology, patients with such symptoms, including paranoia, tending to have a smaller ventricular size.

Others have reported on the presence of third and fourth ventricular atrophy (Pandurangi *et al.*, 1984) and cerebellar atrophy (Weinberger *et al.*, 1979).

Family and twin studies have also been carried out. De Lisi *et al.* (1986) reported that schizophrenic patients show larger ventricles than their well sibs and those with larger ventricular–brain ratios (VBRs) had more head injuries and birth complications, although they suggested, in addition, an independent familial effect. These data are in keeping with the twin studies reported by Reveley *et al.*

(1982), showing that while healthy MZ twins have a higher concordance for ventricular size than DZ twins, when one of the MZ twins has schizophrenia, the discordant one of the pair still has a greater ventricular size than healthy controls, but nonetheless smaller than the affected twin. Reveley *et al.* (1982) speculate that where genetic predisposition is low more environmental insults are required to precipitate the illness; hence the ventricular enlargement tends to occur in those with a low genetic component. However, not all data are concordant with this view (Farmer *et al.*, 1985).

There have been a few negative studies of CT scanning in schizophrenia (for example Jernigan *et al.*, 1982), but perhaps no more than may be expected by chance. However, these studies may also reflect the fact that only a proportion of patients show these findings, and mean values from large samples may obscure the existence of affected subgroups.

One finding that has not been replicated is the suggestion that schizophrenic patients without brain atrophy have reversed brain asymmetries when compared to controls (in normal brain scans, the right frontal and left occipital lobes are wider than their corresponding measurements in the alternative hemisphere) (Luchins *et al.*, 1979).

The relationship to dopamine abnormalities has been examined. Kleinman *et al.* (1982b) reported that the inverse relationship they note between plasma prolactin and psychotic symptoms was only seen for patients who had normal ventricular size. Others have noted a decreased CSF–HVA in those with cortical atrophy or enlarged ventricles (van Kammen *et al.*, 1983).

Follow-up studies suggest that the ventricular enlargement is stable over time, although a proportion of patients (in one study, 40 per cent) tend to show an increase in size (Nasrallah *et al.*, 1986a).

Assessment of brain densities, using CT scans, reveals decreases in both hemispheres, especially in the left frontal region (Golden *et al.*, 1980), confirmed on separate samples (Coffman *et al.*, 1984), and in recent twin studies. Reveley and Reveley (1986) examined eleven pairs of identical twins discordant for schizophrenia and age matched volunteer MZ twins. The schizophrenic twin of the MZ discordant pair had significantly lower left compared with right hemisphere absorption densities than their well co-twins and normal controls. Others report increased densities in the thalamus and caudate nucleus (Dewan *et al.*, 1983) and lower values in the white matter of the left hemisphere (Largen *et al.*, 1984).

Summarizing these data it would seem that most studies, with few exceptions, note that a substantial proportion of patients diagnosed as schizophrenic have evidence of either enlarged ventricles or of dilated cerebral cortical sulci. Some studies separate these two findings as possibly being related to different processes. Some of the clinical features that have been associated with ventricular enlargement are shown in Table 7.

Twin studies support the association between ventricular enlargement and a diagnosis of schizophrenia, the present evidence hinting at interactions between genetic predispositions and environmental insults to explain the findings.

Other abnormalities reported in CT studies include third and fourth ventricular enlargement and cerebellar abnormalities. It should further be noted that several studies of psychotic patients using CT scanning indicate the relative frequency of findings of unsuspected abnormalities, including infarctions, meningiomas, cysts and in particular aqueduct stenosis (Owens *et al.*, 1980; Reveley and Reveley, 1983).

The data do not support the hypothesis that the changes are secondary either to institutionalization or to treatment, and abnormalities are reported in patients who are of early onset and in some cases free of treatment. The importance of the findings, in addition to their clinical relevance, is the obvious support they give to the conclusion that schizophrenia is the outcome of abnormal cerebral pathology, now demonstrable in some cases in vivo.

Recently MRI data in schizophrenia have been reported. Although one early study using blind assessment of scans did not

Table 7 Some features of ventricular enlargement of schizophrenia

---

Early brian damage or birth complication
Poorer premorbid adjustment
More negative symptoms
Less positive symptoms
Cognitive decline
Poorer response to treatment
More minor neurological signs
Decreased CSF–HVA

---

note changes in periventricular appearances with spin echo sequences (Johnstone *et al.*, 1986a), other findings have been more positive. Andreasen *et al.* (1986) reported smaller cranial size and frontal lobes in schizophrenic patients, even when controlled for sex and height. In general, patients with small frontal lobe size or decreased cerebral size had more negative symptoms, although these did not relate to performance on a number of psychological tests including the Wisconsin card sorting test.

Three groups have reported an increase in size of the corpus callosum (Mathew *et al.*, 1985; Nasrallah *et al.*, 1986b; Guenther *et al.*, 1986), even in unmedicated patients, while others note increased width of the fourth ventricle and cortical atrophy (Kojima *et al.*, 1986) and longer septa pellucida (Mathew *et al.*, 1985). Using assessments of proton spin times, increased inversion recovery values have been reported in the white and grey matter anteriorly, and also in the temporal lobes (Smith *et al.*, 1985). Besson *et al.* (1987) reported patients with high negative symptom scores to have increased T1 values in the putamen–globus pallidus and in the left frontal white matter compared with those with low scores, while patients with high positive symptom scores showed increased T1 values in left medial temporal structures compared with those with low scores. However, in this investigation, no overall differences were found between schizophrenic patients and controls. Patients with tardive dyskinesia were shown to have significantly higher T1 values in the basal ganglia than patients without the motor disorder or normal controls. These preliminary data would support the already reviewed findings suggestive of frontal and limbic pathology in patients with schizophrenia.

CBF and PET studies

Ingvar and Franzen (1974) reported that schizophrenic patients have normal mean hemisphere blood flows, but demonstrated a shift in distribution such that higher levels were less common in frontal structures and more common in postcentral structures when compared with controls. This 'hypofrontality' has become an area of controversy with the further investigation of patients using these techniques. However, even in this original investigation, many of the patients had normal distributions, and the hypofrontality was noted more in elder and deteriorated patients.

Several groups have examined regional CBF using the xenon inhalation method. Mathew *et al.* (1982a) reported schizophrenic patients, the majority of whom were medicated or had only one week of treatment washout, to show reduced CBF in both hemispheres in most brain regions. No differences were noted between medicated and unmedicated, chronic and subchronic, and paranoid and non-paranoid patients. Using the Brief Psychiatric Rating Scale, hallucinations correlated inversely with left parietal, left frontal, right temporoparietal and right occipital blood flow. They were unable to demonstrate a hypofrontal pattern.

Ariel *et al.* (1983), again in mainly medicated patients, also noted low values in all brain regions, with relatively greater reduced grey matter CBF values in the anterior regions of the brain.

A number of authors have attempted to activate the brain with various tasks during CBF studies. Franzen and Ingvar (1975) reported left hemisphere activity following such tasks as the Ravens progressive matrices and noted diminished activation of frontal structures in chronic schizophrenic patients. Gur *et al.* (1983a, 1983b), in medicated patients, assessed cerebral activity during verbal and spatial tasks. No hypofrontality was seen, but schizophrenic patients, unlike controls, showed no changes in hemisphere activation during the verbal task, and a greater increase than expected in left hemisphere activity when carrying out the spatial task. Further investigations on unmedicated patients (Gur *et al.*, 1985) showed higher resting left hemisphere flow. Further, more severely affected patients showed decreases of anterior left hemisphere activity during spatial tasks, a pattern rarely found in normals. Their data, they suggested, supported a hypothesis of left hemisphere overactivation in schizophrenia, and the differences between medicated and unmedicated patients suggested that medication helps restore symmetrical blood flow, the main affect being on the left hemisphere.

Weinberger *et al.* (1986) have specifically tested frontal lobe function by administering patients the Wisconsin card sorting task during xenon-133 inhalation. Controlled cognitive tasks, such as a number-matching test, were also used, patients being drug free for a minimum of four weeks. During the number-matching task no differences were noted between patients and controls, but with the frontal lobe task, the clear increases seen in controls were not seen in frontal regions in the schizophrenic patients. The changes were regionally specific, in particular involving the dorsolateral aspect of the prefrontal association cortex. These data, they suggested, indicated that patients with schizophrenia have a specific physio-logical dysfunction of prefrontal cortex. Since, in later studies (Berman *et al.*, 1986), similar results were obtained in patients on medication, and further that schizophrenic patients and controls did not differ on a continuous performance task with regards to CBF, the abnormalities recorded were thought to be independent of medication status and state factors such as attention and mental effort.

The majority of studies of schizophrenia using PET have used the deoxyglucose technique, although one (Sheppard *et al.*, 1983) has reported oxygen-15 data (see Trimble, 1985a; Trimble, 1986a). Hypofrontality has been noted by several groups, although this is not a universal finding, particularly in acute onset medica-tion-free patients (Sheppard *et al.*, 1983). In those studies showing hypofrontality, overlap with normal values is seen, some 30–40 per cent of patients showing the hypofrontal pattern. The hypofrontality does not appear to correlate with ventricular dilata-tion on the CT scan, and is increased by neuroleptic medication (De Lisi and Buchsbaum, 1986). Analysing correlations (coupling patterns) between different regions of interest within the brain, Clarke *et al.* (1984), using patients and controls receiving sensory stimulation, noted different patterns in patients with schizo-phrenia, in particular reporting a paucity of frontal lobe coupling. Also examining patterns of cerebral activity, Volkow *et al.* (1985) reported that schizophrenic patients show high subcortical/low frontal values, normals showing the opposite pattern. Finally, Bustany *et al.* (1985) reported decreased local protein synthesis rates when examining methionine metabolism in hebephrenic schizophrenic patients, involving in particular the frontal lobes.

Evaluation of PET data is difficult at the present time, owing to the limitations of the methodology and the multiple sources of artefact that may occur. Thus, different groups have used different patient populations in different phases of illness and treatment, with different clinical patterns at the time of scanning. Most of the data using glucose has been in patients who are hardly drug free. Since treatment itself increases hypofrontality and as groups that have examined drug-free patients with relatively recent onset ill-ness failed to confirm hypofrontality, the possibility that it may be related to medication cannot be discounted from these studies alone. Nonetheless, they are in keeping with some of the cerebral blood flow studies reported above.

Interestingly, there is more conformity of data with regards to basal ganglia findings in psychotic patients, high values, especially as a ratio to cortical values, being noted by several groups (see Volkow *et al.*, 1985; Gur, 1986), although not all data are in conformity with this (Trimble, 1985a). Using SPECT, Crawley *et al.* (1986) have recently reported increased spiperone binding rates of striatum–cerebellar ratios in schizophrenics free from neuroleptics for at least six months. Wong *et al.* (1986), using radio-labelled spiperone, reported increased D2 receptor densities in the caudate nucleus in schizophrenic patients, even in a group of ten neuroleptic naive patients. Increased values in basal ganglia regions following neuroleptic treatment are reported from several PET studies (De Lisi and Buchsbaum, 1986; Gur, 1986). These data are in keeping with the known high dopamine content of these regions of the brain and their possible abnormalities in patients with psychosis.

The viral hypothesis

As noted in Chapter 6, the possibility that viral infections of the limbic system may be associated with some cases of psychosis has had a long history. There are several reasons to search for viruses, including the known excess of winter births in schizophrenia (Fuller Torrey *et al.*, 1977), the schizophrenia-like presentations of some patients with known encephalitis, the discovery of slow viruses which affect the nervous system, but whose effects are delayed for many years (Fuller Torrey and Peterson, 1973), and the reporting by some authors of evidence for viral activity in schizophrenic patients. Tyrrell *et al.* (1979) reported that CSF from 13 of 38 patients with schizophrenia produced a cytopathic effect on human embryonic fibroblast cultures, the presumed agent being prevented by 50 nm filters. Similar effects were seen in patients with miscellaneous neurological conditions. Innoculation of CSF from patients with schizophrenia intracerebrally into animals has been reported to be associated with some behaviour changes over a period of two to two and a half years, mainly in activity levels in marmosets (Baker *et al.*, 1983).

A second line of evidence has been to examine serum and CSF for abnormal antibody titres, or to seek evidence of impaired immunological function in schizophrenic patients. Scattered early reports of decreased delayed hypersensitivity, prior to the introduction of neuroleptic drugs, are of interest, implying possible immunological dysfunction which cannot be attributed to these agents (De Lisi, 1984). Estimations of lymphocyte characteristics, including the percentages of B and T cells, have produced variable data, as has the quantitative assessment of various immunoglobulin classes. Oligoclonal IgG bands appear normal (Roos *et al.*, 1985). Reports of raised cytomegalovirus antibody levels in CSF in up to 70 per cent of patients (Albrecht *et al.*, 1980) have not consistently been replicated (Shrikhande *et al.*, 1985) and postmortem brain studies using staining for these viruses have also been negative (Stevens *et al.*, 1984).

There is thus minimal evidence that viral illness is aetiologically related to schizophrenia, and the variable findings, in particular the abnormal features of the immunological system, may reflect immunosuppression related to medications. However, viral encephalitis cannot be ruled out as the responsible factor in a subgroup of cases. Crow (1984), following review of the evidence, has attempted to account for the season of birth effect, the genetic factor, the late age of onset of the disease and a viral aetiology by suggesting that retroviruses may be involved. These incorporate their genetic material into the host, altering the expression of the host genome, which may then be passed on to the next generation, the inheritance acquiring Mendelian characteristics.

Associations with neurological disease

The most comprehensive survey of the relationship of schizophrenia-like psychoses to neurological conditions is that of Davison and Bagley (1969). It has already been pointed out (Chapter 6) that a variety of pathologies that affect the limbic system may lead to a disorder with a phenomenological appearance of a schizophreniform psychosis, the most convincing data so far being collected for epilepsy, in particular temporal lobe epilepsy. These data are discussed in Chapter 10.

Table 8 (Davison and Bagley, 1969) lists the neurological conditions that have been associated with a schizophreniform psychosis, giving the expected number and the actual number in the published literature. Taken from Davison and Bagley's review, it indicates a higher than expected frequency, in particular for Huntington's chorea, narcolepsy, cerebrovascular disease, cerebral gliomas and pituitary adenomas. A lower than expected incidence occurs with Parkinson's disease and multiple sclerosis.

Table 8 **Comparison of the relative proportion of CNS disorders with psychosis in the 1958–67 literature and their prevalence in the general population** (from Davison and Bagley, 1969, p.149)

CNS disorder	Prevalence in general population (per 100 000)[a]	Distribution of psychotic cases in 1958–67 literature	
		Expected number	Actual number
Trauma	—	—	532
Epilepsy	548	211	276
Huntington's chorea	4	2	86[b]
Cerebrovascular disease	450	173	42[b]
Parkinsonism	114	44	20[b]
Narcolepsy	—	—	19[b]
Choreoathetosis	—	—	19[b]
Cerebral glioma	8.3	3	19[b]
Benign cerebral tumour	30	12	17
Pituitary adenoma	5.4	2	17[b]
Postmeningitis/encephalitis	—	—	16
Multiple sclerosis	80	30	11[b]
Congenital disorders	—	—	8
General paresis	24	9	5
Hepatic encephalopathy	—	—	5
Wilson's disease	—	—	4
Cerebellar degeneration	7	3	3
Other cerebral degeneration	—	—	3
Cerebral lipoidosis	—	—	3
Hypoglycaemia	—	—	3
Motor neurone disease	11	4	2
Cerebral reticulosis	—	—	2
Torsion spasm	—	—	2
Leber's optic atrophy	—	—	1
Phenylketonuria	—	—	1
Schilder's disease	—	—	1
Friedreich's ataxia	—	—	1
Myotonia congenita	—	—	1

[a]Prevalence figures taken from Brewis, Posanzer, Rolland and Miller (1966).
[b]Indicates probable significant difference.

The conclusion with regards to tumours has already been discussed (p.158), in particular temporal lobe and diencephalic locations being emphasized. Survey of the world literature on psychiatric symptomatology in Huntington's chorea reveals an excess of schizophrenia-like and paranoid conditions, the psychopathology often emerging before the onset of the movement disorder (Trimble, 1981a). It is of interest that this condition is associated with relative overactivity of dopamine function, in contrast to Parkinson's disease, in which the incidence of psychosis is said to be rare, unless provoked by dopaminergic medications such as L-dopa or bromocriptine. The other basal ganglia condition which has been associated with a schizophreniform psychosis is Wilson's disease, the main pathological findings in this condition being multilobular cirrhosis of the liver and cerebral changes maximal in the putamen, caudate nucleus and globus pallidus. Sydenham's chorea and idiopathic basal ganglia calcification (Cummings, 1985) are also sporadically reported to be associated with a schizophreniform psychosis.

The association with narcolepsy is difficult to interpret in view of the widespread use of amphetamine in treatment, although Davison and Bagley (1969) prefer the hypothesis that the psychosis and the narcoleptic syndrome are both manifestations of diencephalic dysfunction.

The decreased association between cerebrovascular disorders and demyelinating disorders and a schizophreniform illness requires further comment. In contrast to some of the other conditions mentioned, multiple sclerosis is a white matter disease affecting in particular periventricular structures, and its psychopathology, which includes emotional lability, affective disorder and a characteristic euphoria (Trimble, 1981a), is markedly different. As emphasized in Chapter 6, it is only occasionally that cerebrovascular accidents are associated with psychosis, which may be related to the sudden onset of the condition in contrast to some of the other pathologies discussed here in which CNS changes develop more slowly.

Davison and Bagley (1969) in particular emphasized diencephalic, brainstem and temporal lobe locations of pathology, and they note that in the majority of cases the onset of the psychosis occurs several years after the onset of the CNS disorder. The shortest interval is seen with brainstem lesions (Davison, 1966). They pointed out that the frequency of premorbid schizoid personalities and family history of schizophrenia is significantly lower in patients who have psychopathology associated with neurological disorders and stressed the similarity of the phenomenological presentations to schizophrenia.

There is an additional literature emphasizing neurological impairments and signs which may be found in patients at risk for schizophrenia or those with the condition. Offspring of schizophrenic parents, thus representing a high-risk group for the later development of the disorder, have an increased number of pregnancy and birth complications. The high-risk subjects who have a psychiatric breakdown have the greatest number of such complications, and show abnormal electrodermal galvanic skin responses with shorter latency, slower habituation and greater resistance to extinction (Parnas et al., 1981). Further, infants at risk for schizophrenia show increased evidence of neurological dysfunction with neurological soft signs, poor motor coordination and perceptual deficits (Marcus et al., 1985). Schizophrenic patients have lower birth weights than expected (Parnas et al., 1981), and cerebral dysfunction, as shown by neurological signs, EEG abnormalities or a history of seizures, are overreported in patients with infantile psychosis (Kolvin et al., 1971).

Patients diagnosed as schizophrenic frequently show neurological abnormalities on routine testing. These affect up to 60 per cent of patients and cannot be solely ascribed to medication or undiagnosed neurological illness (Woods and Short, 1985); they may also be detected in a high proportion of relatives (Kinney et al., 1986). Potential frontal lobe signs, such as the grasp and palmomental reflexes, and perseveration are especially reported (Cox and Ludwig, 1979), while Fuller Torrey (1980) reported abnormal face–hand tests (particularly pronounced in the right hand, suggesting left hemisphere involvement) and graphaesthesia. Minor motor and sensory disturbances, more recognizable choreoathetotic, dystonic and tic-like presentations, gait disturbances, difficulties with coordination and smooth performance of motor activities, reflex changes (increased or decreased) and the presence of infantile reflexes such as the grasp reflex and the palmomental reflexes, mirror movements and variable Babinski responses have all been reported (Quitkin et al., 1976; Keshavan et al., 1979; Tucker and Silberfarb, 1978; Claude and Bourguinon, 1927). These have an inverse relationship to IQ levels (Quitkin et al., 1976), but no apparent association to prognosis.

In a recent comprehensive examination, Manschreck and Ames (1984) assessed neurological and psychopathological features of 53 schizophrenic patients in comparison with affective disorder patients and normal controls. Neurological (motor and sensory) disturbances were seen in 92 per cent of the schizophrenic sub-jects, in comparison with 52 per cent of the affectives and 5 per cent of the normal controls. Motor testing was particularly affected, and right-sided sensory errors were more common in the schizophrenic group. Thought disorder correlated with neurologi-cal abnormalities, in particular motor changes and right-sided grapaesthesia. Further, schizophrenic patients were more inclined to be left handed (a variable finding in other studies; Gur, 1977). In a further investigation of disturbed voluntary motor behaviour in schizophrenia, Manschreck *et al.* (1982) used tests to elicit motor disorders, and examined their relationship to neuroleptic intake, neurological soft signs and features of the schizophrenia. They reported disturbed motor activity in 97 per cent of the schizo-phrenics, in particular clumsiness and a postural disturbance, although stereotypic and manneristic movements, and motor blocking were also common. Elicited motor movement distur-bances detected, for example, by the Luria fist/edge/palm test were also seen in 92 per cent. The role of antipsychotic medication appeared to be to reduce these abnormalities, and medicated schizophrenics showed significantly more impairments than medi-cated affective disorder patients. The authors made the point that many of these motor disturbances may be missed if not carefully looked for, and they cannot solely be ascribed to treatment with neuroleptic drugs.

Abnormalities of eye blinking (Stevens, 1978), either decreased, increased or episodic rapid paroxysms of blinking, have been noted, in schizophrenia, the paroxysms being associated with psychotic episodes. Disturbed eye tracking, including abnormal smooth pursuit eye movements and saccadic eye movements, are also reported. These movements are made as the fovea tracks a moving object. Saccades are fast but ballistic movements that bring the fovea and the target together, while the smooth pursuit eye movements are responsible for fixation of slower moving targets, thus being continuous with the fovea sited on the target. Saccadic movements can be voluntarily executed, whereas smooth pursuit movements require stimulus activation and are maintained by attention to the target. Up to 85 per cent of schizophrenic patients are reported to show abnormal smooth pursuit tracking, similar abnormalities being noted in 34 per cent of relatives (Holz-man *et al.*, 1984). It does not appear to be related to inattention, motivation, or drug effects, and higher concordance for the abnormality is shown for MZ as opposed to DZ twins. Saccadic abnormalities have also been described in schizophrenia (Mialet and Pichot, 1981).

Neuropsychological disturbances in schizophrenia

That patients with schizophrenia have altered neuropsychological performance on a variety of tests has been known for many years and reviewed by several authors (Flor-Henry, 1983; Rogers, 1986). In general, all who have looked for it have noted intellectual decline of some sort in schizophrenic patients, reflecting Kraepelin's (1919) summary that profound dementia occurs in 75 per cent of patients with hebephrenia and 59 per cent of those with catatonia. The Halstead–Reitan test battery, designed to identify patients with brain damage, fails to discriminate between schizophrenic patients and those with known neurological damage (Heaton and Crowley, 1981), and decrements are more likely to be found in those with longer hospitalizations and chronic illness (Goldstein and Halperin, 1977). The decline does not appear to be related to neuroleptic medication; in fact cognitive testing is often seen to improve in patients receiving these drugs (Heaton and Crowley, 1981). Patients with simple schizophrenia show the most markedly dilapidated cognition while those with a delusional form of the disorder may be least impaired (Robertson and Taylor, 1985). Schizophrenic patients demonstrate average reading and spelling abilities in the setting of lower IQ and memory scores, the former tasks reflecting premorbid ability; similar patterns are noted in the dementias (Dalby and Williams, 1986).

Crow and colleagues (Stevens *et al.*, 1978) have drawn attention to age disorientation in chronic schizophrenic patients, affecting approximately 25 per cent, in which they usually underestimate their age. Those with this are more likely to have had a younger first admission to hospital and a longer duration of stay. This same group (Johnstone *et al.*, 1978) have drawn attention to the 'dementia' of dementia praecox. They thus note that there appears to be a subgroup of patients with schizophrenia who not only show intellectual impairment but on CT scan demonstrate evidence of structural brain damage. These patients often display 'negative features' such as poverty of speech, retardation and affective changes, while patients with 'positive features' such as hallucinations, delusions and thought disorder are less likely to show a cognitive decline.

Laterality effects have also been examined. Schizophrenic patients perform abnormally on tests of aphasia. On a battery of neuropsychological tasks including subsets from the Halstead–Reitan and the Luria–Nebraska batteries, schizophrenic patients (the majority drug free) not only displayed marked impairments but had maximal abnormalities on tests related to frontotemporal functions bilaterally (Taylor and Abrams, 1984). In a more comprehensive evaluation, Flor-Henry (1983) compared large numbers of schizophrenic and affective disorder patients and noted asymmetric frontotemporal dysfunction, the left side being more impaired than the right in the schizophrenic sample. When an analysis of covariance was carried out, looking at depression, mania, schizophrenia and control patients, a continuum of increasing cerebral disorganization was seen, depression showing minimal changes, while in schizophrenia it was maximal.

SOME OUTSTANDING ISSUES

The evidence reviewed clearly indicates a significant genetic contribution towards the development of schizophrenia. A reluctance to accept this may well be because it harks back to an earlier generation which emphasized hereditary degeneration as a cause of many neuropsychiatric conditions. These earlier studies were founded on clinical impressions of highly selected cases, while modern research has attempted to dissect out the genetic variables in very precise ways. However, it is clear that the genetic contribution to schizophrenia, while being similar to some other medical conditions, does not explain all the variance, and environmental variables have been persistently sought.

Further, the consensus that what is inherited is a schizophrenia spectrum, as opposed to schizophrenia per se, has gained ground, and certain biological markers, for example platelet MAO activity or dysfunction of eye movements, may reflect upon an underlying genetically determined biochemical propensity to develop psychosis under the right conditions.

With regards to environmental agents, there is evidence that some schizophrenic patients demonstrate increased early brain damage, either through perinatal or uterine insults, which has led to discussion of the interaction between the genetic and epigenetic variables. Murray et al. (1985) advocate it would be useful to divide schizophrenia into familial and sporadic cases. The sporadic cases are thus associated with increased ventricular size as shown on the

CT scan and environmental traumas reflective of perinatal damage or early head injury. The genetic predisposition, if strong, will promote the disorder, while, in the presence of a lesser genetic vulnerability, environmental insult becomes necessary for the full expression of the illness. Where there is no genetic vulnerability, as in, for example, some cases of epilepsy, the cerebral pathology itself directly provokes the schizophrenic symptoms. This is put forward as a continuum model implying interaction between genetic and environmental factors. This and other data reviewed in this chapter would suggest two different forms of the condition, as shown in Table 9. This scheme is of course only illustrative of possible extremes, many cases not falling neatly into one or other group.

Alternative environmental insults have been sought, in particular neurological conditions, head injury or infection, for example with viruses. The emphasis from CNS disorders is on those which affect temporal lobe, basal ganglia and diencephalic dysfunction. Temporal lobe disorders, in particular such conditions as limbic system epilepsy, seem to be more associated with hallucinations (particularly of the Schneiderian type; see Chapter 10) while basal ganglia disorders lead more to disturbances of motoric activity.

Table 9   Two types of schizophrenia

Factors	Type II	Type I
Genetic contribution	Minimal	Maximal
Symptomatology	Negative symptoms	Positive symptoms
EEG	Abnormal	Normal
CT	Atrophy	No atrophy
Intellectual impairment	Present	Absent
Platelet MAO	—	Low
CSF–HVA	Low	Low
Response to neuroleptic drugs	Poor	Good
Associated features	Abnormal involuntary movements (soft neurology)	—
Postulated pathology	Structural brain changes	—
Postulated neurochemistry	Decreased CCK	Increased DA receptors

The pathological studies reviewed reinforce this neuroanatomical distinction, emphasizing medial temporal structures in association with hallucinations, paranoia and thought disorder, and the globus pallidus with negativism and catalepsy. Such findings emphasize the 'anatomy of schizophrenia' (Stevens, 1973) to be predominantly related to subcortical structures, particularly those of the limbic system and the related basal ganglia.

Other authors have drawn attention to the likeness of some schizophrenic symptoms to frontal lobe disorders. In particular this involves the dorsolateral prefrontal cortex, and the symptoms include those seen following frontal injury, such as affective changes, impaired motivation, poor insight and other 'defect' symptoms frequently seen in schizophrenia. Indeed, the evidence for frontal lobe dysfunction in schizophrenic patients is clear, and has been noted not only in the neuropathological studies, but also in EEG, BEAM and evoked potential data, in neuropsychological studies, in testing for soft neurological signs, and more recently using the imaging techniques such as PET and MRI. The blood flow studies clearly show decreased activation in schizophrenic patients on selected frontal lobe cognitive tasks.

The evidence for two distinct syndromes in schizophrenia has been pursued by Crow and colleagues (Crow, 1980). The suggestion is that there is both a neurochemical and neuropathological contribution to schizophrenia, with two syndromes. Thus (see Table 9), type I syndrome (equivalent to acute schizophrenia) is characterized by positive symptoms (delusions, hallucinations and thought disorder) and is related to change in dopaminergic transmission. The type II syndrome (equivalent to the defect state) is characterized by negative symptoms (affective flattening and poverty of speech) and is associated with intellectual impairment and structural changes in the brain. Further, abnormal involuntary movements (Owens et al., 1985) and decreased CCK in the temporal cortex (Ferrier et al., 1984a) have become suggested associated features.

There is certainly considerable evidence that structural changes are likely to be found in some schizophrenic brains and that cerebral atrophy on the whole is related to more negative symptoms. Positive symptoms, in particular first-rank symptoms of Schneider, have been related to abnormal dopaminergic transmission, and the evidence for the dopamine hypothesis has been reviewed in some sections above (see Table 2). Patients with positive symptoms show increased growth hormone responses to apomorphine, decreased baseline prolactin, low CSF–HVA accumulation, minimal heritability (first-rank symptoms) and tend not to have cerebral atrophy. Further, the pathological data reviewed suggests that temporal lobe including parahippocampal gyrus abnormalities may be more related to such symptoms. These data certainly support a relationship between positive symptoms, relatively normal brain structure, abnormalities of dopamine and possibly temporal lobe dysfunction.

In contrast, negative symptoms appear more related to periventricular abnormalities, cerebral atrophy, environmental insults and are less related to dopamine dysfunction. Experimental support for defining two subtypes has derived from intercorrelations of patients symptoms, which indicate generally that positive symptoms correlate positively, as do negative symptoms, although the internal consistency is much greater for negative symptoms (Andreasen and Olsen, 1982).

The contribution of abnormalities of dopamine to schizophrenia has been persistently argued. It is well known that the antipsychotic effects of neuroleptic drugs are not confined to schizophrenia, and they ameliorate psychotic symptoms in mania and acute organic brain syndromes. Further, because such medication alleviates some symptoms of schizophrenia, it does not mean that dopamine itself has the primary role in pathogenesis. While it has been indicated that the dopamine blocking effect of these drugs is the most important for helping the psychosis, it should be remembered that anticholinergic drugs alleviate the symptoms of Parkinson's disease, although the primary pathology in that condition relates to dopamine and not acetylcholine. Other neurochemical hypotheses have obviously been entertained, and as noted involve serotonergic, other catecholaminergic and peptidergic abnormalities. Mackay (1980) has argued that a chronic dopamine deficit is related to schizophrenia, rather than overactivity, highlighting the reported low CSF–HVA levels. This reduced dopamine turnover leads not only to reduced presynaptic dopamine accumulation, but also to a compensatory postsynaptic dopamine receptor proliferation. In his theory, both positive and negative symptoms thus relate to a defect of dopaminergic function, the positive symptoms emerging as a result of a switch from a deficit to an increase in presynaptic release of dopamine, the latter interacting with the excessive number of postsynaptic dopamine receptors and leading to the florid positive symptoms.

In contrast, for Crow, type I and type II syndromes represent different dimensions of pathology, although he does not suggest that they constitute separate disease states. Kety (1980) emphasized the error of referring to acute psychoses as schizophrenia, appealing for a restriction of the term to its original concept of a chronic disorder with an insidious onset. This would correlate more closely with Crow's type II or classical Kraepelinian schizophrenia. This in particular emphasizes the longitudinal course of the condition in many cases, the latter being directed by the underlying, possibly progressive, structural pathology now demonstrated by various methods already noted.

The search for virus infections continues, but to date has not been rewarding. However, one importance of the infective theory relates to some historical considerations of schizophrenia. Thus, it has been suggested that schizophrenia was uncommon in the medical literature prior to the nineteenth century, implying, rather like AIDS encephalitis, that it may have been a new disease, and an environmental agent, such as a virus, must have become prevalent around that time. The alternative is that it is an old condition, which has been ubiquitous and always present. The problem then is to explain its persistence in view of the low fecundity of schizophrenic patients (Hare, 1979).

Finally, substantial evidence has been accumulated which suggests that at least in some forms of schizophrenia, the major disturbance is in the dominant hemisphere (see Table 10).

Because one of the cardinal features of schizophrenia is a disturbance of thought and language and the dominant hemisphere is known to be involved in modulating such activities, it is hardly surprising that the weight of evidence suggests that the dominant hemisphere is primarily involved. Wernicke's aphasia and schizaphasia may be confused clinically, and although schizophrenics do not show a classical aphasic syndrome, some authors, for example Kleist (1969), drew attention to the language disturbances in schizophrenic patients as reflecting left temporal lobe disturbance. While, as emphasized, other areas of pathology, in particular diencephalic, basal ganglia and frontal lobes, are also involved in schizophrenia, the role of the dominant hemisphere is of outstanding importance.

Table 10   Evidence for laterality in schizophrenia

Neurological examination	Increased abnormalities in right-side sensory testing; increased left handedness
Neuropsychology	Association with aphasia, impairment on tests of dominant hemisphere function
EEG	Dominant hemisphere abnormalities on routine testing, power spectra, with telemetry evoked potentials and BEAM studies
CT studies	Density changes
MRI studies	Especially positive symptoms
PET studies and CBF	Variable
Neurochemistry	Increased dopamine left amygdala
Neuropathology	Parahippocampal gyrus abnormalities
Neurology	Epilepsy and head injury studies

CHAPTER 9

Affective disorders

INTRODUCTION

A difficulty in reviewing the literature on affective disorders is the various classifications that have been used by investigators. Although for the present the DSM III seems likely to be influential, much biological information has been accumulated prior to its introduction, and in some areas the lack of consistency of results often reflects lack of similarity of patients. A recurring theme, already referred to, is the confusion between depression as an illness as opposed to a reaction or an ordinary state of misery. Lewis (1934) gave as a definition of the depressive state 'a condition in which the clinical picture is dominated by an unpleasant affect, not transitory, without evidence of schizophrenic disorder or organic disorder of the brain, and in which, moreover, the affective change appears primary. . .' (p.277). This concept, the essential criterion being the disturbance of mood, continues to be embodied in DSM III, the mood being referred to as a prolonged emotion (American Psychiatric Association, 1980, p.205). Episodes of more transient mood change or chronic minor changes of mood are referred to as dysthymic disorder, which replaces depressive neurosis, depressive personality and similar categories. The issue of 'reaction', which has so long pervaded this area, is not discussed.

As Lewis (1934, 1971) has pointed out, the endogenous–reactive dichotomy has had a long but unfruitful history. The concept of endogenicity was linked to that of degeneration, implying an hereditary deterioration and incurability. Its counterpart, exogenous, failed to account for purely psychological traumatic events, such terms as psychogenic, neurotic and reactive filling the void. He noted that these terminologies have a direct bearing on dualistic concepts and could only be justified if they denoted causal distinctions.

Anglo-American attempts to tackle this problem by statistical methods have failed to be conclusive. The results of such investigations are determined by the clinical data used, often in concordance with a priori hypotheses embodied in the choice of information entered into the analysis. Some studies demonstrate bimodality of symptoms, others do not (Kendell 1969), while life event studies fail to show that patients diagnosed as reactive have more antecedent events than those classified as endogenous (Paykel, 1974). In addition, it has yet to be demonstrated that life events cause depressive illness (Tennant *et al.*, 1981), symptom configuration in relation to life events relating more to intrinsic personality characteristics of patients than to the quantitative or qualitative properties of the life event (Uhlenhuth and Paykel, 1973).

Personality factors are rarely taken into account in the assessment of patients with depression. However, patients with premorbid neuroticism, assessed by the EPI, are more likely to have depressive symptoms, usually referred to as neurotic depression with associated anxiety, obsessionality, helplessness, irritability and initial insomnia (Paykel *et al.*, 1976). In one follow-up study of a hundred patients classified as neurotic depression, 24 showed a characterological tendency to react to normal stress with a depressed affect. Subsequent psychiatric illnesses suffered were quite heterogeneous, including one-third that went on to develop an endogenous pattern, reflecting on the fragility of neurotic depression as a diagnostic entity (Akiskal *et al.*, 1978).

Winokur (1985), whose own classification of depression distinguishes a primary (bipolar/unipolar) from a secondary depression, has recently given support for the concept of neurotic depression, citing positive criteria for its diagnosis. These include younger age, poorer response to treatment, family history of alcoholism and personality problems. These then are patients with lifelong personality disorders who recurrently display depressive symptoms, more often than not DSM III dysthymic disorder. They represent an entirely different problem from those in whom the depressive process is referred to as endogenous depression. As such, the latter is not a common disorder, and probably one of the most overdiagnosed conditions in clinical medicine.

Anxiety states are often confused with depression. While anxiety almost invariably accompanies depressive illness, and, particularly in chronic anxiety, a dysphoria or some depressive symptoms intervene, clear distinctions are desirable. Although there have been advocates for blurring the distinction between the two, including Lewis, and it is noted that in many patients, particularly in a primary care setting, an admixture of anxiety and depressive symptoms are found, the phenomenology, treatment, outcome and biological associations of the two are different (Roth, 1977). Again, failure to identify patients with a depressive illness can only confuse research data and obfuscate the results of therapeutic trials.

A more widely accepted distinction, adopted by the DSM III and originally made by Leonhard (1957), is that between unipolar and bipolar forms of affective illness. While the latter is readily identifiable, biological diferences between the two are emerging, and the failure to identify manic episodes in the patient's history may provide a further source of error.

In summary, there is still much confusion regarding the nosological status of subtypes of depressive illness, although the entity referred to as endogenous depression seems well recognized and more homogeneous than others. The DSM III has disbanded the concept of neurotic depression, the evidence for which emphasizes the importance of personality vulnerabilities for its expression, but confusion with the endogenous form still abounds in clinical practice and research. This confounds attempts to expose the biological substrates of the depressive process, and often leads to inappropriate treatments. This is not to say that patients with other forms of depressive symptoms do not require treatment, or are not meaningful subjects for research. In fact, so numerous are these patients, and so chronic often are their disorders, that more effective remedies for them urgently need to be sought, particularly psychotropic agents.

GENETICS

As with most other conditions reviewed in this book, the affective disorders have an important genetic component to their pathogenesis. This is particularly so for bipolar illness.

Family studies reveal that the risk for affective illness is increased severalfold in first-degree relatives of probands over that expected by chance (Gershon, 1983). Further, while bipolar patients often have relatives with unipolar illness, the converse is uncommon. Recent estimates, based on combined data from several studies, put the risk at 20 per cent for first-degree relatives of bipolar probands and 7 per cent for first-degree relatives of unipolar patients (McGuffin, 1984b).

Winokur (1982) has identified three types of unipolar illness based on familial patterns: familial pure depression disease (FPDD), with a family history of depression, depressive spectrum disease (DSD), with a familial history of alcholism or antisocial personality, and sporadic depressive disease (SDD), with negative family history.

The concept of a genetic spectrum for bipolar disorders emerges with the reporting of an increased frequency of schizoaffective disorder and cyclothymic personality in relatives of probands (Gershon, 1983). Studies of schizoaffective patients tend to show both affective illness and schizophrenia in the relatives (Angst *et al.*, 1979), greater for affective illness, and Perris (1974) reported that in cycloid psychosis an increased frequency of the same condition was seen in relatives.

Twin data give a concordance rate, by combining studies, of 69 per cent for monozygous and 13 per cent for DZ pairs (McGuffin, 1984b). Most of these investigations were carried out prior to the acceptance of the unipolar/bipolar distinction, but Bertelsen *et al.* (1977) calculated the pairwise concordance rates for MZ twins to be 0.43 for unipolar and 0.74 for bipolar illness, the corresponding figures for DZ pairs being 0.19 and 0.17. The concordance was particularly noted for females, and the differences between the unipolar and bipolar rates were significant, supporting the familial data that the bipolar form carries the greatest heritability.

Price (1968) reported 67 per cent concordance in twelve pairs of MZ twins raised apart. This and the adoption study of Mendlewicz and Rainer (1977), in which the rate of affective illness was significantly greater in biological (28 per cent) as opposed to adoptive (7 per cent) parents of probands separated in early life, further support the genetic contribution to the illnesses.

A single autosomal dominant gene with reduced penetrance and variable expressivity was supported by Slater (Slater and Roth, 1969), while others have suggested X-linked (Winokur and Tanna, 1969) and multifactorial models, implying underlying quantitative liability to an affective disorder, being greater for bipolar illness (Gershon, 1983). The X-linked hypothesis seems unlikely, in that father–son transmission of affective disorder is frequently seen, although it received initial support from linkage studies with colour blindness and glucose-6-phosphate dehydrogenase deficiency (Mendlewicz *et al.*, 1980), known to be sex linked. These data have not been consistently replicated (Gershon, 1983). Recently studies using restriction fragment length polymorphisms have suggested that genes on chromosome 11 are closely linked to a locus conferring a strong predispositon for bipolar illness (Egeland *et al.*,

1987), although this is not confirmed in other studies. HLA studies have been inconsistent.

SOMATIC VARIABLES

Kretchmer's pyknic body build, corresponding to Sheldon's endomorphy, was reported to be associated with both the cyclothymic temperament and affective psychoses, although the relevance of this is unclear. Some patients, particularly those with bipolar illness, show muscle endplate abnormalities as reported in schizophrenia (Crayton and Meltzer, 1976).

METABOLIC AND BIOCHEMICAL FINDINGS

Early metabolic studies found abnormalities of electrolyte distribution in affective disorder. In particular, retention of sodium intracellularly (including bone) during depressive episodes (Coppen and Shaw, 1963), with increased loss during recovery. In mania even more marked changes were reported (Coppen et al., 1965). Some interpreted these data as a reflection of dietary changes consequent to the change of mood. No evidence has shown that the brain is also involved, or that the changes somehow lead to an alteration of cell membrane excitability.

Naylor et al. (1970) examined erythrocyte electrolytes in affective disorder and reported falling sodium levels with recovery. The activity of sodium/potassium-activated ATPase, thought to reflect sodium pump behaviour, is lower in the depressive phase of a manic depressive psychosis, and possibly in the manic phase as well, with increased activity on recovery. Glen et al. (1968) measured the concentration of sodium in the saliva, finding it raised in depression, suggestive of a failure of membrane transport. These data do suggest impaired handling of electrolytes in association with affective disorder, reflected in part by alteration of membrane transport. Studies of calcium suggest this is not influenced by the illness, and data on magnesium are inconsistent.

The essential trace element vanadium has been studied in relation to the electrolyte changes. It is an inhibitor of Na^+/K^+ ATPase. It is reported to be raised in hair, but not blood, in mania, and in blood and serum in depression, with a fall on recovery. Substances that lower vanadium concentration, such as ascorbic acid and EDTA, are therapeutic in mania and depression (Naylor et al., 1984). Lithium responders are reported to have lower erythrocyte Na^+/K^+ ATPase and to show the greatest increases in activity when on lithium compared with non-responders (Naylor *et al.*, 1976).

Platelet MAO activity has been reported in affective disorders, although results show variability. It is of interest, however, that several groups have reported increased values, particularly in unipolar (Reveley *et al.*, 1981) as opposed to bipolar patients in which reduced values are more frequently reported. This seems a trait as opposed to a state finding, and low levels are also noted in first-degree relatives of bipolar patients (Leckman *et al.*, 1977). However, there are reports of significant positive correlations between scores on depressive rating scales and MAO activity (Mann, 1979). Some authors report an increase in MAO activity with age and link this to the increasing incidence of depressive disorders in later life. MAOI drugs lower MAO activity, the effect of lithium treatment is unclear, whilst ECT has no effect (Mann, 1979). The variability of results, especially with bipolar patients, presumably reflects different patient populations and different techniques of measurement of MAO with differing substrates.

Sandler *et al.* (1975) gave a tyramine conjugation test to untreated patients with severe depression. Following an oral load, most tyramine is degraded by MAO to its main metabolite *p*-hydroxyphenylacetic acid but some 15 per cent is conjugated. In the patients the secretion of conjugated tyramine was significantly low, suggesting increased MAO activity. They have since gone on to suggest that the tyramine test may be a possible biological marker of depressive illness, useful in diagnosis. This deficit persists after recovery from illness, and is noted in both bipolar and unipolar patients (Harrison *et al.*, 1984).

With regards to central monoamines, in contrast to the literature on schizophrenia, that on the affective disorders has been dominated not by dopamine, but by noradrenaline and 5-HT.

The 5-HT (serotonin) hypothesis

The main biochemical hypotheses relating to the affective disorders were inspired by the revolution in psychopharmacology of the 1960s. Early observations were that reserpine, a drug that depletes monoamines, led to a depressive illness in some 20 per cent of patients taking it (mainly hypertensives); that MAOI drugs, initially used to treat tuberculosis, were noted to be mood elevating and increased monoamine levels; and that the other class of antidepressants, the tricyclic drugs also, by a different mechanism, elevated functional levels especially of noradrenaline and 5-HT. One emerging hypothesis was therefore that depletion of monoamine levels related to depressive illness. While investigators in the United States provided much data on catecholamines, in Europe the serotonin (5-HT) hypothesis was more vigorously pursued.

Pharmacological evidence

Experimentally it was shown that tertiary amines were more powerful at inhibiting 5-HT uptake whereas secondary amines influenced more noradrenergic uptake (Carlsson, 1977). However, clinically, patients taking tertiary amines, such as imipramine or amitryptiline, rapidly metabolize them to secondary amines and, if anything, with chronic treatment, have higher secondary amine levels. Recently highly selective 5-HT uptake inhibitors, such as fluoxetine and paroxetine, have been developed, which minimally influence catecholamine activity. Although as yet still in an early phase of investigation, they do seem to possess antidepressant potential (see Chapter 12).

In order to test the 5-HT hypothesis, patients were treated with amine precursers, notably tryptophan and 5-hydroxytryptophan (5-HTP). In normals, both compounds lead to elevation of mood, minimal with the former and most dramatic with 5-HTP (Trimble et al., 1977; Wirz-Justice, 1977). In depressed patients, L-tryptophan has a limited antidepressant effect, enhancing that of either clomipramine (a relatively selective inhibitor of 5-HT uptake) (Walinder et al., 1976) or an MAOI (Coppen et al., 1963) when given together. 5-HTP has antidepressant properties alone, or when given with clomipramine (van Praag et al., 1974) or an MAOI. In contrast, parachlorophenylalanine, a drug that selectively depletes 5-HT, reverses the antidepressant effect of both tricyclic and MAOI antidepresants, but such an effect was not observed with the catecholamine depleter alpha-methyl-paratyrosine (Shopsin et al., 1976).

Tryptophan in the plasma has been measured by several groups. It exists in a free and bound form (unlike other amino acids that are not bound to plasma protein), and entry across the blood–brain barrier is competitive with other amino acids. Since the rate-limiting enzyme for 5-HT formation, tryptophan-5-hydrolase, is not saturated under ordinary conditions, the level of tryptophan in the plasma can influence central 5-HT synthesis. Results of plasma tryptophan studies are not consistent, with reports of decreased total (Riley and Shaw, 1976) or normal total but reduced free (Coppen and Wood, 1978) and normal free levels (Moller et al., 1979), even when unipolar and bipolar patients were examined separately (Moller et al., 1979). A seasonal variation exists, possibly related to the seasonal variations of depressive illness. Studying the ratio of plasma tryptophan to that of five other amino acids, Meyer et al. (1981) reported lower ratios, but mainly in samples taken within 72 hours of admission in unipolar depressed patients. Improvements in depression, rated with the Hamilton scale, correlated significantly with an increasing ratio, suggesting lowered brain availability of tryptophan in the depressive phase.

Using radioactively labelled tryptophan, Shaw et al. (1978) investigated two tryptophan pools (intra- and extracellular) using multicompartmental analysis. Unipolar patients showed reduced extracellular tryptophan concentrations, interpreted as a response to stress (the procedure was stressful), which may reflect alterations of cortisol levels, which induce liver enzymes that metabolize tryptophan.

In summary, there is a suggestion that lower plasma tryptophan levels are associated with some aspect of depressive illness, but further investigations are required to establish its significance.

Another way to examine this issue has been using platelet binding studies. Platelets take up and store 5-HT in a manner thought similar to synaptosomes, and have therefore been used as a model for central 5-HT terminals. Early reports found decreased V_{max} (maximum transport rate) through the platelet membrane in manic depressive, depressive, unipolar, bipolar and schizoaffective patients (Meltzer et al., 1981). It is unclear from the data whether values return to normal with recovery or the relationship to response with tricyclic drugs. Imipramine and related compounds are potent inhibitors of the active transport of 5-HT into platelets (Todrick and Tait, 1969), although the site of this action may not be identical to that of 5-HT under all conditions. Decreased imipramine binding sites (B_{max}) have also been reported in several studies in a variety of depressive subgroups (Briley et al., 1980; Lewis and McChesney, 1985), including unipolar, bipolar and FPDD patients, although considerable overlap with control values is seen, and it is unclear whether this is a state or trait-dependent marker.

Brusov *et al.* (1985) have recently identified plasma low molecular weight compounds that inhibit both the imipramine binding and 5-HT uptake of platelets, suggesting possible endogenous compounds that may regulate 5-HT platelet and synaptosome activity and play a role in affective illness. The issue is more complex, however, since seasonal variations of both 5-HT uptake and platelet binding have been reported, with lower levels in the winter and spring, accounting for some of the variability in the results (Egrise *et al.*, 1986).

The data from these platelet studies have some consistency, and imply, if the platelet receptor resembles the neuronal receptor, and the animal data suggest this is a reasonable assumption, that the central 5-HT store is depleted in some patients with affective disorder.

Another haematological marker is red blood cell choline. This is reported elevated in some unipolar patients, possibly those that do not show altered imipramine binding (Wood *et al.*, 1983).

Attempts to identify changes in urinary metabolites of 5-HT in depression have not been consistent. Only about 5 per cent of urinary amine metabolites are of central origin, with the exception of the catecholamine derivative MHPG, the urine being too remote from CNS activity to provide meaningful data. Further evidence for the 5-HT hypothesis from CSF and brain binding studies are discussed below.

The noradrenaline hypothesis: pharmacological evidence

Although most antidepressant drugs influence catecholamine uptake (there are exceptions, for example iprindole or mianserin), the evidence that precurser loading with, for example, dihydroxy-phenylalanine and L-dopa in depression improves the response of other drugs, or is antidepressant, is poor. Further, alpha-methyl-paratyrosine does not reverse the antidepressant effect of imipramine (Shopsin *et al.*, 1976). However, L-dopa may switch a patient from the depressive to the manic phase of a bipolar illness, and alpha-paramethyltyrosine does the opposite (Murphy *et al.*, 1971). Some antidepressants are reported to be selective for noradrenergic systems (for example maprotiline), although this does not necessarily reflect on their mode of antidepressant action.

Biochemical evidence

Tyrosine levels in blood have been evaluated, but there is little consistency between studies.

Plasma noradrenaline levels have been reported as increased in affective disorder by several groups (Lake et al., 1982; Roy et al., 1985b), notably those with major affective disorder, especially those unipolar patients with melancholia (Roy et al., 1985b). The increased levels fall with ECT (Cooper et al., 1985). Esler et al. (1982) measured the rate of entry of noradrenaline to plasma from sympathetic nerves ('norepinephrine spillover') with tritiated noradrenaline and showed higher levels and spillover in patients with endogenous depression characterized by retardation or agitation. This suggested increased sympathetic tone, although interestingly, in this and some of the other studies, the raised levels were not accompanied by elevated blood pressure. In a small number of patients, tricyclic drugs led to a drop in both noradrenaline levels and spillover. Plasma adrenaline (Esler et al., 1982) and dopamine beta hydrolase (Friedman et al., 1984) tend to be normal.

Various strategies have been adopted to test catecholamine receptor function. These include the tyramine pressor test, clonidine challenge, estimation of the alpha adrenergic receptor on platelets and the beta receptor on lymphocytes.

The tyramine test involves assessing changes in blood pressure after a tyramine load. The blood pressure is elevated in depressed patients in some studies (Ghose et al., 1975) but not others. Clonidine, an alpha-2 adrenergic agonist, leads to a fall in blood pressure by acting on central alpha-2 receptors, and also lowers plasma noradrenaline and MHPG. Results in depressed patients are variable, although one group (Siever and Uhde, 1984) has reported decreased response of the MHPG decrement in major depressive disorder. This is compatable with other evidence of blunted alpha receptor activity reported in clonidine studies (see below). Tricyclic antidepressants attenuate the physiological responses of clonidine on MHPG and blood pressure (Charney et al., 1981), one postulated mechanism being that the increased synaptic neurotransmitter levels after treatment lead to negative feedback and reduction of neuronal firing and subsensitivity. Interestingly, similar effects were not observed with mianserin, indicating that not all antidepressants act in this way (Charney et al., 1984b).

Platelet alpha receptors have been examined using agonist ligands such as clonidine, and antagonists such as dihydroergocryptine or yohimbine. Of the studies to date, some show a difference, with increased binding (Garcia-Sevilla et al., 1981; Healy et al., 1983), although the majority are negative.

Using an alternative technique, that of examining the functional response of platelets, Garcia-Sevilla *et al.* (1986) studied platelet aggregation to adrenaline hydrochloride and found it increased in patients with major affective disorder, the effect being diminished by lithium. In contrast, Siever *et al.* (1984) reported decreased prostaglandin-E_1-stimulated cyclic AMP production in platelets, an indication of subsensitivity, while others have reported no change.

Antidepressants (long-term), lithium and ECT reduce the sensitivity of the alpha-2 receptor in both animal models and patient studies (Healy *et al.*, 1983). These attempts to find alteration of alpha-2 function in depressive illness and changes with treatment stem from hypotheses that implicate the receptor in the aetiology of depression, at least in a subgroup of patients, enhanced alpha-2 receptor activity being associated with reduced noradrenaline output. However, while there is some evidence to support these ideas, results are not reliably consistent. Further, the platelet data presupposes that the platelet alpha-2 receptor replicates the CNS receptor. This is unlikely, as centrally the alpha-2 receptor is both pre-and postsynaptic.

Studies of the beta-receptor, using lymphocyte binding, are also inconclusive, although decreased responsiveness of cyclic AMP or adenylate cyclase to isoprenaline challenges have been reported in manic and depressed patients (Pandy *et al.*, 1979; Extein *et al.*, 1979). This suggests down-regulation of the receptor, possibly a response to high circulating noradrenaline levels.

Increased urinary noradrenaline and normetanephrine and lower DOPAC levels have been reported in unipolar depressed patients (Roy *et al.*, 1986a). However, the main urinary metabolite studied has been MHPG, some 20–60 per cent deriving from central sources. The earlier studies, particularly from Schildkraut *et al.* (1984), found low levels, especially in a subgroup of patients with the depressed phase of a bipolar illness, and higher levels in manic or hypomanic episodes. Similar findings were not found with VMA, adrenaline or normetadrenaline. Estimates of MHPG levels in unipolar depression have been variable, some authors reporting low levels (Maas *et al.*, 1972), others finding no change but a wide variation suggesting subtypes with both high and low levels (Schildkraut *et al.*, 1984). Patients with low excretion rates have been found to be particularly responsive to treatment with tricyclic drugs (Maas *et al.*, 1972; Hollister *et al.*, 1980). This is more consistent for imipramine, nortryptiline and desipramine than for amitryptiline, for which higher excretion rates are reported in responders (Modai *et al.*, 1979), possibly reflecting pharmacological differences between the drugs, especially on noradrenergic systems.

Wiesel *et al.* (1982) reported on urinary excretion values of MHPG, HVA, 5-HIAA and dihydroxyphenylacetic acid (DOPAC) in healthy volunteers. Those with a family history of psychiatric morbidity had increased variance of MHPG levels. This correlated positively with CSF levels, and suggested that altered noradrenergic metabolism may be related to vulnerability to psychopathology.

Other biochemical hypotheses

In addition to the above hypotheses that have dominated depression research in recent years, both dopamine and choline hypotheses have had supporters. Further, biochemical findings relating to other systems have been reported and are of interest.

The dopamine hypothesis has been strongly supported by Randrup *et al.* (1975). It is based on pharmacological evidence that neuroleptic drugs block dopamine receptors and are effective antimanic agents; that a 'depression' is not infrequently seen in patients on these drugs; that some neuroleptics, especially in small doses, may be antidepressant; the fact that nearly all antidepressants act, at least to some extent, on dopamine uptake systems; that L-dopa, in some patients, may be antidepressant or may precipitate a manic phase; and animal pharmacology that links certain behaviours (especially stereotypy) to increased central dopamine activity.

Some support for this derives from CSF data and the association of depressive illness with Parkinson's disease (see below), although there is, to date, relatively little direct evidence to implicate dopamine in the primary pathogenesis of affective disorders.

Cholinergic mechanisms have been implicated by Janowsky *et al.* (1980). In particular they discuss the relative balance between cholinergic and adrenergic tone, with depression representing a cholinergic and mania an adrenergic excess. The evidence is as follows: animal data show that cholinergic agents inhibit self-stimulation; many, especially of the older, first-generation, antidepressants, have considerable anticholinergic properties; cholinomimetics such as physostigmine produce an 'inhibitory syndrome' of lethargy and psychomotor retardation, and may reverse mania, sometimes provoking a switch to a depressed phase; and precursors such as deanol and choline may provoke depressive symptoms (Tammingar *et al.*, 1976). Patients with affective disorder are reported to be more sensitive to the behavioural effects of physostigmine (Janowsky *et al.*, 1980), and some show elevated levels of red cell choline (Wood *et al.*, 1983) or reduced acetylcholinesterase levels (Mathew *et al.*, 1982b).

GABA has recently been implicated following observations that the anticonvulsant sodium valproate may have antimanic properties (Emrich *et al.*, 1984) and that some precursor drugs, such as progabide, possess antidepressant properties (Morselli *et al.*, 1980). Plasma GABA has been reported low in euthymic bipolar patients and CSF data offer some support for these findings (Berrettini *et al.*, 1983).

Urinary cyclic AMP has been reported to be decreased in depression and increased in mania (Paul *et al.*, 1971b), and in rapid cycling patients there appears to be an increase in cyclic AMP levels during the switch from depression to mania (Paul *et al.*, 1971a). With treatment, values tend to return to normal (Abdulla and Hamadah, 1970). It is difficult to interpret these data since some 50 per cent of urinary cyclic AMP derives from the kidneys. However, they may reflect altered receptor function in affective disorders, a suggestion supported by observations that antidepressant drugs and lithium decrease noradrenaline-stimulated cyclic AMP. The inhibition of ADH-activated cyclic AMP is a possible explanation for one of the side effects of lithium, namely polyuria.

The phenylethylamine hypothesis states that this compound, structurally related to amphetamine and the catecholamines, is a neuromodulator which is deficient in depressive illness. It is excitatory in animals, and is degraded by MAOB to phenylacetate. The latter and beta-phenylethylamine are reported low in patients with major depressive disorders (Sabelli *et al.*, 1983).

Peptides have recently become a focus of interest. Initial observations that some, for example TRH or beta-endorphin (Kline *et al.*, 1977), may possess antidepressant properties have not led as yet to any therapeutic advances. Plasma beta-endorphin levels have been reported as normal in patients with unipolar major affective disorder (Alexopolous *et al.*, 1983).

Low levels of folic acid have been reported in association with a variety of neuropsychiatric conditions, especially in patients with epilepsy. There are several reports of depressive illness being associated with low levels (Trimble *et al.*, 1980), not explained away in terms of diet or institutionalization, and reported in out-patients and in community studies (Edeh and Toone, 1985). Reynolds *et al*. (1984) have drawn attention to the fact that the methyl donor SAM (see p.205) is antidepressant, that folate mega-loblastic anaemia is more frequently associated with affective dis-order than is B_{12} deficiency and that folic acid is reported to improve mood, notably in patients with folate deficiency. The fact that SAM and folate are intimately connected with monoamine metabolism may mean that CNS methylation is intimately involved with the regulation of mood.

Hormonal data

With the development of new techniques for the accurate mea-surement of small quantities of hormones, a plethora of data have recently appeared assessing neurohormonal function in affective disorders. Most interest has centered around cortisol and the dexamethasone suppression test (DST). Indeed, there are already over 500 publications relating to this alone, and reviews are readily available (Arana and Baldessarini, 1985; Braddock, 1986).

Raised plasma cortisol levels and corticosteroid excretion rates had been observed in patients with depression, and an early report of abnormal dexamethasone suppression came from Butler and Besser in 1968. They reported failure of suppression with up to 8 mg of dexamethasone in severely depressed patients, results returning to normal after treatment of the depression. They emphasized the similarity of the results to those found in Cushing's disease.

Following investigation of over 400 patients, Carroll *et al*. (1981) defined a standardized protocol, and suggested that the test may be 'a specific laboratory test for the diagnosis of melancholia'.

The object of the test is to suppress ACTH with a dose of dexamethasone, and most laboratories have adopted a schedule as shown in Table 1, or a variant of it.

Normal subjects show a diurnal rhythm of secretion, with inhibi-tion during the noctural hours. They suppress cortisol for 24–48 hours after dexamethasone.

The use of 1 mg of dexamethasone gives the most sensitivity, although doses up to 8 mg have been used in some studies. The most practical time to take the sample for cortisol measurement is at 1600 hours, although the use of additional times may increase the rate of positivity. Using a plasma cortisol criterion value of

Table 1   Schedule for the dexamethasone suppression test

Day 1		Day 2		
2300		0800	1600	2300
↑		↑	↑	↑
Dex 1 mg				
oral		Cortisol determinations		

Non-suppression: cortisol >5µg per 100 ml (157 nmol/l)

>5 µg per 100 ml, Carroll *et al.* (1981) gave an overall test sensitivity (true positive rate) of 43 per cent and a specificity (true negative rate, that is false positive rate minus 100 per cent) of 96 per cent. The diagnostic confidence for a diagnosis of melancholia with values above this level was 96 per cent, although that for ruling out melancholia at levels below this was only 54 per cent. In other words, a positive result had much more significance than a negative result.

In a review of over 5000 cases, Arana and Baldessarini (1985) found the sensitivity to be 44 per cent, and the specificity 93 per cent when distinguishing major depression from normal controls, but the latter fell to 76.5 per cent in comparison to all other psychiatric disorders. However, it remained high when major depression was compared with bereavement (90.5 per cent), anxiety and panic (88.2 per cent), schizophrenia (86.9 per cent) and alcoholism not active or in acute withdrawal (80.0 per cent).

In contrast to these data, other authors have been more critical, and in particular have noted high levels of positivity in other psychiatric conditions. Some of these are shown in Table 2.

Age and sex do not seem related to the results, although higher levels of positivity are reported in older patients. It is not affected by the use of antidepressant or neuroleptic medications or lithium. There are a number of conditions that give false positive results, shown in Table 3.

False negative results are seen in Addison's disease and hypopituitarism.

The data with some psychiatric populations other than depression are often confused by the inclusion of patients with associated affective symptoms which increase the rate of positivity. The

Table 2 Abnormal DST results and psychiatric diagnoses

Psychiatric condition	Result (%)	Reference
Melancholia	45	Caroll *et al.* (1981), Arana and Baldessarini (1985)
Mania	0–40	Rabkin *et al.* (1985)
Schizophrenia	0–20	Coppen *et al.* (1983), Munro *et al.* (1984)
Panic disorder	25	Roy-Byrne *et al.* (1985b)
Obessive compulsive	2	Checkley (1985)
Anorexia nervosa	36–100	Rabkin *et al.* (1985)
Bulimia	35–67	Lindy *et al.* (1985)
Borderline personality	8	Krishnan *et al.* (1984)
Normals	4–27	Carroll *et al.* (1981), Braddock (1986)

results in schizophrenia are influenced by acute psychosis and hospital admission, both of which increase the non-suppression rate.

Although no specific clinical features of the melancholia have been associated with the positive result, some appear to be emerging. There are several reports that the DST reverts to normal after treatment, and that failure to do so, or reversion back to a positive response after normalization, is a bad prognostic (Arana and Baldessarini, 1985) and may signal an increased risk of suicide (Targum *et al.*, 1983a). Coppen *et al.* (1985) have suggested that if higher cut-off points (for example 10 μg per 100 ml) are taken, then prediction of response may be improved. In addition, endogenicity, as assessed by the Newcastle scale, may be relevant (Coppen *et al.*, 1983), as may be severity of depression as measured by the Hamilton rating scale (Meador-Woodruff *et al.*, 1986). Patients with psychotic depression and bipolar illness have higher levels of non-suppression (Arana and Baldessarini, 1985), as shown in Table 4.

Some have reported that abnormal DSTs are associated with a family history of depression (Mendlewicz *et al.*, 1982), although others do not find this (Rudorfer *et al.*, 1982). There are several reports suggesting that patients with secondary depression have

Table 3   False positive DST

Medications	Benzodiazepines
	Anticonvulsants
	Barbiturates
	Reserpine
	Alpha-methyl dopa
	Methadone
	Morphine
	Spironolactone
	Indomethacin
	Cyproheptadine
Drugs	Alcohol; excess caffeine
Diseases	Diabetes mellitus
	Dementia
	Cerebral tumour
	Cardiac failure
	Cushing's disease
Metabolic	Dehydration
Other	Pregnancy
	Acute medical illness or trauma

lower rates of suppression than those with primary depressive illness, and, in a smaller number of studies, psychotic depressives yield a higher rate than non-psychotics (Rabkin *et al.*, 1985).

Table 4   Non-suppression in DST and affective state (from Arana and Baldessarini, 1985)

	Non-suppression (%)
Normal control	7.2
Acute grief	9.5
Dysthmic disorder	22.9
Major depressive disorder	43.1
Melancholia	50.2
Psychotic affective, includes bipolar disorder	68.6
With suicide intent	77.8

The abnormal responses are not due to an unusually rapid clearance of the dexamethasone by patients with melancholia (Carroll *et al.*, 1981) and the circulating half-life of the cortisol is normal (Butler and Besser, 1968). Depressed patients seem to have an increased number of cortisol secretory episodes with an increased time per day of release (Sachar *et al.*, 1973).

ACTH levels are higher and dexamethasone plasma levels lower in DST positive patients, in spite of the normal dexamethasone clearance (Arana and Baldessarini, 1985). One explanation of the raised ACTH levels is that the hypothalamic–pituitary–adrenal axis is 'set' at a higher level in the non-suppressors. In preliminary investigations, Holsboer *et al.* (1985) have given corticotrophin releasing factor (CRF) to non-suppressing depressed patients, and repeated the investigation on recovery when suppression was normal. No differences in the profiles of ACTH, cortisol or corticosterone output were noted in the two conditions. This implies that the hypersecretion of steroids in depression is not the result of excessive hormonal reserves in the pituitary or adrenal glands. Whalley *et al.* (1986) measured the number of glucocorticoid receptors on lymphocytes in patients with depression, schizophrenia and controls. The number of receptors was significantly lower in the depressed patients, even in those who had not received psychotropic medication. This suggests that in depression there may be changes in steroid receptor sensitivity, which if it also occurred in the brain would lead to dexamethasone non-suppression.

In relation to other biological markers, patients with dexamethasone non-suppression have higher platelet MAO activity (Schatzberg *et al.*, 1985) and higher plasma MHPG (Jimmerson *et al.*, 1983).

Sherman *et al.* (1984) followed the circadian patterns of plasma cortisol in suppressors and non-suppressors before and after a dose of dexamethasone. They noted that, generally, non-suppressors show a temporary drop in values after dexamethasone (1 mg at 11 p.m.), but in some the escape was later than 8 a.m., and thus false negative results may be obtained dependent on the time of the sampling (see Figure 1). In contrast, for suppressors, the levels are low throughout the day and the timing of sampling was less likely to influence the classification of the patient. Their study suggested that major surges of pituitary activity occur at 3 to 4 hour intervals in non-suppressors, beginning at about 8 a.m., and that sampling at two times, either widely spaced (8 a.m. and 4 p.m.) or separated by an hour, will minimize the likelihood of sampling during a trough.

Among the factors that may influence the DST must be included the method of cortisol analysis and patient compliance. Thus part

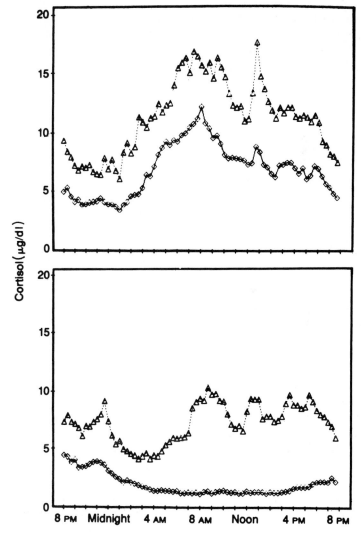

Figure 1. Top: mean 24-hour plasma cortisol concentration for suppressors ($N = 17$, diamonds) and non-suppressors ($N = 8$, triangles) during 24 hours before dexamethasone administration. Bottom: results for 24 hours during which 1 mg of dexamethasone was given at 11 p.m. (From Sherman *et al.*, 1984. (Reproduced with permission. Copyright 1984, American Medical Association.)

of the variation in the data may reflect the use of radioim-munoassay as opposed to a competitive protein binding assay, the latter appearing to be more reliable (Meltzer and Fang, 1983). HPLC and mass spectrometry are rarely used, but will be even more accurate. Poor compliance may be a reason why in-patient studies show higher rates of non-suppression than out-patient investigations, although severity of the illness is a more likely explanation. Some authors have suggested that weight loss is a critical variable, although others have failed to replicate this (Keitner et al., 1985).

The abnormal suppression has been interpreted in terms of a simple response to stress, although an alternative is that it reflects abnormal limbic–hypothalamic function. The lower levels of abnormality in association with anxiety disorders and bereave-ment are against this being a non-specific stress response. Further, an abnormal DST does not relate to an excess of life events as assessed by the Bedford College Life Events and Difficulties Schedule, although patients with severe life events in a six month period prior to the onset of depression have higher urinary-free cortisol levels than those without (Dolan et al., 1985a) and acute stress will elevate postdexamethasone cortisol levels (Baumgartner et al., 1985). It is unlikely that the raised cortisol levels have a causative role in the depressive illness since cortisol itself tends to provoke euphoria or mood elevation when given to patients, and in Cushing's disease, although depression is com-mon, it is not universal, being severe in less than 20 per cent of patients (Cohen, 1980).

A more attractive hypothesis is that the abnormal DST reflects altered CNS function, especially neurotransmitter action in hypo-thalamic and related limbic pathways, and is thus a marker of some more fundamental biological change. This has been explored by Carrol et al. (1980), whose data suggest a cholinergic mechanism. They noted that physostigmine, an inhibitor of anticholinesterase, allowed normal subjects to escape from suppression, an effect that could be blocked by atropine.

Patients with organic mental disorders have been investigated, and generally high levels of non-suppression are reported. In particular, the DST does not seem to reliably differentiate between depressive illness and dementia (Spar and Gerner, 1982). It is abnormal in patients after the acute phase of a cerebrovascular accident, and this relates both to the presence of major depression and greater lesion volume on CT examination (Lipsey et al., 1985).

Some conclusions regarding the ever-accumulating information on the DST are given in Table 5.

Cortisol plasma levels may also be stimulated by amphetamine and methylamphetamine. As this can be blocked by alpha adrenergic antagonists, the effect is thought to be mediated noradrenergically. This response seems blunted in depressed patients (Checkley, 1979). Clonidine appears to normalize the hypercortisolaemia of depression (Siever and Uhde, 1984), providing support for a role of adrenergic mechanisms.

Other neurohormonal data

Several other neuroendocrine responses in depression have been assessed. These include the thyroid stimulating hormone (TSH) response to thyroid releasing hormone (TRH), and growth hormone responses to dopamine agonists, insulin, L 5-HTP and clonidine.

In the TRH test, 200–500 μg of IV-TRH are given, and blood samples are taken over the next hour for the assessment of TSH values. Some 40–50 per cent of patients with depression show blunted responses (Extein et al., 1981; Calloway et al., 1984). One group, studying 145 medication-free depressed patients, gave the specificity of the test as 93 per cent with a sensitivity of 56 per cent, and predictive value of a maximum TSH response (the peak level after infusion−baseline) of <7 μ IU/ml as 91 per cent for major unipolar depression (Extein et al., 1981). The response tends to normalize with treatment (Extein et al., 1982). Claims that this test may distinguish different subgroups of affective disorder have not been upheld. Further, although cortisol excess itself leads to

Table 5   Some conclusions regarding the DST in psychiatry

1. An abnormal DST is found in some patients.
2. This suggests hypothalamic–pituitary axis dysfunction.
3. It is most abnormal in anorexia nervosa.
4. It is often abnormal in depression, especially endogenous, melancholic and psychotic subtypes.
5. It is state rather than trait dependent.
6. It may help differentiate anxiety disorders from depression.
7. It may predict relapse after treatment.

impaired TSH release, not all patients with blunting on this test are dexamethasone non-suppressors. About 30–40 per cent of patients are abnormal on both dexamethasone and TRH tests, although this does not identify any particular diagnostic group. Interestingly, a subgroup of patients with blunted responses have an elevated free thyroxine index (FTI), some, while not being clinically hyperthyroid, having values in the hyperthyroid range (Calloway *et al.*, 1984). Abnormal responses are also reported in alcoholism, anorexia nervosa and acute starvation.

Because of the observed endocrine changes in depressed patients, other investigators have given multiple neuroendocrine challenges to look for a more generalized hypothalamic–pituitary defect in the disorder. Brambilla *et al.* (1978) gave TRH and LH RH to sixteen patients with primary affective disorder, and 79 per cent had some demonstrable abnormality. Winokur *et al.* (1982), using TRH, LH RH, DST and insulin challenge tests in patients with primary unipolar depression and controls, reported abnormalities in 96.2 per cent of patients and only 29 per cent of controls.

Both growth hormone and prolactin have been studied because of the relationship of their release to underlying neurotransmitters. Growth hormone is affected by a number of factors including stress, fasting and diet, but is thought to be released under the influence of growth hormone releasing factor (GHRF, somatostatin) from the hypothalamus. Release of growth hormone is altered by drugs that act on the adrenoceptor, being stimulated by clonidine, methoxamine and phenyephrine (alpha agonists), an effect potentiated by propanolol. This suggests that alpha receptors are excitatory and beta receptors inhibitory. The growth hormone response to apomorphine is related to dopamine receptor stimulation, and it can be blocked by dopamine antagonists such as chlorpromazine. Other neurotransmitters also probably involved in growth hormone release include 5-HT and GABA, although their influence is weaker.

Growth hormone responses have been studied in depression. Impaired release is reported after metamphetamine (Checkley, 1979), insulin hypoglycaemia (Mueller *et al.*, 1969), clonidine (Checkley, 1985; Siever and Uhde, 1984) and desmethyl-imipramine (Glass *et al.*, 1982), a tricyclic drug that selectively blocks the re-uptake of noradrenaline. Responses to apomorphine are not reliably altered, supporting a major role for alpha adrenergic mechanisms in affective disorder with decreased alpha receptor responsiveness, probably at the hypothalamus. Katona et al. (1985) have reported that patients with blunted growth hormone responses to clonidine are more likely to be DST nonsuppressors, suggesting a common underlying mechanism for these changes.

Prolactin release, regulated by prolactin inhibitory factor (PIF), itself thought to be dopamine, is stimulated by dopamine antagonists and inhibited by dopamine agonists. 5-HT and GABA also stimulate its release. Baseline prolactin levels are consistently normal in depressed populations. In one study, the degree of suppression following apomorphine has been reported impaired in major depression and schizoaffective disorder, the degree of depression as rated on the Hamilton scale correlating with the degree of suppression (Meltzer et al., 1984), although in this investigation, baseline levels were elevated. While this may suggest a role of dopaminergic systems, blunted prolactin responses have also been reported after methadone (Judd et al., 1982) and tryptophan (Heninger et al., 1984), suggesting both peptide and serotonergic abnormalities.

A summary of some of these neurohormonal findings in affective disorder is found in Table 6. In general, taking into consideration the methodological problems associated with these data (see Table 7), they offer support for adrenergic involvement in major affective disorders, the most robust findings relating to studies of the alpha receptor in depressive disorders.

NEUROCHEMICAL INVESTIGATIONS

There has been a considerable number of investigations of CSF in the affective disorders, the majority examining the noradrenergic

Table 6 Summary of neurohormonal data

Hypersecretion of cortisol
Loss of normal circadian cortisol cycle
Increased urinary excretion of cortisol and metabolites
Abnormal response to dexamethasone
Blunting of growth hormone output to alpha adrenergic stimulants
Blunting of TSH responses to TRH
Blunted prolactin responses to several agents

Table 7   Some important methodological considerations

Influence of age and sex
Influence of circadian, monthly and annual cycle of hormone
    activity
Influence of stress, diet and associated illness
Many hormones are released in a pulsatile fashion
Influence of nicotine and alcohol intake
Influence of psychotropic drugs
Variability of assay procedures

or the 5-HT hypotheses. In contrast to the studies in schizophrenia, the neuropathological studies are few in number.

CSF

The main metabolites investigated, in studies with or without the
probenecid technique, have been 5-HIAA and MHPG. Overall,
more studies report lower levels of 5-HIAA than no differences
compared with controls. Many of the early studies did not use the
probenecid method, and were dismissed on account of methodological problems. First, much 5-HIAA released from the brain
is removed from the CSF by an active transport system, giving a 3
to 1 gradient from ventricular to lumbar fluid. Secondly, factors
such as diet, time of day and patient height and posture were often
not taken into account. Thirdly, the spinal cord was known to
contribute to the 5-HIAA pool, further diminishing the relevance
of lumbar fluid findings.

Using the probenecid technique, several groups have shown
diminished accumulation of 5-HIAA, further diminished by the
administration of antidepressants (Post and Goodwin, 1978) but
elevated by L-tryptophan and 5-HTP (Takahashi et al., 1975). In
addition, the low levels seem to persist on clinical recovery, in both
baseline (Coppen et al., 1972) and probenecid studies (van Praag,
1980a). In a series of investigations, van Praag (1980a), using the
probenecid method, reported low levels of 5-HIAA to characterize some 40 per cent of cases, although he did not report any
psychopathological differences between these and other patients.
In contrast, Banki et al. (1981) reported anxiety, insomnia, retardation, fatigability and suicide to be more prevalent in a subpopulation of patients with low 5-HIAA. The low levels are noted

in patients with an absence of significant adverse life events in six months prior to onset of their illness (Roy *et al.*, 1986b).

A relationship between suicide and low 5-HIAA has been replicated by all studies except two that have examined it. Åsberg and colleagues (Åsberg *et al.*, 1976; Lidberg *et al.*, 1985) reported 5-HIAA as lower in those who attempt suicide, even in non-depressed subjects, and in those who have murdered sexual or familial partners or their children. They have also reported in a follow-up study of depressed patients that those with low values are more likely to die from suicide in the ensuing twelve months. Since similar findings are reported in schizophrenics who attempt suicide (Ninan *et al.*, 1984), in alcoholic impulsive violent offenders (Linnoila *et al.*, 1983b), and in patients with aggression who have borderline personality disorders without depressive illness (Brown *et al.*, 1982), one interpretation is that the low 5-HT turnover is related to impulse control and aggression, rather than to depression per se.

There is one investigation of ventricular fluid metabolites in depression. Bridges *et al.* (1976), in a study of patients having psychosurgery, with chronic or persistently resistant depression, reported severely depressed patients to have the lowest and agitated patients to have the highest 5-HIAA levels respectively.

In contrast, results of 5-HIAA levels in mania have been contradictory, some studies reporting increased and others decreased values.

CSF catecholamine or catecholamine metabolite levels have been studied with less consistent results. In keeping with the urine investigations, some authors report low levels of MHPG (Post *et al.*, 1973) and others show normal results (Post *et al.*, 1985) and no relationship to suicide. Low HVA levels have been reported in subgroups of patients, notably those with retardation (van Praag, 1977a). This observation is consistently reported in probenecid studies, and seems robust. In contrast, agitation and psychosis are reported to be related to increased HVA levels (Banki *et al.*, 1981).

Estimates of noradrenaline levels have produced inconsistencies, although there are two reports of elevations in mania (Gerner *et al.*, 1984; Post *et al.*, 1985) associated with paradoxically decreased dopamine beta-hydroxylase levels (Post *et al.*, 1985). Lower adrenaline levels have also been reported in depressed patients, returning to normal with recovery (Christensen *et al.*, 1980).

Recently there are several reports of CSF data combining with other biological markers. In particular, DST non-suppressors show lower HVA (Banki *et al.*, 1983) and a poor association with adverse life events (Roy *et al.*, 1986b).

Lower CSF GABA has been noted in several studies (Gerner *et al.*, 1984; Berrettini *et al.*, 1983), as has lower CSF somatostatin (Rubinow *et al.*, 1985), especially in dexamethasone non-suppressors (Doran *et al.*, 1986). This suggests a functional interdependence of CRF on somatostatin, possibly at the level of the hypothalamus, and receives some support from observations of higher CSF cortisol in depression (Träskman *et al.*, 1980), associated with non-suppression of the DST (Banki *et al.*, 1983).

Brain neurochemistry

The CSF data provide limited support for changes in catecholamines in depressive illness, especially in relation to motor activity. The data from brain neurochemical studies in this area are minimal. Those reported lend weight to changes in the 5-HT system, and are largely derived from studies of brains of patients who have committed suicide. These data are difficult to interpret methodologically, especially since psychotropic drugs are often the main cause of death in such patients, and there are difficulties of controlling for post-mortem degradation.

One of the earliest reports was that of Shaw *et al.* (1967), who found significantly lower 5-HT concentrations in the hindbrains of seventeen depressed and eight suicide patients compared with controls. Low 5-HT has also been reported in the substantia nigra and amygdala (Birkmeyer *et al.*, 1977) and hypothalamus (Korpi *et al.*, 1986). Others reported lower 5-HIAA (Bourne *et al.*, 1968), changes being especially noted in the raphe nuclei (Lloyd *et al.*, 1974).

In contrast to these findings, Stanley and Mann (1983, 1986) reported increased 5-HT_2 receptors, measured by 3H-spiroperidol binding, in the frontal cortex of suicide victims. They were all deaths by violent non-overdose means, and, since antidepressant drugs decrease 5-HT_2 receptor binding, it is unlikely that this represents a drug effect. This same group has reported reduced presynaptic imipramine binding to the frontal cortex in similar patients, also found by others in the hippocampal and occipital cortex (Perry *et al.*, 1983). These data suggest decreased presynaptic and increased postsynaptic 5-HT function, compatible with decreased synaptic levels of 5-HT in depression.

In other studies, brain MAO, noradrenaline levels and muscarinic cholinergic binding have been studied with negative results, but one group has reported low dopamine levels in the caudate nucleus (Birkmeyer *et al.*, 1977), and another has shown significantly increased beta-adrenergic receptor binding to frontal cortex (Mann *et al.*, 1986).

NEUROPHYSIOLOGICAL AND NEUROLOGICAL DATA

Electrophysiological studies

Some of the earliest reports of EEG traces in affective disorder found a higher than expected incidence of abnormalities. For example, Finlay and Campbell (1941) found abnormalities in 33 per cent of 137 manic depressive patients, similar data being given by others (Davis, 1941). As with schizophrenia, attention was drawn to the presence of abnormally fast (20–50 Hz) frequencies.

Abrams and Taylor (1979) analysed the records of 27 schizophrenic and 132 affective disorder patients , noting that in contrast to the more extensive and temporal location of the abnormalities in schizophrenia, the affectives had more parieto/occipital changes (24 per cent). In cases where the abnormalities were lateralized, 71 per cent were right sided. This did not relate to age, severity of illness or medication.

Two waveforms in particular have been associated with affective symptoms. The six-per-second rhythmic waves, also referred to as rhythmic midtemporal discharges (RMTD), are associated with an increased risk for psychopathology, including high hypochondriasis and depression scores on the MMPI (Hughes and Hermann, 1984) (see Figure 2). Small sharp spikes (SSS), brief-duration small amplitude spikes that are sometimes exclusively temporal in location and manifest in drowsy states or light sleep, have been associated with neurovegetative symptoms, affective disorders and a tendency to suicide (Small, 1970) (see Figure 3). In particular, related symptoms included mood swings, anxiety, insomnia, concentration difficulties and feelings of hopelessness. Further, in patients with bipolar affective disorder, 43 per cent show SSS, which may be significantly related to a family history of affective disorder (Small *et al.*, 1975).

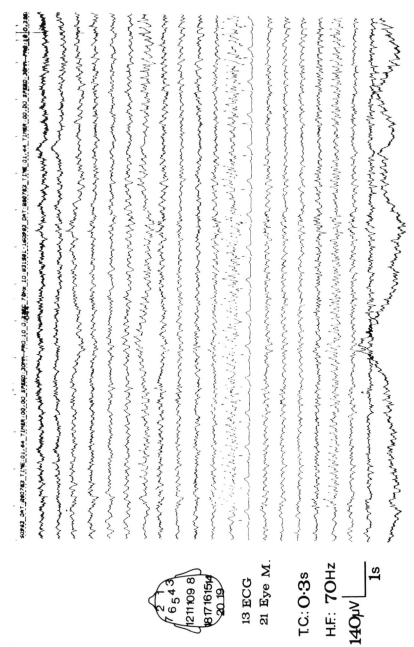

Figure 2. Rhythmic midtemporal discharges. Note trains of notched waves, maximal in the left temporal regions (leads 7, 12 and 18). (Kindly supplied by Dr Colin Binnie, Institute of Psychiatry.)

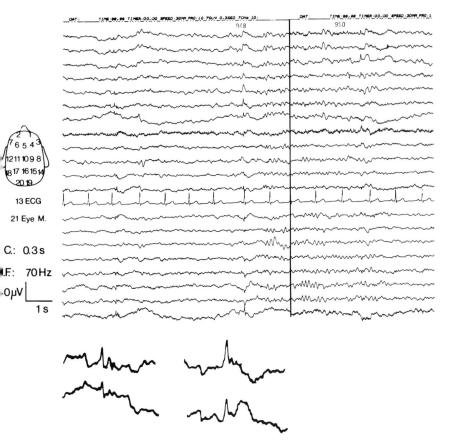

Figure 3. Small sharp waves (benign epileptiform transients of sleep). Note the short duration spikes. A magnification of those from channels 6 and 7 is shown below. These are predominant in the temporal regions and seen during drowsiness or stages one and two sleep. (Kindly supplied by Dr Colin Binnie, Institute of Psychiatry.)

Struve *et al.* (1979) reported a highly significant positive relationship between paroxysmal EEG abnormalities and suicidal ideation and acts, and assaultive/destructive acts, unrelated to medication. Both SSS and RMTD were included in the paroxysmal events that were associated with suicide. The relevance of these findings for such conditions as episodic dyscontrol (see p.302) and the association between epilepsy and affective disorder and suicide (p.303) is not clear. However, they do emphasize the importance of paroxysmal electrophysiological events beyond epilepsy, and that 'all that spikes is not fits' (Stevens, 1979).

Data from power spectra analyses have been reported in detail by Flor-Henry (1983). He confirms the increased amount of 20–50 Hz activity, notably bilaterally in the temporal regions for both mania and depression, and in the left parietal region in mania. In his studies there was a significant reduction of right parietal alpha energy in both states, thought to reflect abnormal activation of the non-dominant hemisphere. Examining interhemispheric organization by means of an EEG measure of left/right hemispheric energy oscillations, at rest and during certain cognitive tasks that activated one or other hemisphere, he reported that the organization is most disturbed and bilateral in schizophrenia, is intermediate and in the dominant hemisphere only in mania and is normal in depression.

The evoked potential literature is confused and difficult to interpret. Shagass *et al.* (1981), in studies where potentials were evoked by four different kinds of sensory stimuli, claim to show differences between psychotic depressives and schizophrenics. They report that the amplitudes of earlier peaks are higher in the latter, while later peaks (P90, N130 and P185) were higher in depressives. However, in both groups most amplitudes were lower than controls. The data were interpreted as suggesting some impairment of sensory processing in depression, although less than that seen in schizophrenia.

Others maintain there are differences between bipolar and unipolar affective disorder patients. Buchsbaum *et al.* (1971) reported that bipolars tend to be augmenters and unipolars reducers. Laterality differences have been reported, but the results are inconsistent, some suggesting non-dominant (Flor-Henry, 1983) and others dominant hemisphere (Shagass *et al.*, 1979) abnormalities.

Sleep studies

One biological marker of depression that has become of interest in recent years is polygraphically defined sleep changes. Some disorder of sleep has long been held to be a key symptom of depression, notably early morning waking and nocturnal restlessness in endogenous depression. The major changes of sleep in depression are shown in Table 8.

One consistent observation is the shortening of the time from the onset of sleep to the first REM period (REM latency). This falls by about 30 per cent, and is associated with an increase in the length of the first REM period and decreased stages 3 and 4 sleep.

Table 8 Sleep and affective disorder

Patient symptoms	Difficulty getting off to sleep Poor sleep Early morning waking Increased waking
Duration	Decreased total time
Non-REM sleep	Increased stage 1 Decreased stages 3 and 4
REM sleep	Decreased REM latency Increased REM time in early hours Decreased REM in late hours
Treatment	Sleep deprivation Selective REM deprivation Some antidepressants suppress REM

The REM period is said to be more dense, with an increased number of eye movements per minute. Patients show increased waking during the night, and will complain of both early morning wakening and poor sleep quality.

The shortened REM latency does not seem specific for depression, and has been reported in such conditions as narcolepsy, anorexia nervosa, some schizophrenics and in normals following artificial REM deprivation (Gillin *et al.*, 1985). However, in depression it has good sensitivity (60–70 per cent) and high specificity (80–97 per cent), and is associated with some other biological markers. Latencies are briefer in patients who are cortisol non-suppressors (Rush *et al.*, 1982; Mendlewicz *et al.*, 1984).

The meaning of these changes is unclear. They seem to identify a pattern of depression referred to as endogenous, and may be presumed to be a reflection of the underlying biochemical abnormality associated with the condition. Manipulation of sleep, for example deprivation, has an antidepressant effect, and, in patients switching from depression to mania, a change in sleep pattern heralds the change in mood and motoric behaviour. Several hypotheses have been advanced (Gillin *et al.*, 1985). Since REM sleep is regulated by monoamines and is influenced by cholinergic medications (REM latency can be shortened by physostigmine), one suggestion is that it reflects a disturbed cholinergic/aminergic balance. Another is that the short latency represents a 'phase advance', a shift of diurnal rhythms.

Radiological studies

In contrast to the now-extensive data accumulated in schizophrenia, radiological investigations of the affective disorders are limited. However, there does seem to be a subgroup of patients in whom abnormalities can be demonstrated, mainly relating to ventricular dilatation and cerebellar atrophy (Nasrallah et al., 1982a). Rieder et al. (1983) found no differences in the degree of abnormality between schizophrenic, schizoaffective and bipolar affective disorder patients, all groups containing some patients with ventricular enlargement, sulcal prominence or cerebellar atrophy. Increased ventricular size has been reported in patients with manic depressive illness (Pearlson and Verloff, 1981), psychotic depression with delusions (Targum et al., 1983b), mania (Nasrallah et al., 1982a), young manics (Nasrallah et al., 1982b), those with associated hypothyroidism (Johnstone et al., 1986b) and elderly depressives (Jacoby and Levy, 1980c).

Dolan et al. (1985b), in a study of over a hundred patients meeting the RDC criteria for depression, reported significantly greater VBRs compared with volunteer controls, which was not related to family history, treatments or course of the illness. In a series of studies, using age-matched volunteer controls, Jacoby and colleagues have studied elderly patients with affective disorders (Jacoby and Levy, 1980c; Jacoby et al., 1981). There appears to be a subgroup of patients with late-onset depressive illness, characteristically endogenous in character, with enlarged ventricles. These patients have a greater mortality on follow-up.

In a longitudinal study of their normal controls, a subgroup were identified that went on to develop a depressive illness. The patients had significantly higher VBRs on initial and follow-up scans, compared with the rest (Bird et al., 1986).

Using MRI, Rangel-Guerra et al. (1983) reported that bipolar patients had higher T_1 values than normal controls in frontal and temporal lobes, which returned to normal after treatment with lithium.

CBF and PET studies

CBF has been reported to be reduced in major depressive disorder, maximally in the frontal regions (Mathew et al., 1980b), normal (Gur *et al.*, 1984), and increased in the left frontal region (Uytdenhoef *et al.*, 1983). It is normal in mania (Silfverskiöld *et al.*, 1985).

Studies with PET using the glucose method tend to support the conclusion that some patients with affective disorders have hypo-frontality. Baxter *et al.* (1985) reported that bipolar depressed patients showed globally reduced metabolic rates, especially marked in all cortical areas, cingulate gyrus, caudate nucleus and thalamus. They identified a small number of rapid cycling patients in whom the metabolism increased in the hypomanic phases, and a subgroup with distinctly lower metabolic rates in the left lateral inferior frontal cortex. Similar results, especially with regards to the frontal cortex and the basal ganglia, have been reported by Buchsbaum *et al.* (1986).

Neurological data

It is clear that depression can be associated with a wide range of somatic illnesses, including endocrine disorders, malignancy, viral disorders, hepatic and pancreatic disease, electrolyte disorders and the collagenoses (Hall, 1980). Further, many people with chronic illness become despondent and demoralized. These states, often associated with some symptoms of a major depressive illness, are sometimes referred to as secondary depression or depressive reactions, but in most instances their phenomenology has not been well specified, and their response to conventional antidepressant treatments not evaluated. Again it is of importance to understand the definition of a depressive illness, and to differentiate it from understandable reactions to adverse circumstances, and human misery. Failure to do so leads to confusion over biological data collected in supposed major affective disorder and to unnecessary prescription of antidepressant drugs, which themselves carry morbidity.

Secondary mania, although rarer, has been noted with several CNS conditions, including postencephalitic states, Huntington's chorea, tumours, in epilepsy, following head injury and with cerebellar atrophy (Krauthammer and Klerman, 1978; Yadalam *et al.*, 1985). Euphoric mood changes were commonly described in GPI, and a 'eutonia' and empty euphoria accompanies the periventricular demyelination of multiple sclerosis.

A number of drugs may precipitate, provoke or exacerbate a depressive illness, and the role of reserpine in originally providing an insight for the biochemical theories has been mentioned. A short list of commonly used drugs associated with the condition is shown in Table 9; more extensive reviews are available (Whitlock and Evans, 1978; Hall, 1980).

Depressive illness is common with neurological disorders, and the literature has been reviewed elsewhere (Trimble, 1981a; Whitlock, 1982; Cummings, 1985). The association is more than just an accompaniment to chronic illness, and touches upon the biochemical and neuroanatomical underpinnings of affective expression. The conditions most considered are head injuries, cerebrovascular disease, epilepsy, multiple sclerosis and Parkinson's disease. Depressive symptoms in dementia are discussed in Chapter 11, and head injury and tumours in Chapter 6. It is germane to note that head injuries, often of a relatively trivial nature, may provoke depressive symptoms, often in the setting of a

Table 9   Some drugs commonly associated with affective disorders

Depression
  Alcohol
  Barbiturates
  Benzodiazepines
  Butyrophenones
  Digitalis
  Disulfiram
  Fenfluramine and appetite suppressants
  Methyl dopa
  Metronidazole
  Non-steroidal anti-inflammatory drugs
  Oral contraceptives
  Phenothiazines
  Propranolol and other beta blockers
  Reserpine

Mania
  Amphetamine and other stimulants
  Bromocriptine
  L-dopa
  MAOI antidepressants
  Steroids
  Tricylic antidepressants

post-traumatic neurosis. The contributions of neuronal, personality and psychosocial influences to the final picture have been discussed elsewhere (Trimble, 1981b).

With regard to tumours, meningiomas, especially frontal meningiomas, are notoriously liable to induce a picture of typical major depressive disorder (see Figure 5 in Chapter 5). Both temporal and frontal lobe tumours are likely to present with changes of affect, including euphoria, hypomanic-like features, lability, depression and irritability, with a tendency for this to be commoner with dominant hemisphere pathology (Lishman, 1978; Cummings, 1985). However, parietal and diencephalic tumours are also reported to lead to affective change, especially hypomanic swings with diencephalic lesions (Greenberg and Brown, 1985).

The association between basal ganglia disorders and depression is of particular interest. In Parkinson's disease some 30–60 per cent of patients have a depressive illness, not entirely due to the limitations of the chronic disability. Robins (1976) compared patients not on L-dopa to controls with physically disabling conditions using the Hamilton scale and reported the Parkinson's patients to have significantly higher depression scores, especially on items of suicide, work and interest, retardation, anxiety, somatic symptoms and loss of weight. Mindham et al. (1976) also reported a high incidence of affective symptoms in patients with Parkinson's disease, but in contrast to Robins found a correlation of depressive symptoms to severity of the motor impairment. However, he also noted that improvement in motor symptoms with treatment was not associated with corresponding improvements in mood, and that L-dopa may precipitate depression, especially in those with a prior history of affective disorder.

The association between basal ganglia dysfunction and affect has been explored more intimately by studying patients suffering from the 'on–off' phenomenon (Brown et al., 1984). In this condition, after treatment with L-dopa, the motor state fluctuates from normal to severe disability over short periods of time, thought to be related to fluctuations of dopamine activity in the basal ganglia. When the affective state was compared between on and off states, it was found that the latter was associated with a marked deterioration. Similar results have been reported with the 'end of the dose deterioration' phenomenon, temporary immobility being associated with adverse changes of mood (Cantello et al., 1986).

The depression associated with Parkinson's disease is often reported to occur prior to the onset of the motor disorder, responds to ECT, and has been associated with decreased CSF 5-HIAA levels (Mayeux *et al.*, 1984).

Huntington's chorea also often presents with disorders of affect, including psychotic depressive and hypomanic pictures. Again this can be dissociated from the motor disability, and may be seen prior to the onset or diagnosis of the chorea. Further, a high frequency of suicide is reported, even in those with no knowledge of their diagnosis. In a comparison of the frequency of major affective disorder in this condition and Alzheimer's disease, Mindham *et al.* (1985) reported that the Huntington's disease patients showed twice the incidence, emphasizing some special relationship, as opposed to the depressive symptoms merely being a prodrome to the dementia.

Other basal ganglia disorders associated with affective change, either depressive or euphoric, include Wilson's disease, Sydenham's chorea and the blepharospasm–oromandibular–dystonia syndrome (Bruegel's or Meige's syndrome) (Trimble, 1981a).

Cerebrovascular accidents (CVA) regularly leave neuropsychiatric sequelae, and depression is common. A controlled study in comparison with similarly disabled orthopaedic controls revealed a significantly higher level of depression in the CVA patients (50 per cent as against 13 per cent for controls), suggesting the mood change is not a simple reaction to disability (Folstein *et al.*, 1977).

In a series of studies, Robinson and colleagues have explored this, using CT evaluation of lesion extent and site (Robinson and Szetela, 1981; Robinson *et al.*, 1984). Of 103 cases of CVA they noted 27 per cent to have a major depressive disorder and 20 per cent a dysthymic disorder. They found that location in the dominant hemisphere, and the nearer the lesion to the frontal pole, the more severe the depression. In the non-dominant hemisphere, the further away from the frontal pole the higher the frequency of the depression. There was no association with aphasia, although others have noted depression to be more prevalent in association with Broca's aphasia (Benson, 1979). In a six month follow-up, the major depressive disorder persisted in the majority, and others developed a new depressive syndrome. The correlation to the left frontal pole persisted. A similar relationship was confirmed in a series of only left-handed patients and in brain-injured non-stroke patients. They speculated on the possible reasons for the association of lesion site to severity of depression, citing their own animal work. They produced experimental stroke lesions in rats and noted greater postlesion decline in catecholamine levels with anterior as opposed to posterior cortical lesions. They suggested that a frontal lesion interrupts more arborizing monoamine projection pathways than does a posterior lesion, leading to greater destruction of axones and more catecholamine depletion.

Patients with affective disorder have been examined for clinical neurological abnormalities. Generally these are noted with a lower frequency than in schizophrenia, and no specific pattern emerges (Manschreck and Ames, 1984).

Neuropsychological disturbances in affective disorder

There is no doubt that a marked cognitive impairment can accompany depressive illness, and that complaints of poor memory, impaired concentration and difficulty with planning, decision making and abstracting abilities by patients are common. The term pseudodementia has been used to specify this (Wells, 1979; Caine, 1981). It can be argued that this state is better referred to as one of 'reversible dementia', and categorized as a subcortical dementia (see Chapter 11).

The presentation can so resemble dementia that many patients are misdiagnosed as having Alzheimer's disease, and left untreated. The importance of the recognition of pseudodementia is that it is a reversible state of cognitive decline, and improves in association with improvement of the depressive illness.

Although there are other causes of pseudodementia, which include hypomania, hysteria and schizophrenia (Trimble, 1981a), that associated with depression is the commonest, and some degree of cognitive impairment is found in most cases. Important clues to help distinguish it from dementia include a past history of affective disorder; the relatively acute onset, with little evidence of decline prior to the development of affective symptoms; the patient's distress and complaints about cognitive function (as opposed to the lack of insight often seen in dementia); the response to questions in the mental state examination (patients often using 'don't know' as an answer, whereas in dementia the answers are more evasive, skirting the correct but lost answer); and the performance on more structured psychological tasks which do not reveal the focal deficits of Alzheimer's disease and produce patchy inconsistent impairment.

Pseudodementia is one of the most frequent problems leading to an inappropriate diagnosis of dementia, and follow-up studies of patients with dementia often reveal a subgroup that has not declined or has even improved over time. In retrospect, depressive illness is then often diagnosed (Marsden and Harrison, 1972; Ron et al., 1979).

In addition to the clinical features, CT and EEG evaluation are essential, both often being within normal limits. However, since a subgroup of patients with depressive illness has cerebral atrophy, confusion will occur if only CT data are taken in isolation.

There is no clear pattern of cognitive impairment that emerges, but often the patients' subjective complaints are worse than their performance on objective tests. When patients with depressive illness are compared with controls on cognitive test batteries they tend to show impairments of attention, lack of speed in mental processing, poor attention to detail (Caine, 1981), difficulty in abstraction and memory difficulties, especially on tasks that require effort, motivation and active processing.

There is some suggestion of more non-dominant hemisphere dysfunction, with greater impairment of performance as opposed to verbal abilities, especially for spatial information (Weingartner and Silberman, 1985). Although not entirely consistent, the literature from investigations adopting different testing strategies does suggest predominantly non-dominant frontotemporal dysfunction in depressive illness (Taylor and Abrams, 1984; Flor-Henry, 1983). These impairments seem greater with more severe depression, and improve with treatment and clinical response of the depression.

SOME OUTSTANDING ISSUES

It seems clear that much biological information about the affective disorders has been accumulated in recent years. Although there are many conflicting data, there is also a growing body of consistency, and some of the earlier difficulties have been overcome by improved technology, better patient selection and clarification of hypotheses to be tested. However, new problems have arisen with the wealth of investigations now available to the investigator, and the complexities of interpreting empirically derived data, often collected without reference to any clear underlying hypothesis.

Classification is still quite unsatisfactory, and continues to be a potential source of data conflict. Although the DSM III has provided a reasonable attempt to unify the researchers' ideals, it fails, perhaps in the sense of being too broad for identifying truely homogeneous groups. The loss of the reactive–endogenous dichotomy is welcomed, not only because of the inconsistency and confusion surrounding the word reactive, but because it has falsely assumed a classification based on aetiology. Unlike the original scheme of Mobius, in which endogenous was contrasted with exogenous, on grounds of causation, the evidence that depressions are somehow either provoked by external circumstances or are the result of a mysterious internal process does not stand up. There are many studies employing life event methodology which show that antecedent life events do not predict clinical pattern (Paykel and Hollyman, 1984), although the fact that human adversity may lead to depressive symptoms hardly requires scientific validation. The important question is why some people develop a depressive illness, and what are the constitutional, neurophysiological and neurochemical correlates of vulnerability and presentation.

Most authors seem to identify a core of patients that suggests a biological syndrome, and in the past the term endogenous has been used to describe them. DSM III major depression is a substitute, and the reintroduction of the word melancholia is welcomed for a most severe form. The relationship to bipolar disorder depression still requires clarification. While clinically they are identical in phenomenology, there may be important biological differences. Further, the filiation with dysthymic disorder should be questioned. The important confusion that continually arises when mood changes based primarily on underlying personality disorders are confused with depressive illness has already been discussed.

The relative lack of data in mania is immediately obvious. This stems in part from the fact that it is less common, and manic patients, because of their clinical state, are often poor research subjects. Much information is hidden under bipolar disorder, patients occasionally being examined in both a depressed and a manic phase. The main hypotheses tested, as in depressive illness, relate to the various monoamine hypotheses.

The initial monoamine theories were simple, depression relating to a deficit of catecholamine or 5-HT activity or turnover. In the United Kingdom the data have concentrated more on the latter, while in the United States it is the catecholamine hypothesis that became predominant. As shown in Table 10, evidence reviewed in this chapter provides support for the involvement of both transmitters, but this is hardly surprising. Few would uphold any suggestion that neurotransmitters act in isolation, and the various feedback and regulatory events that exist between them, now including the neuromodulators, are gradually being unravelled.

Schildkraut and Kety's (1967) original hypothesis was that some or all depression was associated with 'a relative deficiency of noradrenaline at functionally important adrenergic receptor sites in the brain, whereas elations may be associated with an excess of such amines' (p.8). Maas went on to suggest two types of depression, A and B, the former having disordered noradrenaline and the latter abnormal 5-HT systems. Another catecholamine, dopamine, has also been involved, although there has been less enthusiasm to develop a 'dopamine hypothesis'. After careful consideration of all the data, van Praag (1980b) concluded that dopamine deficiency characterizes vital depressions, and was linked to the motor features of the illness. This is consistent with the observed associations with Parkinson's disease, common neurotransmitter abnormalities being implicated in both conditions. He further accepted that 'within the group of vital depressive patients with central monoamine disorders, it is either the

Table 10 Evidence for the serotonin and catecholamine hypotheses

	5-HT	Noradrenaline
Precursor drug studies	+	−
Reversal by inhibitors	+	*
Chemistry of antidepressants	+	+
Selective uptake inhibitors	+	+
Plasma precursors	?	+
Platelet studies	+	?
Urine studies	*	+
Hormone release studies	*	+
CSF data	+	−
Post-mortem studies	+	−
Association with neurology	+	+

+ = reasonable supportive evidence
− = little supportive evidence
* = inadequate or no data

5-HT system or the noradrenaline system that is predominantly disturbed' (p.51).

Others have speculated on the role of catecholamines in relation to brain reward systems, deficiencies thus leading to lack of pleasure, the clinical counterpart being anhedonia, or have invoked animal evidence that links learned helplessness, an animal model of depression, to catecholamine systems (Willner, 1983).

Van Praag (1980a, 1985) has also considered in detail the role of 5-HT. He pointed out the substantial evidence for at least a subgroup of patients having a 5-HT deficiency syndrome that seems to persist when the depressive illness has abated. It is thus a trait factor, linked to susceptibility to develop depression and with poor control over aggression. The 5-HT deficiencies are unlikely to be secondary to increased sensitivity of the postsynaptic 5-HT receptor. First, the precursor loading studies with increased 5-HT function alleviate depressive symptoms, and secondly, the limited binding studies of brain or platelets do not support the hypothesis.

Other transmitter hypotheses have been put forward. The 'permissive amine hypothesis', originally suggested by Prange *et al.* (1974), stated that central 5-HT deficiency related to a vulnerability to affective illness, and lowered catecholamines correlated with depression raised values with mania. Cholinergic mechanisms have been implicated (Janowsky *et al.*, 1980), and a cholinergic–adrenergic imbalance suggested. Depression was seen as a state of cholinergic dominance, mania one of adrenergic excess. The evidence for involvement of the cholinergic system at present is very limited, being mainly of an indirect nature from the effects of drugs that influence the choline system and mood.

Recently attention has shifted from interest in neurotransmitter levels and turnover to the role of receptors, both pre- and postsynaptic. The investigations of Sulser (1984) revealed that nearly all treatments effective in depressive illness lead to decreased activity ('down-regulation') of the postsynaptic noradrenergic receptor. This applies to antidepressant drugs and relates to the adenylate cyclase linked beta receptor. This down-regulation is dependent on an intact presynaptic serotonergic neuronal input, and can be reversed by 5-HT depletion. Further, the time course of these effects correlates better with the known clinical effects of antidepressants, emerging over days rather than acutely. Much of the receptor binding and neurohormonal data reviewed above has been aimed at testing hypotheses relating to alteration of monoamine receptor activity in depressive illness. At the present time interpretation is difficult. The blunted growth hormone responses, especially to clonidine, support decreased alpha-2 noradrenergic receptor activity (the growth hormone effect is probably mainly mediated by postsynaptic hypothalamic receptors), which could be accounted for by increased presynaptic noradrenergic output but decreased efficiency of the noradrenergic system. The decreased receptor sensitivity may explain some of the other neurohormonal findings, including the abnormalities of cortisol and failure to suppress with dexamethasone. However, the way in which different receptors may interact, the primacy of any changes, in other words whether a receptor modification succeeds or leads to synaptic changes of neurotransmitter activity, and the whole area of linking more traditional monoamine hypotheses to receptor theories are unresolved.

Laterality has been discussed in relation to affective disorder, as it has for schizophrenia. Generally the evidence is less convincing, but important observations have been made. Flor-Henry (1983), starting from his own observations that patients with psychosis and epilepsy awaiting temporal lobectomy are more likely to have a manic depressive picture if they have a non-dominant hemisphere focus, has persistently argued for a role of that hemisphere in the regulation of mood. The most persuasive data come from the EEG and psychometry studies of patients with depressive illness, but some observations of patients with CVA affecting either one or the other hemisphere (Gainotti, 1972), studies of split-brain patients, and direction of gaze in response to stimuli (to the left in affective disorder in contrast to the right in schizophrenia, the direction implying activation of the opposite hemisphere; Myslobodsky *et al.*, 1979) have all been used to support the concept. Certainly the proposition that the non-dominant hemisphere in health is concerned with emotional behaviour is convincing (Bear, 1986a), and its link to affective disorders is thus a reasonable postulate. However, not all findings support this, especially the recent data on CVA and further studies in epilepsy (see p.304).

CHAPTER 10

Epilepsy

INTRODUCTION

The longstanding relationship between epilepsy and psychiatry has already been discussed in the introductory chapter. The links have been explored by a number of authors (Temkin, 1971; Hill, 1981) and stem back to at least the ancient Greek tradition. Although the modern era may be said to begin with the introduction of the EEG into clinical practice and the work of, for example, Gibbs (1951), it should be recalled that the nineteenth century physicians classified epilepsy as a neurosis and introduced the concept of epileptic equivalents, or masked epilepsy, namely the idea that epilepsy could manifest in forms other than pure seizures. Kraepelin (1923) recognized three major categories of insanity, one of which was epileptic insanity (Blumer, 1984). He further emphasized intellectual and personality changes which may be noted in patients with epilepsy, a source of much discussion today (see below).

Guerrant *et al.* (1962) have suggested that concepts regarding the relationship between epilepsy and psychiatry may be divided into four periods as shown in Table 1.

The late nineteenth century view, associated with the concept of hereditary degeneration, assumed that patients with epilepsy would automatically show personality change and deterioration. A modern version is that only patients with psychomotor seizures, and hence temporal lobe epilepsy, are susceptible to such changes. This view is contrasted with the position of others who would support the concept that patients with epilepsy do not develop any

Table 1   Recent periods of history relating epilepsy to psychiatry (after Guerrant *et al.*, 1962)

1. Period of epileptic deterioration	−1900
2. Period of epileptic character	1900–1930
3. Period of normality	1930–
4. Period of psychomotor peculiarity	1930–

psychopathology, except that brought about by structural brain damage, uncontrolled seizures, anticonvulsant medications or psychosocial stigma.

It is only in this century that chronic epilepsy has become more the province of neurology than psychiatry. The large psychiatric hospitals in the last century contained many patients with obvious neurological disease and epilepsy was particularly common. The efficacy of anticonvulsant medication and the introduction of the EEG have markedly influenced the diagnosis and management of epilepsy over time, and now the more extreme psychiatric manifestations are seen in a smaller proportion of patients.

There are four reasons why psychiatrists need to know about epilepsy and its complications. First, the history of its association with psychiatry emphasizes the changing nature of ideas with regards to neuropsychiatric conditions, both as to their supposed pathogenesis and their psychopathological manifestations. Secondly, in any psychiatric setting, patients with epilepsy, particularly chronic epilepsy with continuing uncontrolled seizures, are still seen. Thirdly, some forms of epilepsy, particularly temporal lobe epilepsy, are associated with cognitive and emotional sequelae which closely resemble psychopathology seen in non-epileptic patients. Finally, virtually all drugs used in the management of epilepsy have also been used to treat psychopathology, for example the bromides, barbiturates, benzodiazepines, and more recently carbamazepine.

CLASSIFICATION, PREVALENCE AND CLINICAL CHARACTERISTICS

Defining epilepsy is, as with schizophrenia, difficult. The often-quoted definition of Jackson (Taylor, 1958), of 'occasional, sudden, rapid and local discharges of grey matter' (p.100), emphasizes the acute paroxysmal nature of the disorder, but fails to distinguish it from other similar disorders such as migraine or acute panic attacks. While it is accepted that the cardinal clinical symptom of epilepsy is the seizure, and it is usual to accept that epilepsy requires recurrent seizures as opposed to a single seizure before the diagnosis can be made, it has to be emphasized that epilepsy refers to a heterogeneous group of conditions, and, like schizophrenia, clear evidence for organic brain dysfunction becomes evident the more it is looked for. However, in a number of cases, even with modern technology, recurrent seizures are found in the absence of identifiable neuropathology.

CLASSIFICATION

It is important to distinguish the classification of seizures from that of epilepsy. Recently, several classifications of seizures have emerged, an abbreviated version of the latest one being shown in Table 2.

Partial seizures are those in which the clinical and EEG changes suggest a focal onset, and the classification is based mainly on whether or not consciousness is impaired in the attack. In a simple partial seizure, consciousness is retained. Various forms are recognized, for example focal motor seizures (when accompanied by a march are referred to as Jacksonian); with somatosensory or special sensory symptoms; with autonomic symptoms; or associated with psychic symptoms such as dysphasia, dysmnesia (for example déjà vu), cognitive, affective, illusory or hallucinatory experiences. In general, this last group of symptoms is usually accompanied by impairment of consciousness, and therefore is often associated with complex partial seizures. In these, the impairment of consciousness is often the first clinical sign, although simple partial seizures may evolve into the complex variety. In patients presenting to psychiatric clinics, complex partial seizures are the commonest seizure type, and they usually, but not inevitably, give a history of progression to generalized motor seizures on occasions.

Table 2   Revised ILAE classification of epileptic seizures (1981)

 I   Partial (focal, local) seizures
   A   Simple partial seizures (consciousness not impaired)
   B   Complex partial seizures (with impairment of consciousness; may sometimes begin with simple symptomatology)
   C   Partial seizures evolving to secondarily generalized seizures (this may be generalized tonic–clonic, tonic or clonic)

 II   Generalized seizures (convulsive or non-convulsive)

III   Unclassified epileptic seizures

Generalized seizures are those in which the first clinical changes suggest bilateral abnormalities with widespread disturbances of both hemispheres. Absence seizures (petit mal) are usually associated with regular 3 Hz per second spike and slow wave activity on the EEG, although variants of this with 2–3 Hz activity may be seen. Myoclonic seizures typically present with myoclonic jerking, and these are sometimes associated with clearly delineated EEG changes. Tonic–clonic seizures are the classical grand mal attacks with associated EEG abnormalities.

Finally, seizures that cannot be classified into the above groupings are included as unclassified seizures.

It should be noted that in this classification the term complex has been altered from earlier classifications. In the 1969 version, complex had been used to refer to alteration of higher cortical function and had some neuroanatomical logic, in the sense of implying altered function to the integrative cortices of the brain.

Classic tonic–clonic seizures are unmistakable. There is sudden loss of consciousness, often without warning, and tonic muscular contractions are followed by clonic ones. The patient falls to ground, during which time self-injury may occur and tongue biting or urinary incontinence may be noted. Following the attack, the patient is unrousable for a time, and there follows a period of postictal confusion. If the attack has a focal origin prior to its generalization, then the patient may experience an aura, namely a brief feeling or sensation immediately before the attack, which represents the origin of the epileptic activity. These auras need to be distinguished from prodomata, which occur several hours or even days before a seizure, and serve to warn the patient about a forthcoming seizure. Prodromal symptoms are often changes of mood, but may also be headaches or changes of appetite.

Generalized seizures that present as absence attacks impair consciousness briefly and are virtually unaccompanied by motor signs. They occur primarily in children and in many cases cease before the age of 20, although in about 50 per cent of patients this form of seizure is replaced by generalized tonic–clonic seizures. In the generalized absence seizure there is sudden arrest of attention, some blinking and eye fluttering and perhaps pallor with subsequent amnesia.

The symptoms of focal attacks correspond to the site of origin of abnormal electrical activity, the commonest disturbances seen in psychiatric practice relating to a temporal lobe location. There may be disturbance of thought, perception, behaviour, affect and, in complex partial attacks, consciousness. Hallucinations may be formed and complex, as opposed to those that arise from seizures of primary sensory cortex which are usually simple, for example a flash of light. Characteristically in epilepsy the hallucination is constant and with repeated episodes is carefully reproduced. Any recognized emotion may occur, although the commonest experience is fear, which is intense, and is often associated with a fear of death. Depression is uncommon, but well documented (Robertson and Trimble, 1983), although rage and outbursts of anger are rare. Cursive seizures refer to running during attacks; gelastic seizures are laughing attacks. In uncinate seizures, the patient experiences an unpleasant smell or taste and this may be accompanied by chewing movements and lip smacking.

Automatisms, which may occur with partial or generalized seizures, refer to 'all kinds of doings after epileptic fits, from slight vagaries up to homicidal actions' (Jackson, see Taylor, 1958, Vol. 1, p.122). Characteristically, the motor activity is automatic and occurs during a state of altered consciousness, for which time there is amnesia. Automatisms may either be perseverative, in which patients continue actions they were involved in prior to the attack, or they may herald the initiative of a completely new behavioural sequence. During automatisms, which generally last less than 15 minutes, patients carry out complex quasi-purposeful behaviour; violence is unusual, but, if the patient is interfered with during the automatism, aggression may result. The neurophysiological basis for automatisms is thought to be bilateral involvement of the amygdaloid–hippocampal region (Fenton, 1972).

Myoclonic seizures are sudden, brief jerk-like contractions which may be generalized or confined to one or more muscle groups. They may be solitary or repetitive, and may be triggered by action. They commonly occur late at night or early in the morning, and in some people herald a generalized tonic–clonic seizure.

Status epilepticus denotes recurrent epileptic seizures without return of consciousness between attacks. Persistent focal seizures are referred to as epilepsia partialis continua, and when complex partial seizures are continuous (complex partial seizure status), prolonged states of behaviour disturbance may be seen. These occur with detectable but minimal alteration of higher cognitive function, and associated hallucinations and delusions may closely resemble those of schizophrenia. In contrast, during absence status, prolonged alteration of cognitive function occurs with intermittent prolonged stupor. Occasionally it may present as a psychotic illness, with hallucinations and delusions, intermingled with a fluctuating confusional state and associated EEG changes.

Although approximately one in twenty people may have a seizure during their lifetime, the prevalence of epilepsy is far less, being around 0.5 per cent for the general population. A provisional classification of the epilepsies has recently been published (ILAE, 1985). This is essentially a classification of syndromes rather than diseases, and, rather as with classification in psychiatry, the concensus of opinion as to the most appropriate way to classify epilepsies has yet to be reached. An abbreviated version of the classification of epilepsies is shown in Table 3.

Terms found in earlier versions such as primary and secondary have been omitted and the main dichotomy separates epilepsies with generalized seizures from those with partial or focal seizures, the latter being referred to as localization related partial or focal epilepsies. Of particular relevance for psychiatrists are the localization related symptomatic seizures, further designated by the area of localization affected. For example, frontal lobe epilepsies often present as brief episodes of behavioural change with minimal or no postictal confusion. There may be deviation of the head and

Table 3 Classification of epilepsies (ILAE, 1985)

---

1. Localization related (focal, local, partial) epilepsies and syndromes
   Idiopathic with age-related onset (e.g. benign epilepsy of childhood)
   Symptomatic, e.g. frontal lobe, temporal lobe

2. Generalized epilepsies or syndromes
   Idiopathic
   Idiopathic and/or symptomatic (e.g. West's syndrome)
   Symptomatic

3. Epilepsies and syndromes undetermined as to whether they are focal or generalized

4. Special syndromes (e.g. febrile convulsions)

---

eyes, sometimes referred to as an adversive seizure. Under temporal lobe epilepsies there is a category of limbic epilepsies, with particular emphasis on hippocampal and amygdala pathology. These epilepsies characteristically present with partial seizures, alteration of consciousness and often automatisms.

Some distinctive syndromes are included in the classification of epilepsies. West's syndrome (infantile spasms) consists of a characteristic picture of infantile spasms in association with hypsarrhythmia on the EEG. The onset is in the first year of life, and the spasms are flexor or extensor or both. Males are affected more commonly than females, and a symptomatic subgroup is recognized with clear evidence of preexisting brain damage. The Lennox–Gastaut syndrome occurs in children up to the age of about eight and presents with a variety of seizures, focal, myoclonic, atonic and absence, with a markedly disturbed EEG and associated mental retardation.

Benign childhood epilepsy is a syndrome that affects children between three and sixteen years of age. It has a good prognosis, and presents with simple partial seizures, which may or may not lead to secondary generalized attacks, and an EEG with characteristic centrotemporal spikes.

The prognosis of epilepsy is dependent upon the aetiology, the age of onset of the condition and the setting in which outcome is examined. If children are followed into adulthood, some one-third will be seen to have considerable epilepsy-related problems (Harrison and Taylor, 1976). The mortality is approximately 10 per cent, a further 10 per cent requiring institutional care, either in mental handicap or psychiatric hospitals. Continuing seizures occur in some 25 per cent of survivors, and only half of these patients are self-supporting in the community. For newly referred adult patients, successful treatment will abolish seizures in over 70 per cent of patients, although the remainder have continuing seizures. The most striking association with failure of treatment to control the attacks is the presence of additional neurological or psychiatric illness (Shorvon and Reynolds, 1982). In particular, patients with combined partial and generalized seizures and those with symptomatic epilepsy show a poor prognosis.

Why patients have seizures when they do is not clear, although 'reflex epilepsy', where seizures are provoked by sensory or motor events, has been described (Fenwick, 1981). Visually evoked seizures, by photic stimulation, and musicogenic seizures, in which attacks are triggered by patterned tones, are well-known examples. 'Psychogenic seizures', where seizures are evoked by specific mental activity, also occur. Fenwick (1981) divides these into primary and secondary types. In the former, a direct act of will precipitates seizures, for example intense concentration or sudden alteration of attention. In secondary psychogenic seizures, there is precipitation by a mental act without the deliberate intention of the patient. Examples include attacks brought on by mental arithmetic.

GENETIC CONSIDERATIONS

The division of epilepsy into idiopathic and symptomatic groups recognizes that in many patients there is no known or suspected aetiology other than potential hereditary disposition. It has been shown that there is an increased incidence of seizures in siblings of epileptic patients (6–12 per cent) (Andermann, 1980), and the concordance rate for monozygotic (12–100 per cent) is higher than for dizygotic (0–35 per cent) twins (Newmark and Penry, 1980). Further, an abnormal EEG is common in close relatives of epileptic patients, particularly showing generalized spike and wave discharges (Newmark and Penry, 1980).

The hereditability of epilepsy depends to a considerable extent on the seizure type of the proband, being greatest for generalized seizure disorders and least for partial and symptomatic seizures. However, most studies suggest a slight increase in positive family histories of patients with symptomatic seizures, emphasizing an environmental–genetic interaction.

Of particular interest has been the discovery of a specific pathological lesion, namely mesial temporal sclerosis, in some patients who have simple and complex partial seizures. It is often unilateral, and specifically there is sclerosis of the hippocampus and related structures of the temporal lobe, with neuronal loss and increased glial elements. Many patients who develop this have a history of febrile convulsions in childhood, and similar lesions can be produced in primates by experimentally provoking seizures (Meldrum, 1976). It has been suggested that the pathology represents damage to the temporal lobe which occurs secondary to anoxic episodes at vulnerable periods during life. Since children with febrile convulsions are likely to have a positive family history for epilepsy (Newmark and Penry, 1980), it seems they inherit a lowered seizure threshold. This renders them prone to febrile convulsions and to the resulting structural damage. The latter then leads to an even greater chance of the development of complex partial seizures in adult life, emphasizing the complexities of environmental and genetic interactions in these conditions.

HLA studies have so far been inconsistent, and both autosomal dominant and polygenic inheritance models are compatible with the genetic data (Andermann, 1980).

SYMPTOMATIC EPILEPSY

Some of the underlying pathologies and metabolic defects related to seizures and epilepsy are outlined in Table 4.

There is variation with age. Neonatal seizures may be caused by prenatal events such as cerebral malformations, rubella embryopathy, toxoplasmosis and perinatal birth damage from hypoxia or trauma. Postnatal events include metabolic changes such as hypoglycaemia, hypocalcaemia, hypomagnesaemia, infections such as meningitis, and a number of inborn errors of metabolism which become expressed early in life.

Early childhood epilepsy (starting around the age of three) is more likely to be idiopathic, while in adult life, tumours and

Table 4 Some causes of epilepsy (from Trimble, 1981a, p.169)

Metabolic causes:	Hypoglycaemia, hypomagnesaemia, fluid and electrolyte disturbances, acute intermittent porphyria, amino acid disorders
Trauma:	Head injuries, especially penetrating wounds and birth injuries
Neurological causes:	Tumours, cerebrovascular accidents, degenerative and storage disorders, demyelinating diseases, Sturge–Weber and other malformations, tuberose sclerosis; infections, e.g. cytomegalovirus, toxoplamosis, meningitis, cysticercosis, syphilis
Drug withdrawal:	Especially alcohol and the barbiturates
Vitamin deficiency:	Pyridoxine
Poisons:	Lead, strychnine
Temperature:	Fever

cerebrovascular disease become prominent causes. Head injury is a common cause at any age, and is most likely to be responsible if the dura is penetrated or if the injury produces coma and a post-traumatic amnesia of more than 24 hours. Early seizures following injury increase the probability of the later development of epilepsy (Jennett, 1975), and the usual pattern is of focal or secondary generalized attacks. Fifty per cent of patients who develop post-traumatic epilepsy have their first attack within 12 months of injury, although in some patients onset is delayed for several years. Genetic factors may be important here, but evolving neurophysiological and neurochemical events are presumably also involved. This model has relevance for schizophrenia, where the interaction of genetic and early environmental insults does not necessarily lead to the expression of the clinical condition for a number of years.

Kindling is a phenomenon in which repeated subthreshold electrical stimulation leads to the subsequent development of seizure activity, and has been well demonstrated in animal models. The underlying neurophysiological change related to the kindling process is not clear (Racine and McIntyre, 1986), although it leads to a permanent increase in epileptogenicity within the brain. Kindling is most readily produced from limbic system structures, in particular the amygdala and hippocampus. Although the relevance for human epilepsy is not clear, the kindling phenomenon may well help explain such important biological phenomena as memory, and in addition be related to neuronal changes that underlie behavioural patterns seen in various psychiatric illnesses where acceleration of the disease process appears to occur with each succeeding bout of illness.

BIOCHEMICAL FINDINGS

In contrast to affective disorder and schizophrenia, there have been relatively few clinical investigations relating to the biochemical underpinnings of the epileptic process. Experimental investigations have concentrated on alterations of monamine and acetylcholine activity, while more recently GABA and the excitatory amino acids such as glutamate and aspartate have attracted attention.

In general, catecholamine agonists raise the seizure threshold, while antagonists lower it (Trimble and Meldrum, 1979). In particular, drugs such as chlorpromazine may precipitate seizures, although dopamine agonists such as apomorphine are not therapeutically valuable. A number of anticonvulsant drugs increase CNS 5-HT levels experimentally, although data from patients are variable, reflecting either an increase, no change, or a decrease of activity (Reynolds, 1981). The evidence for the role of GABA is more substantial, although it largely derives from animal studies. Some anticonvulsants such as sodium valproate are GABA agonists, and the benzodiazepines interact with GABA receptors, explaining some of their antiepileptic properties. Both glutamate and aspartate provoke excitatory neuronal activity and they can be inhibited by certain anticonvulsants (Chapman *et al.*, 1983). Recent evidence has suggested that these amino acids may be endogenous neurotoxins, increased release of which may provoke neuronal damage. The relevance of this for both the development of an epileptic focus and progressive neuronal damage in recurrent seizures has yet to be established.

INVESTIGATION AND DIFFERENTIAL DIAGNOSIS

Following history taking and neurological examination, it is customary to request routine haematology and electrolytes, also estimating calcium and serology. A plain skull X-ray is requested infrequently these days and the technique of choice is the CT scan. An EEG is very helpful, not only to help further with diagnosis, but to form a baseline for any future investigations.

Any suggestion from clinical examination or the EEG that the seizures are focal should alert the clinician to the possibility of an intracranial lesion being present, and CT scanning for such patients is mandatory. The finding of intracranial pathology will obviously require further investigation under the appropriate specialist, using more sophisticated radiological techniques.

Where there is doubt about the epileptic nature of the seizures, the possibility of non-epileptic (pseudo)seizures arises. Further psychiatric exploration will become necessary to rule out psychopathology, and possibly admission to a specialized unit where prolonged observation with videotelemetry or ambulatory monitoring can be carried out.

With careful neuropsychiatric investigations it is possible to reach a diagnostic conclusion in the majority of patients who present difficulties. However, there are patients, especially amongst those seen at special referral centres, where diagnosis is difficult and where a primary psychiatric diagnosis is most likely.

Current estimates suggest that up to 20 per cent of patients in a chronic epilepsy clinic and diagnosed as epileptic suffer from alternative conditions.

PSEUDO-SEIZURES

The term itself is problematic. The seizures are real, both to the patients and the observing physician, but they do not have an epileptic origin. A preferred term is non-epileptic seizures, which is less pejorative than either pseudo or hysterical seizures. Although some patients with epilepsy have non-epileptic seizures, the majority of patients with the latter are not epileptic patients. The diagnosis rests on good clinical descriptions of the attacks and good history taking. Patients with non-epileptic seizures are more likely to have a family or past history of psychiatric illness, to demonstrate current affective disorder on examination, to be sexually immature and to have attempted suicide more than epileptic controls (Roy, 1977).

The attacks themselves may have a dramatic quality, and in many cases are obviously dissimilar from epileptic seizures. However, some attacks resemble almost entirely epileptic attacks, and in these patients, even ambulatory monitoring and video telemetry may be unhelpful, particularly if the EEG record is obscured by muscle artifact during the attack.

Prolactin levels may be helpful taken 15–20 minutes after the episode. In the majority of patients with epilepsy, particularly generalized tonic–clonic seizures, a marked postical rise of this hormone is seen, in contrast to patients with non-epileptic seizures (Trimble, 1978a).

Diagnosis should include not only negative neurological criteria but positive signs and symptoms. The history may thus reveal other episodes suggestive of conversion phenomena or a personality disorder with a propensity to seek medical help. Some patients will be found who have histories of several surgical interventions, and whose complaints, when carefully probed, all seem to indicate episodes of abnormal illness behaviour. The most florid form of this is Briquet's hysteria, a condition which characteristically affects females, who are polysymptomatic, and give a history of an excessive number of hospitalizations, vague complaints, surgical operations and gynaecological problems (DSM III somatization disorder).

While it may be possible to detect secondary gain in patients with non-epileptic seizures, this may only become apparent later in the course of the illness, and at best is only based on a value judgement of the investigating physician. The diagnosis of non-epileptic seizures should never be based solely on the assumption of a secondary gain.

Of the positive neurological criteria, the presence of hemi-anaesthesia or clearly defined anaesthetic patches is relevant. Interestingly, these have been described in hysteria for over a hundred years. As noted, they are more commonly found on the left side of the body, and may be associated with other stigmata of hysteria, such as constriction of the visual fields and occasionally contractures (Trimble, 1981c).

Other conditions to be considered in the differential diagnosis are panic attacks, rage attacks, fugue states and syncope. With panic attacks, the onset is often more gradual, with a growing dysphoria, and after the episode, which usually terminates slowly, feelings of apprehension still exist. Some patients present with phobic anxiety and depersonalization, the episodes often appearing suddenly without precipitating events. The depersonalization in particular may suggest a simple partial seizure, and associated clinical features such as déjà vu and perceptual disorders may further confuse the diagnosis. In one study (Harper and Roth, 1962), a phobic group were distinguished from a control epileptic group by being somewhat older, their first attack often being related to a traumatic experience, particularly bereavement. Depersonalization in the phobic patients was often associated with fear, and was never associated with aphasia or evidence of clouding of consciousness. Déjà vu and jamais vu were equally common in the two groups, although in epileptic patients the experience was more vivid, and in the phobic anxiety–depersonalization syndrome it continued for long periods of time. The attacks themselves occurred with greater frequency in the neurotic patients, and while they were as abrupt in onset as epileptic seizures, they tended to terminate more slowly. Mild or non-specific abnormalities of the EEG, particularly over the temporal regions, were not of value in differentiating the two groups.

Rage attacks, as ictal events, are rare, but aggression may occur postictally. The issue of episodic dyscontrol is discussed below. Fugue states are prolonged episodes of amnesia associated with wandering, which may be seen with a variety of psychopathologies, particularly depression. The amnesia lasts hours, weeks or occasionally years, but the patient remains in contact with his environment, being able to manipulate it successfully.

Additional conditions that cause non-epileptic attacks are syncope, particularly vasovagal syncope, migraine, especially basilar artery migraine, vertebrobasilar ischaemic attacks, especially in the elderly, transient ischaemic attacks, hypoglycaemia and sleep disorders such as narcolepsy and cataplexy.

Although 'borderlands of epilepsy' have been recognized for years, it was Gowers (1907) who clearly formulated the idea, and included vasovagal attacks, vertigo and migraine within the boundaries. The area continues to attract attention (Trimble and Reynolds, 1986), especially the overlap with psychiatric disorders such as aggression and the psychoses. Recently, the finding that carbamazepine has mood stabilizing properties has led to attempts to compare the paroxysmal symptoms of patients with simple and complex partial seizures to those of the affective disorders and no known epilepsy (Post and Uhde, 1986). It has been found that psychosensory and psychomotor (paraepileptoid) symptoms are commonly reported by psychiatric patients, considerably more so than in control groups, for example with hypertension.

PSYCHIATRIC DISORDERS IN EPILEPSY

Classification

It is logical to classify the psychiatric disorders of epilepsy in relation to the seizure itself. Ictal (peri-ictal) disorders are directly related to the seizure, while interictal disorders are unrelated in time to the seizure. A third category, discussed by Pond (1957), is of disorders which, due to brain disease, lead to both seizures and psychiatric illness. In this would be included many causes of mental handicap, and some epileptic syndromes such as those of West and Lennox-Gastaut. It would also cover organic mental disorders such as autism and the disintegrative psychosis of childhood, and cerebrovascular disease and Alzheimer's disease in adults.

Ictally related psychiatric disorders

No one doubts that acute disruption of cerebral activity, as occurs with the electrical events of the seizure, may disturb cortical function sufficiently to provoke acute psychiatric syndromes. Many of the manifestations of simple and complex partial seizures outlined above are psychological symptoms which, in other settings, would clearly be described as psychopathology. In addition, prodromal symptoms, predominantly affective, and the psychiatric presentations of both generalized absence and complex partial seizure status are included in this category.

Postictal disorders occur immediately following the seizures when there is usually still disruption of the EEG, mainly with diffuse slow frequencies and little normal activity. Patients present with a variety of behavioural syndromes, the underpinnings of which are clearly defined confusional states. These are short-lived, but occasionally persist for days or even weeks, and when long-lasting the psychopathology may be seen in the setting of relatively clear consciousness.

Williams (1956) studied 100 patients who had ictal emotional experiences. Fear and depression were the commonest. The severity of the latter ranged from mild to severe, and in five patients suicidal ideation occurred. Ictal depression lasted longer than other ictal epileptic experiences, and in several cases lasted for longer than 24 hours.

Ictally driven psychoses may be schizophrenia-like, especially in complex partial seizure status, although more often represent a more obvious organic brain syndrome with a variety of hallucinatory and delusional experiences and evidence of cognitive disruption in association with a disturbed EEG.

Although the division of these psychopathological states into ictal and interictal is convenient, it should be noted that the distinction between them is not always so clear. Thus, in some patients, prolonged ictal psychotic states merge into an interictal condition with a psychosis in the setting of clear consciousness and little disturbance of the EEG. In addition, as already noted (p.220), patients with schizophrenia may demonstrate EEG abnormalities in limbic system structures. These observations place doubt on a classification based purely on clinical and crude surface EEG recordings. Further, it fails to take into account such phenomena as 'forced normalization' (see below) and alternating psychoses, in which some antagonism between seizure events and psychotic symptoms is seen, the psychotic behaviour being relatively short-lived but occurring in seizure-free interludes.

Interictal psychiatric disorders

Prevalence

There are few epidemiological studies of the psychopathology of epilepsy. Pond and Bidwell (1959) noted that nearly 30 per cent of patients have 'psychological difficulties', 7 per cent having been in a psychiatric hospital before or during the survey year. A temporal lobe group had a higher rate of admission to a psychiatric hospital, and of severe personality change and psychosis. Gudmundsson (1966), in a survey of Iceland, noted 25 per cent of epileptic patients to show neurotic symptoms and 50 per cent of epileptic patients to show some form of abnormal personality; 8 per cent were psychotic, and again the frequency of psychopathology was greater (50 per cent) for those with temporal lobe epilepsy, compared to those without (25 per cent). In a survey of Poland, Zielinski (1974) reported 58 per cent of epileptic patients to show some 'mental abnormality' and 3 per cent to have psychotic symptoms. Again temporal lobe epilepsy was overrepresented with psychopathology, particularly those with secondary generalization.

One of the more careful studies has been that from Rutter *et al.* (1970). They gave standardized and validated rating scales to children living on the Isle of Wight. They reported the prevalence of psychiatric disorders to be 8 per cent in the general population, nearly double in patients with chronic disability not involving the brain, and doubled again in those with uncomplicated epilepsy. Although numbers were small, those classified as temporal lobe epilepsy fared worse.

There are some hints therefore that psychopathology is increased in epileptic populations and that patients with temporal lobe epilepsy may be the most susceptible, especially to severe disorder.

Personality disorder and epilepsy

This is one of the most controversial issues. As noted in the introduction, the main arguments revolve around whether personality changes are secondary to an organic brain syndrome, preferentially affecting the temporal lobes, or whether they are due to secondary factors such as recurrent head injuries, social stigmatization and the long-term prescription of anticonvulsant drugs.

Much of the literature in this area has failed to distinguish clearly between personality and illness, and the whole concept of 'the epileptic personality' fell into disrepute in the early part of this century with the introduction and extravagant use of Freudian psychopathology in psychosomatic medicine (period of the epileptic character).

Many studies in this area have used the MMPI to detect personality change, and while some show differences between epileptic patients and a normal population, many fail to show statistical differences between temporal lobe and generalized epilepsy subgroups (Trimble and Perez, 1980). Interestingly, several of these 'negative' results show non-significant but higher levels of psychopathology in a temporal lobe group, raised paranoia or schizophrenia scales being quite common. In some studies, scores for psychotic behaviour are higher in those with combined psychomotor and generalized seizures or those with bilateral foci. In addition, in a recent report (Hermann and Whitman, 1984), a meta-analysis of MMPI studies in the literature was carried out, and patients with epilepsy were compared to others with chronic medical disorders. Epileptic patients who were classified as abnormal by the MMPI showed more severe psychopathology than other groups, suggesting that while chronic illness may be one variable, patients with epilepsy were more susceptible to severe problems.

To overcome the shortcomings of the MMPI, Bear and Fedio (1977) developed a rating scale of eighteen behavioural features, drawn from the literature, thought to be associated with temporal lobe epilepsy. Their scale was given to epileptic patients with a temporal lobe focus, neurological control patients and healthy controls. They reported that the temporal lobe group scored significantly higher on several subscales, notably humourless sobriety, dependency, obsessionality, and religious and philosophical concerns. This study has had partial replication from other groups (Hermann and Riel, 1981; Hermann et al., 1982) who also highlighted a sense of personal destiny, dependence, paranoia and philosophical interests in patients with a temporal lobe origin of attacks when compared with those with generalized seizures. Psychopathology has been reported to be especially overrepresented in patients with auras of ictal fear, being more often classified, using Goldberg's sequential diagnostic system for the MMPI, as psychotic. An aura of ictal fear immediately suggests a periamygdaloid, and hence limbic, focus for the onset of the seizure.

Other evidence that patients with limbic-related epilepsies may be more prone to psychopathology derives from Nielsen and Kristensen (1981). They also gave the Bear–Fedio scale to patients with temporal lobe epilepsy, and noted that those with a medio-basal EEG focus showed significantly more hypergraphia (a tendency towards extensive and compulsive writing), elation, guilt and paranoia than those with a lateral focus. They also reported that patients with left-sided abnormalities scored higher than those with right.

Rodin and Schmaltz (1984) gave the Bear–Fedio inventory to 148 patients with epilepsy, 18 pain patients, 15 psychiatric in-patients and 40 volunteer controls. Patients with temporal lobe epilepsy scored higher on anger, humourlessness, aggression, emotionality and paranoia, and cluster analysis revealed a 'hyper-emotional–dysphoria' cluster on which the temporal lobe group scored higher.

Ounsted and Lindsay (1981) have reported careful follow-up data on children with temporal lobe epilepsy. In 1964, demographic data on 100 children were collected, and in 1977 they were followed up. Generally a poor outcome with regards to psychopathology was associated with low IQ, early age of onset, frequent temporal lobe and grand mal seizures, a left-sided EEG focus, and presentation with hyperkinesis or cataclysmic rage in childhood. 14 per cent had antisocial behaviour as adults, notably court convictions or aggression, commonly associated with a dominant hemisphere focus. Interestingly, a grossly disordered childhood home had no predictive effect on adult outcome.

Rutter *et al.* (1970) have also commented on the increased psychiatric disability associated with temporal lobe epilepsy in children and Stores (1977) reported that behaviour disturbances in temporal lobe epilepsy were most common in male children with a left-sided focus.

Generally, the data suggest that patients with epilepsy do show abnormal personality profiles, although the main argument relates to whether a subgroup with temporal lobe epilepsy may be identified. While the results do not support the concept that a specific 'epileptic personality' exists in all patients with temporal lobe epilepsy, they do suggest that patients with temporal lobe lesions, particularly those with medially sited, limbic lesions, are more susceptible to severe psychiatric disturbances, notably scoring high on such parameters as religiosity, emotionality and paranoia. This should be seen as representing the outcome of an organic process in the limbic system.

The view that there is a specific interictal syndrome of temporal lobe epilepsy receives most support from clinical evidence and has been most strongly made by Geschwind and colleagues (Geschwind, 1979; Waxman and Geschwind, 1975). They have drawn attention in particular to disorders of sexual function, religiosity, hypergraphia, philosophical concern and irritability. Bear (1986b) defined three subgroups of behaviours that contribute to the interictal behaviour syndrome. The first relates to alteration of physiological drives, such as sexuality, aggression and fear. These are alterations that reflect a change in the range of stimuli that elicit responses. Plasticity of sexual behaviour is highlighted rather than hyposexuality, and disturbances of mood, often short-lived, are noted. Secondly, there are 'nascent intellectual interests' (p.24), with preoccupation with religious, moral and philosophical themes. Finally, there are altered interpersonal dispositions which include increased preoccupation with detail (obsessive), circumstantiality of speech and a tendency to prolong social encounters, referred to as viscosity.

The hypergraphia of this syndrome frequently leads to a written output that is meticulous, obsessional and carried out with a compulsion. The content is often moral or religious. Repetition of words and sentences may be seen and variants include excessive drawing or painting or the hiring of a third party to write down information (see Figure 1). There is some suggestion that hypergraphia is associated with non-dominant hemisphere temporal lobe disturbances (Trimble, 1986e).

Aggression and epilepsy

As emphasized in Chapter 4, neurophysiological studies in aggression strongly point to alteration of the limbic system, in particular amygdala function. Since this area of the brain is frequently damaged in patients with temporal lobe epilepsy, it may be expected that they would display more aggression than those with other forms of epilepsy. This is an area of considerable controversy. While ictal violence, recorded using videotelemetry, has been clearly described (Delgado-Escueta et al., 1981), the problems of recording and quantifying interictal aggressive behaviour, almost entirely seen in an interpersonal setting, has led to considerable variability of results in clinical studies. Kligman and

302

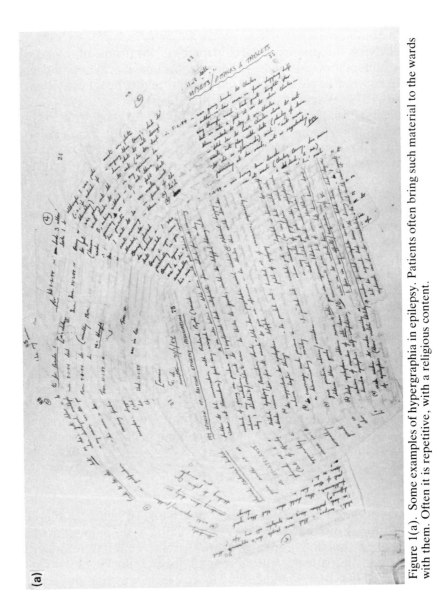

Figure 1(a). Some examples of hypergraphia in epilepsy. Patients often bring such material to the wards with them. Often it is repetitive, with a religious content.

Goldberg (1975) examined eight controlled studies where the relationship between aggression and epilepsy had been investigated, and noted only two that supported the link. Hermann and Whitman (1984) note the high risk factors for aggression in epilepsy which include organic cerebral disease, low socioeconomic status and poor environmental upbringing. Fenwick (1986), in a more recent review, notes the evidence from intracranial implanted electrode studies which suggests that the amygdala is involved in the mediation of aggression in man, further commenting that an amygdalectomy improves aggressive behaviour in those series where it has been tried. In addition, patients with temporal lobe epilepsy who undergo temporal lobectomy show improvement of seizures and improvement of behaviour, most notably aggression. His conclusion was that a relationship between seizure discharges and aggressive behaviour had been shown, although the relationship was more between poor impulse control and brain damage than necessarily to the seizure process itself.

A related condition is the episodic dyscontrol syndome (Monroe, 1970; Fenwick, 1986). This presents as sudden episodes of spontaneously released violence, often in the setting of minimal provocation, which tend to be short-lived. They may be provoked by small amounts of alcohol, and after the events, patients may feel remorse. Generally, the condition is associated with non-specific variables which are also seen in epilepsy, for example evidence of brain damage, low socioeconomic status and a disturbed upbringing. Evidence of minimal neurological damage, with soft neurological signs and abnormal EEGs, are often found, although there is no evidence that these episodes have the same pathophysiology as epileptic seizures. Their paroxysmal nature, however, has led them to be associated with epilepsy, and the possibility that they are somehow 'epileptic equivalents' has been frequently suggested.

Affective disorders

Many people with epilepsy are miserable and unhappy, but this does not equate to a depressive illness. Further, many patients suffer from a chronic dysphoria, often provoked or exacerbated by the long-term administration of anticonvulsant drugs. However, interictal depressive states are frequent in epileptic patients. Several authors have shown, using the MMPI, that the depression scale is elevated in epileptic patients compared with controls (see

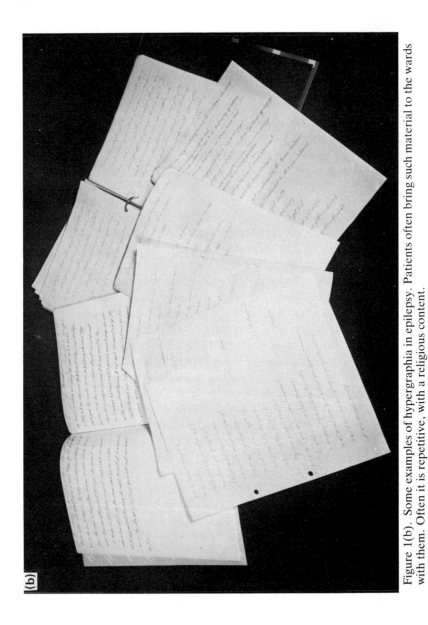

Figure 1(b). Some examples of hypergraphia in epilepsy. Patients often bring such material to the wards with them. Often it is repetitive, with a religious content.

Trimble and Perez, 1980), with a tendency for temporal lobe epilepsy patients to score higher than patients with generalized epilepsy. Standage and Fenton (1975) used the PSE to examine the mental state in chronic epilepsy compared with controls with locomotor disorders. They found somatic symptoms of depression in approximately 60 per cent and depressive mood in 75 per cent of the epileptic sample. More recently, Kogeorgos *et al.* (1982) examined the psychiatric morbidity of epileptic patients using the General Health Questionnaire and the Crown Crisp Experiental Index, comparing profiles with non-epileptic neurological controls. Nearly half of the epileptic patients were rated as probable psychiatric cases, and the morbidity was more prevalent and more severe than in the comparison group. Depression, anxiety and hysterical symptomatology were the commonest characteristics. Betts (1974) studied 72 patients with epilepsy in a psychiatric hospital and found that depression was the commonest diagnosed condition, affecting 31 per cent of the patients. It was classified as endogenous in 17 per cent and reactive in 14 per cent. Gunn (1977) reported depression to be the most common psychiatric finding in prisoners with epilepsy.

In order to explore in more detail the phenomenology of interictal depression, Robertson (1986) examined 66 consecutively referred cases, using standardized and validated rating scales. The severity of the depression was described as moderate, and in 42 per cent was endogenous. High anxiety, neuroticism and hostility were recorded features.

Several authors have commented on the frequency of suicide in epileptic patients (Barraclough, 1981), the risk being approximately five times that expected, highest ($\times 25$) for those with temporal lobe epilepsy. In patients assessed for self-poisoning, epileptic patients are overrepresented (Mackay, 1979), and frequent use of barbiturates for this purpose is noted.

With regards to the interrelationships between epileptic variables and depressive symptoms, some authors have suggested that depression is commoner in late-onset epilepsy (Serafetinides, 1965) and that a decline in fit frequency occurs prior to hospitalization for treatment of depression (Betts, 1974). This latter finding may represent one variant of forced normalization (see below). Flor-Henry (1969, 1983) examined 50 patients with temporal lobe epilepsy awaiting temporal lobectomy who at one time had been psychotic, and compared them with 50 non-psychotic cases with the same form of epilepsy. Where the lateralization could be determined, he noted that 18 per cent were lateralized to the right hemisphere and the majority of these had manic depressive psychoses. He suggested that affective disorders were more likely to reflect non-dominant hemisphere pathology. While generalized tonic–clonic seizures were more often the only ictal manifestations in the affective disorder group, the occurrence of psychomotor seizures was lowest. Flor-Henry suggested this implied that infrequently released seizures were somehow related to the expression of the psychopathology. This is in keeping with the observations of decreased seizure frequency prior to the onset of a depressive illness (Betts, 1974), a finding noted in 43 per cent of patients in the study of Robertson (1986).

The suggested link of affective disorder with the non-dominant hemisphere in Flor-Henry's studies has been criticized not only on the grounds that the patients selected were all awaiting temporal lobe surgery, but also because of the small numbers. It has received partial support from some studies (for example Taylor, 1975), but was not confirmed by Robertson (1986).

Low serum, red cell and CSF folate levels have been reported in a high proportion of patients with epilepsy (Reynolds, 1976) associated with the taking of anticonvulsant drugs, in particular, phenobarbitone, phenytoin and sodium valproate. While the deficiency rarely leads to a megaloblastic anaemia, there are several studies which show a high incidence of low folate levels in epileptic patients with mental symptoms (Reynolds, 1976). Psychoses and dementia are often reported, but in three studies in adults and one in children (Trimble *et al.*, 1980; Rodin and Schmaltz, 1983; Edeh and Toone, 1984; Robertson, 1986) the association has been with depression. Reynolds (1986) has pointed out that folate deficiency and depression have also been reported in non-epileptic patients, not wholly explained by poor diet, and that *S*-adenosylmethionine (SAM) has antidepressant properties (see p.205).

In summary, fewer studies have been carried out on the relationship between affective disorder and epilepsy than, for example, personality disorder. While it is possible that for some patients a neurophysiological explanation exists for an association, particularly relating to laterality (non-dominant hemisphere) and suppressed seizures, this is not entirely clear. However, many patients with epilepsy report depressive symptoms, and attempted suicide and suicide are common.

Psychosis and epilepsy

A difficulty with the literature on psychosis and epilepsy is that few authors specify their precise diagnostic criteria for psychosis, and recognized research criteria are rarely quoted. Many continental authors refer to organic brain syndromes in the context of epileptic psychosis, whereas British authors tend to use it to refer to a psychosis in the setting of clear consciousness. Generally authors distinguish between schizophrenia-like presentations and those with manic depressive presentations. Further, a clear dissociation between ictal and interictal psychoses is not always clear, and issues such as forced normalization must be accommodated in any overall concept of understanding the psychoses of epilepsy.

Perez and Trimble (1980) used the present state examination (PSE) of Wing to document the phenomenology of 24 patients prospectively referred with a psychosis in clear consciousness. Of the sample 50 per cent were categorized as having a schizophrenic psychosis, 92 per cent having a profile of nuclear schizophrenia (NS), the diagnosis being based on the first-rank symptoms of Schneider. The syndrome profile of patients with schizophrenia-like symptoms and epilepsy, when compared to those with schizophrenia and no epilepsy, showed few significant differences, emphasizing the similiarity of the clinical presentation of these two disorders. Similar findings have been reported in a retrospective study by Toone et al. (1982b).

Some differences between process schizophrenia and the schizophrenia-like psychoses of epilepsy were emphasized by Slater and Beard (1963), who noted the retention of affective warmth in the latter, patients showing less personality deterioration. They reported on 69 patients with a schizophrenia-like illness and epilepsy, and suggested, on statistical grounds, that the association was more than just coincidence. They noted an absence of premorbid schizoid personality traits and an absence of family history of psychiatric disturbance that might suggest a predisposition to schizophrenia. Forty-six had a psychosis that was highly typical of paranoid schizophrenia, and twelve had a hebephenic presentation. Eleven of their series had a chronic psychosis that had been preceded by recurrent short-lived confusional states. The mean onset of the psychosis was 29.8 years, which occurred after the epilepsy had been present for a mean of 14.1 years. In 25 per cent of the cases, the psychotic symptoms appeared as the frequency of generalized seizures was falling and there was a preponderance of temporal lobe abnormalities on neurological investigations.

Risk factors

Since only a minority of patients with epilepsy develop psychosis, attempts have been made to define the risk factors in more detail. Stevens and Hermann (1981) suggested the following important variables: age of onset, an abnormal neurological examination, automatisms and visceral auras, sphenoidal spike activity on electroencephalography and the presence of multifocal spikes. While some of these may reflect merely more cerebral disturbance, the automatisms with specific auras and the high incidence of sphenoidal spike activity would suggest involvement of medial temporal structures in the psychosis. In particular, the study of patients with auras of fear by Hermann *et al.* (1982) (see above) showed that patients with temporal lobe epilepsy and such auras displayed markedly raised elevations of the MMPI scales, especially for schizophrenia.

Age of onset in late childhood and early adolescence emerges from several studies (see Toone, 1981), while other data suggest that the relationship is not with temporal lobe epilepsy and partial seizures, but with temporal lobe pathology and complex partial seizures that lead to secondary generalized attacks.

Laterality

Flor-Henry (1969) suggested that a left-sided temporal lobe focus was more likely to be associated with a schizophrenia-like psychosis, contrasting this with the right-sided abormality linking with an affective disorder. The evidence for the former is more substantial than the latter.

In the follow-up study of Ounsted and Lindsay (1981), nine patients developed a schizophreniform psychosis with first-rank symptoms of Schneider, and seven had a left-sided focus.

Trimble and colleagues, using EEG criteria for lateralization of the focus, compared the PSE syndrome profiles of patients with temporal lobe epilepsy with left-sided and right-sided lesions. Patients with a dominant focus had significantly more nuclear schizophrenia (NS) and ideas of reference than those with non-dominant hemisphere abnormalities. The former group also had a non-significant increase in delusions of persecution, delusions of reference, fantastic delusions and auditory hallucinations (Perez *et al.*, 1984). Sherwin (1982), examining patients awaiting temporal lobectomy, had the laterality of the focus established by depth recording of ictal episodes and cessation of seizures following the operation. He reported that patients with left-sided temporal lobe foci were at special risk for the development of a schizophrenia-like psychosis and that psychosis was a rare complication of patients with other focal (non-temporal) abnormalities.

Using PET and oxygen-15, Trimble and colleagues (Trimble, 1986b) have reported data on patients with complex partial seizures, comparing a psychotic with a non-psychotic subgroup. Generally, psychotic patients showed lower values for oxygen metabolism, but in particular, maximal differences were seen in the left hemisphere, across the entire temporal cortex. The majority of this sample had schizophrenia-like psychoses with Schneiderian symptoms.

Summarizing these data, it appears that several authors, using independent samples and differing techniques, show a link between dominant hemisphere pathology in patients with temporal lobe epilepsy and a schizophrenia-like psychosis. It should be noted that the emphasis is on Schneiderian symptoms, presentation being with positive symptoms, and lack of deterioration and negative features. Authors who have failed to detect such a relationship tend to use different diagnostic criteria for the psychotic states, although, even so, emphasize the relevance of limbic system dysfunction to the development of psychopathology (Kristensen and Sindrup, 1978).

Antagonism and the concept of forced normalization

An earlier idea that schizophrenia and epilepsy had an inverse relationship has caused confusion. Essentially, this antagonism, observations of which led von Meduna to introduce convulsive seizures as the therapy for schizophrenia, was between seizures and the symptoms of psychosis, rather than between epilepsy and schizophrenia (Wolf and Trimble, 1985). Landolt (1958) recorded changes in the EEG during preseizure dysphoric episodes and during limited periods of frank psychosis lasting days or weeks in epileptic patients. He noted improvement in EEG activity during such episodes and referred to this as 'forced normalization'. He suggested that similar changes could be provoked by anticonvulsant drugs, and noted that, at the end of a psychotic episode, the EEG returned to being abnormal. Although initially he discussed this in relation to temporal lobe epilepsy, later he drew attention to its occurrence with generalized epilepsies, in particular the precipitation of psychosis in patients with generalized absence seizures by ethosuximide. Although forced normalization is generally associated with psychosis, variant forms including prepsychotic dysphorias, depressive, manic, hypochondriacal and twilight states (Wolf and Trimble, 1985).

The clinical counterpart of forced normalization is referred to as alternative psychosis, in which less attention is paid to EEG phenomena and more to the presence or absence of seizures, in association with the psychosis. Clinically, such states can be very problematic, since control of seizures leads to an even more disturbing and often difficult to control problem, namely the development of a psychosis. This sometimes has a schizophrenia-like presentation, but more often it appears as a paranoid or even manic psychosis. In lesser forms, the problem may merely present as an exacerbation or precipitation of behavioural problems as seizures remit.

Mechanisms

There appears to be some association between the development of an epileptic focus in one or other temporal lobes, expressed around early adolescence, and the development of a later psychiatric illness. The evidence implicates the dominant hemisphere in patients who develop a schizophrenia-like psychosis with positive symptoms, and suggests that in some patients there is an inverse relationship between the expression of the seizures and the expression of the psychosis. The latter is not only noted with forced normalization, but also is seen in patients with chronic psychosis, some of whom develop the psychosis as their seizure frequency declines. The latter holds for affective disorder (Flor-Henry, 1969) and for the schizophrenia-like conditions (Slater and Beard, 1963).

Most authors have used EEG criteria for assessing the side and site of the epileptic focus associated with psychopathology, which implies some disturbance of CNS function. This is supported by the inverse relationship to seizures and by the observations of authors such as Heath (1962) and Kendrick and Gibbs (1957) of abnormal EEG discharges from deep limbic sites in patients who have psychosis, whether or not epilepsy is present. Heath has emphasized the involvement of the septal region for the development of psychosis, and showed that, while during interictal periods epileptic patients show paroxysms of abnormal activity, particularly in the hippocampus and amygdala, as psychosis becomes apparent these spread to involve the septal region. Schizophrenic patients also show spiking and slow wave activity, primarily in the septal region, but to a lesser extent in the hippocampus and amygdala. The spiking is relatively infrequent in schizophrenic patients, but in epileptic psychosis there are dramatic high amplitude spikes frequently associated with pronounced slow wave activity. Thus, although differences were noted in the electrical patterns, the same anatomical regions are involved in psychosis, whether or not the patient has epilepsy.

There are two main contrasting hypotheses to explain the development of the psychosis. The first, supported by the above, suggests that they are truly epileptic in origin and should be referred to as 'epileptic psychoses'. The second is that they are a manifestation of organic neurological damage, and not specifically of epilepsy. The former view has been most strongly expressed by Flor-Henry (1969), supported by the observations of the link between seizure frequency and psychosis and the depth electrode data. Slater and Beard (1963) advocated the second hypothesis, noting a significant proportion of psychotic patients to have a defined organic basis for their epilepsy; a similar view was taken by Kristensen and Sindrup (1978).

CT studies do not add further information. Thus, patients with epilepsy tend to show a high frequency of abnormalities, as do those with psychosis. Toone et al. (1982a) reported a tendency towards the reporting of more left-sided structural abnormalities in patients with schizophreniform psychosis of epilepsy, and hallucinations were exclusively reported in those with left-sided CT lesions. Trimble and colleagues (Perez et al., 1984) quantitatively evaluated the CT scans of ten patients with epileptic psychosis and first-rank symptoms, ten patients with non-nuclear psychoses of epilepsy and eight with schizophrenia who were not epileptic. All these psychotic groups showed high values for the bilateral septum–caudate distance, and the size of the third and fourth ventricle compared with expected normal data. However, no laterality differences were noted on such indices, nor on measures of cortical abnormality.

Studies with PET lend further support to the concept that the psychoses are associated with disturbed function as opposed to structure. There have been several studies of PET in epilepsy (see Trimble, 1986b) using either oxygen-15 or glucose. In general, patients with localization related epilepsies, in particular temporal lobe epilepsy, show hypometabolic areas at the site of the seizure focus as demonstrated on the EEG. However, the extent of the underlying pathology, assessed during temporal lobectomy, tends to be much smaller than the zone of hypometabolism. This suggests a widespread functional disturbance in the associated brain regions of such patients. Further, these hypometabolic areas become hypermetabolic during an ictus. They do not appear to be dependent on seizure frequency, duration of seizures or the clinical expression of the seizures. In epileptic psychosis, these functional disturbances tend to be greater, and with schizophrenia-like presentations to predominantly involve the left side.

Neuropathological data (Stevens, 1986) do not clarify the situation much further. Thus, a common finding in epilepsy is mesial temporal sclerosis, with pyramidal cell loss in the CA1 area of the hippocampus. Although most common in patients with temporal lobe epilepsy, it is also seen following status epilepticus. It is suspected to be aetiological for partial seizures with a temporal lobe origin, but may also occur as a secondary consequence of recurrent seizures. Mesial temporal sclerosis has been reported in brains from schizophrenic patients who have never had seizures, and in epilepsy is associated with pathology elsewhere, such as Purkinje cell loss in the cerebellum. Patients with epilepsy and psychosis are reported to have gliosis and degenerative changes in such areas as the pallidum, the brainstem, the tegmentum and the periaqueductal and periventricular regions of the basal forebrain, similar to the changes observed in patients with schizophrenia (see Chapter 8). Thus, mesial temporal sclerosis alone is insufficient for the development of psychosis, and other areas, in particular periventricular and forebrain sites which receive projections from the amygdala and hippocampus, would seem important. Further evidence for this stems from clinical observations that patients who have had temporal lobectomy sometimes develop psychosis postoperatively, which clearly implicates other areas of the brain than the medial temporal structures in the overall pathogenesis of the psychoses (Jensen and Larsen, 1979).

Symonds (1962) pointed to the 'epileptic disorder of function'. It was, he suggested, not the loss of neurones in the temporal lobe that was responsible for the psychosis, but the disorderly activity of those that remain. One possibility is that chronic temporal lobe ictal lesions lead to kindling of activity in other regions of the brain, especially forebrain limbic areas—changes which lead to the gradual development of the psychosis. Such a hypothesis fits in with the intracerebral recording studies of Heath (1962), as well as observations that it is difficult to kindle epileptic seizures in certain parts of the limbic system, particularly those that are catecholaminergic such as the dopamine-rich areas of the limbic forebrain. In such sites, kindled behaviour changes rather than seizures are seen (Stevens and Livermore, 1978). These data are important for understanding the pathogenesis of schizophrenia since the temporal lobe epilepsy model of schizophrenia-like psychosis is one for the 'positive symptoms' of psychosis, and draws attention to the medial temporal lobes and forebrain limbic system in the development of some schizophrenic symptomatology.

COGNITIVE DETERIORATION AND EPILEPSY

It has long been recognized that some patients with epilepsy undergo dilapidation of their intellect, in particular showing disturbances of memory, which later may progress to intellectual deterioration and dementia. In some cases this may be related to a progressive encephalopathy. This may reflect an underlying neuropathology, such as a lipid storage disorder, which leads to both seizures and intellectual deterioration. Alternatively, recurrent head injuries, bouts of anoxia and intracranial bleeds may over time lead to deterioration. More recently, attention has been drawn to anticonvulsant-induced encephalopathies.

Most studies of non-institutionalized epileptic patients show a near-normal distribution of the IQ with skewing at the lower end of the scale. Memory disturbance, particularly for more recent events, may be impaired, and there is some evidence of a laterality effect, patients with left-sided foci having memory deficits for verbal material and right-sided lesions for non-verbal material (Iversen, 1977). Other selective deficits include impairment of attention, poor perceptuomotor scores, deficient arithmetical and reading ability, and a generalized slowing of cognitive processes. References to the latter have been long noted, and described as viscosity and stickiness of thought, referring to the prolonged speed of cerebration noted in some patients with epilepsy (Trimble and Thompson, 1985).

Factors influencing cognitive performance in epilepsy include an early age of onset of seizures, an increasing frequency of seizures and associated neuropsychiatric handicaps such as depressive illness. With regard to seizure types, generalized absence seizures seem less damaging than generalized tonic–clonic seizures, and patients with partial seizures seem more likely to show impairments of memory function.

In recent years, the adverse effects of anticonvulsant drugs on neuropsychological abilities have become appreciated (Trimble and Reynolds, 1984). Phenobarbitone and phenytoin have been the drugs most implicated and carbamazepine the least. Polytherapy itself, particularly with older anticonvulsants, would appear detrimental, and significant improvements in both cognitive performance and affective symptoms can be brought about in patients by rationalizing polytherapy, or by substituting patients on polytherapy with more sedative compounds for some of the newer anticonvulsants such as carbamazepine (Thompson and Trimble, 1982). These data on carbamazepine are in keeping with its known psychotropic properties (Post and Uhde, 1986), and serve to emphasize the role of careful choice of medications in chronic conditions generally, but in epilepsy in particular.

Diagnosing an anticonvulsant-induced encephalopathy can be difficult, since it may produce a typical picture of dementia, sometimes associated with focal neurological signs and dyskinesias, in association with a raised CSF protein. Since this represents one possible reversible cause of dementia, it should always be considered in patients who, for unclear reasons, are slowly becoming cognitively impaired.

CHAPTER 11

The dementias

The dementias are assuming an increasing importance in psychiatry in recent years, and progress with classification and their neuropathological and neurochemical bases has been dramatic. However, at once the very subject presents one of those paradoxes that seem to pervade psychiatry, namely the obvious organicity of the conditions and the expected role of the psychiatrist in diagnosis and management. Several fundamental discoveries were originally made by neuropsychiatrists. These range from the early separation of a group of conditions in which the changes in mental state were seen early—dementia praecox—by Morel, to the elegant pathological studies of Alzheimer. Since then, the pathological findings associated with several varieties of dementia have been well recorded, and in recent years modern investigation techniques have become available to help distinguish dementia from other conditions. However, it often seems the case that obvious investigations such as CT scanning and EEGs are not provided for those who would most require them, and many patients still receive a final diagnosis of dementia with little more than routine blood tests and a chest X-ray being performed. Further, in a situation almost unique to medicine, as the neuropathological basis of the condition becomes better defined, it is expected that one group of physicians should diagnose the condition, while another group carries out management. The latter are generally psychiatrists, and, while expected to carry the burden of care for several years, are seemingly sometimes denied ready access to the relevant technology for fundamental investigation.

DEFINITION

Dementia is not a disease; like epilepsy and schizophrenia, it is a syndrome. Over the years, many have attempted definitions, and most agree on the following characteristics. It is acquired and chronic, thus distinguishing it from mental retardation and acute organic brain syndromes, and is in most cases irreversible, being secondary to structural changes in the brain. Further, it is distinguished by a decline in intellectual capabilities, in addition to other areas of behaviour, notably emotional and motor changes. The emphasis is on social decline and failure to cope with an independent life.

Lishman (1978) defined dementia as 'an acquired global impairment of intellect, memory and personality but without global impairment of consciousness' (p.9). Alternatively the DSM III suggests the following as criteria for primary degenerative dementia:

1. A loss of intellectual abilities of sufficient severity to interfere with social or occupational functioning.

2. Memory impairment.

3. At least one of the following: (a) impairment of abstract thinking; (b) impaired judgement or impulse control; (c) other disturbance of higher cortical function; (d) personality change.

4. Failure to meet the criteria for 'intoxication' or 'delirium', although these may be superimposed.

5. Either of the following: (a) evidence from physical examination, laboratory tests or history of a specific organic factor judged to be causally related to the disturbance; or (b) in the absence of such evidence, the assumption of the existence of an organic brain syndrome (American Psychiatric Association, 1980, p.112).

Cummings and Benson (1983), whose own definition is 'an acquired persistent impairment of intellectual function with compromise in at least three of the following spheres of mental activity; language, memory, visuospatial skills, emotion or personality, and cognition (abstraction, calculation, judgement etc.)' (p.1), are critical of the DSM III definition. They suggest that it confuses one form of dementia (Alzheimer's disease) with a dementia syndrome that has many causes, and is thus too restrictive.

One feature of the various definitions is their descriptive nature, the concept being, initially at any rate, clinical. Another is the global nature of the impairments. This distinguishes dementia from persistent focal brain syndromes such as aphasias or amnesias. Although several of the dementias present with signs of focal brain damage, their resulting incapacity is clearly much more extensive than purely focal dysfunction would allow.

PREVALENCE

Most agree that dementia is posing one of the most rapidly increasing medical problems of the Western world. This is on account of the rising age of the population, the tendency towards a nuclear family structure, leaving many elderly people without the support of the extended family, and an increased awareness of diagnosis.

Prevalence rates rise with age, some 10 per cent of the population over 65 being affected (Kay *et al.*, 1970). Over 75 the prevalence increases rapidly to around 40 per cent by the age of 95. In geriatric units, over one-third of patients show evidence of mental impairment, and many in retirement communities and residential homes are affected. The incidence rate is variously estimated around 0.5 to 2.0 per cent per annum.

Although the majority of cases, between 22 and 60 per cent, are diagnosed as Alzheimer's disease (Cummings and Benson, 1983), these estimates are invariably made on selected referral patients, the diagnosis being clinical and rarely supported by post-mortem confirmation. The second commonest diagnosis is multi-infarct dementia (MID), accounting for around 10 per cent of cases.

DIAGNOSIS AND CLASSIFICATION

Not all dementias show the same presentation, and one of the advances in recent years has been the identification of different subtypes, based on clinical presentation, that appears to conform to underlying pathological processes. In the classical picture, memory disorder is the initial complaint, especially for new events. This emerges gradually, although the family may report a dramatic event early on in the condition which signalled to them that something was wrong with their relative. Over time, other features of intellectual impairment become apparent, including a lack of spontaneity, concrete thinking and an impairment of abstract reasoning. Disorientation is a frequent early cognitive sign, patients easily losing their way in often familiar surroundings.

As the disorder progresses thought disorder may emerge, with delusions, often of persecution, and illusions or hallucinations, usually of a fleeting nature. Ultimately patients may become floridly psychotic.

Affective symptoms are present early in many cases, with lability of affect, tearfulness, withdrawal and frank depressive symptoms. In some presentations, the distinction with major affective disorder may be difficult (see below). Hypochondriacal complaints, often with bizarre presentations, may arise.

Focal symptoms such as aphasia or apraxia are common, and as the disorder progresses abnormal neurological signs may appear. Motor signs, in particular Parkinsonism, can lead to a poverty of facial expression and postural disorders, and add to the slowness of movement and impaired ability to act. Premorbid personality traits are exaggerated, irritability and aggression common, but the focal deficits may give rise to a more clearly defined change of personality, for example frontal lobe pathology leading to disinhibition and perseveration. As time progresses, apathy, personal neglect and vacuousness come to dominate the clinical picture.

Identification of dementia in its early stages can be difficult. Often the patient is well supported by a relative, who, while noting the failing powers of their companion, cover up for any deficits. The loss of such support, for example with the death of a spouse, may lead to a crisis, but by this time the disorder is well advanced. Sim (1979) outlined some of the early behavioural patterns seen in Alzheimer's disease in response to questions. These were:

1. Perseverative movements, such as snapping of the fingers, indicating the answer to a question is on the tip of their tongue.
2. The offering of entirely irrelevant answers.
3. They may simply smile in response to a question in the hope that they may then receive an alternative, less demanding one.
4. Anger may be displayed, or a reply given such as 'I'm not a child to be asked these silly questions'.
5. Tearfulness.
6. A full catastrophic reaction, patients acting violently with anger or tearfulness.

Wells (1979) noted such features as overexpression of satisfaction with trivial achievements, the increased reference to diaries and calendars for everyday events, and the abandonment of interest in hobbies and other topics, noting how it is for others, for example the younger generation, to keep up with them.

It is clear that in the diagnosis of dementia, especially in the early stages, the witness account of a third party, especially one who knows the patient well, is essential. A full mental status and neurological evaluation are then followed by a series of special investigations. These include psychometry, with assessment of both the premorbid and current level of functioning, skull and chest X-ray, and now CT scanning, EEG investigations and, where necessary, more specialized techniques such as angiography, air encephalography and isotope cisternography. Laboratory investigations include haematology and electrolytes, B_{12} and folate levels, serology, thyroid, liver and renal function tests, and an ESR. CSF is rarely of value, usually showing only elevation of proteins. However, it may help exclude an inflammatory process. In the future it is likely that evoked potential techniques and MRI will assume an increasing importance in the evaluation of the dementias.

SPECIFIC DEMENTIAS

Alzheimer's disease

This is the most commonly diagnosed of the dementias. Although the patient originally described in 1907 by Alzheimer probably did not have that which we refer to as Alzheimer's disease, the eponymous term is now used by many to refer to a dementia of either the presenile (arbitrarily taken as 65) or older age group. Thus parenchymatous senile dementia is included, some preferring dementia of the Alzheimer type (DAT) as the notation. In life, the diagnosis is made by exclusion, there being no confirmatory test. It is the commonest of the dementias diagnosed, and its prevalence rises with age.

Familial cases have been described suggesting an autosomal dominant inheritance, and there are several reports of identical twins with the disorder, confirmed histologically (Kilpatrick *et al.*, 1983). In such reports the cases usually present in the presenile period. There tends to be an increase in cases among relatives of probands, especially with a presenile onset, and, further, the relatives have an excess of Down's syndrome, lymphoma and immune system disorders (for example rheumatoid arthritis, lupus erythematosus) compared to that expected from a control group (Heston *et al.*, 1981). The link with Down's syndrome is the more interesting in that it is now established that, if patients with the Trisomy 21 survive long enough, they will almost certainly develop a dementia, the pathological features of which are typical for Alzheimer's disease.

Although it may present in the fourth decade, the disease typically comes on later, and is commoner in females. It progresses slowly over five to ten years, with early signs of amnesia and lack of spontaneity. The course is steady, with the emergence of additional intellectual deficits, and finally extrapyramidal signs, seizures and advanced dementia. Focal neuropsychological disorders are prominent, and the presentation with aphasia or disorientation is seen. Depressive symptoms, irritability and aggression may be early signs, and slight infections or centrally active medications may provoke an acute organic brain syndrome.

The memory disturbance in Alzheimer's disease has recently been studied in detail by Kopelman (1985). He compared this condition to Korsakoff's psychosis and normal controls on a battery of memory tasks, and provided evidence that in the dementia, primary (short-term) memory was impaired, and there was also an increase in the rate of forgetting. Secondary memory (long-term) was also impaired, Alzheimer's patients showing a higher rate of false positive errors. However, like Korsakoff's patients, those with the dementia, if allowed, could acquire memory by prolonged exposure of the stimulus material. Thus the Alzheimer's disease patients showed defects in both memory systems, notably primary memory capacity and retention, and secondary memory acquisition. One interpretation given by Kopelman was that these data support the clinical impression that the forgetfulness of these patients is due to a failure to take in information. Further, the existence of these multiple memory deficits may explain the failure of cholinergic replacement therapy, which primarily acts on secondary memory systems. The retrograde amnesia that patients develop remains unaccounted for.

Language disturbances are almost universal. Anomia is the commonest impairment, followed by comprehension difficulties. Speech is characterized by being fluent but irrelevant, with a high incidence of semantic jargon (Appell et al., 1982). A consistent relationship has been reported between the impairment of language and severity of the dementia, but not to duration of symptoms (Cummings et al., 1985). The pattern of the aphasia resembles transcortical sensory aphasia, albeit usually with a diminished output, being fluent, paraphasic and with the ability to repeat remaining intact. In the later stages of the illness, echolalia, palilalia and verbigeration may occur, and finally mutism.

The personality in Alzheimer's disease remains relatively preserved in the early phases of the illness, and patients may retain social graces, in spite of severe impairments. This may be quite deceptive, the patient making good cognitive deficits by employing polite replies to questions and avoiding further interrogation.

Gradually changes become obvious, and in the later stages, features of frontal lobe or temporal lobe disease appear. Fragments of the Kluver–Bucy syndrome may be recognized.

The EEG is invariably abnormal, with reduction of alpha rhythm, and later rhythmical theta and delta discharges, particularly over frontal and temporal regions, or diffuse slowing, being recorded. There is some correlation between the degree of the dementia and the degree of slowing of the background rhythms (Gordon and Sim, 1967). Of importance is the observation that, with the exception of some conditions such as Pick's disease, the EEG tends to deteriorate over time in most forms of dementia. The investigation is thus essential for assessing difficult cases with regards to clarifying diagnosis over time, and may give an impression of the rate of the progression of the disease (Gordon, 1968). There are several reports that the P300 of the evoked potential shows increased latency and diminished amplitude, greater than that seen in aging (St Clair *et al.*, 1985), although to date no diagnostically specific findings have been noted.

The CT scan usually, but not always, reveals enlarged ventricles and enlarged cortical sulci. Nonetheless, as with the EEG, the CT scan is an essential technique in investigating the disorder. First, it reliably will rule out many other causes of dementia (see below), some of which are potentially reversible. Secondly, it is of help in assessing the course of the condition in difficult to diagnose or established cases. Thirdly, a normal scan in the presence of a severe dementia should alert the physician to the possibility that the problem is a pseudodementia, still one of the commonest causes of a misdiagnosis of dementia.

Earlier PEG studies suggested that the size of the lateral ventricles more accurately predict outcome at follow-up (Mann, 1973), although correlation to psychological testing was poor. Generally, brain atrophy as shown on the CT scan and the degree of dementia tend to correlate, although using planimetric measurements considerable overlap is seen when comparing patients with Alzheimer's disease and age-matched controls (Jacoby and Levy, 1980b). Again, with this technique, correlations to cognitive tasks vary. Roberts and Caird (1976) showed a negative correlation between memory and orientation scores and maximum ventricular area, and Jacoby and Levy (1980b) noted the digit symbol test to negatively correlate with two estimates of ventricular size. Interestingly, in the latter study, the presence of paranoid delusions was negatively correlated with estimates of cortical atrophy, emphasizing perhaps the necessity of a relatively integrated cortex for the development of such symptomatology. Some authors have drawn attention to the width of the third ventricle as providing a good correlate to cognitive decline (George *et al.*, 1981), while others have examined parenchymal attenuation values. Although the results of the latter have been inconsistent, there is a suggestion of decreased values in the patients with dementia, notably in the temporal and frontal cortices and the caudate nucleus (Bondareff *et al.*, 1981a).

Dementia associated with more severe atrophy has a poorer prognosis (Fox *et al.*, 1975), especially with marked parietal atrophy (Jacoby and Levy, 1980b). The latter is in keeping with the clinical data, implying a shorter survival in those with low scores on parietal tests (McDonald, 1969) and lower attenuation densities in the right parietal region (Naguib and Levy, 1982).

MRI studies in dementia are few. Besson *et al.* (1985) compared patients with Alzheimer's disease to those with MID and age-matched controls. The T_1 values increased with the dementia score in both groups, especially in white matter, and proton density measurements differentiated the two dementia groups, being significantly greater in the Alzheimer patients. While this study draws attention to possible white matter changes in the disease, further studies are required before MRI can be used diagnostically.

CBF and PET have also yielded interesting data. Mean hemisphere CBF flow is decreased with increasing cognitive deterioration, especially grey matter flow (Hagberg and Ingvar, 1976). Further, some correlations to cognitive tasks have been detected, with decreased temporal CBF with impaired memory scores, and a reduction in occipito-parieto-temporal areas with verbal and symbolic language defects. In addition, a positive correlation between rCBF reduction in the postcentral areas and increasing EEG abnormalities has been shown in patients with post-mortem histological confirmation of their diagnosis (Johannesson *et al.*, 1977). However, no correlation seems to exist between rCBF and ventricular dilatation or cortical atrophy as seen on CT scan (Melamed *et al.*, 1978). Gustafson and Risberg (1979) compared the flow values of patients with Alzheimer's disease, Pick's disease and MID and noted similar low flow values in all three. In Alzheimer's disease, the abnormalities were maximal in the postcentral region, predominantly in the area of the parietal lobes.

The PET studies confirm the decreased CBF, but also note low oxygen and glucose uptake. In general they confirm that the extent of the abnormalities reflects the degree of the dementia (Frackowiak *et al.*, 1981), and in Alzheimer's disease reveal early abnormalities in the parietotemporal regions and later frontal lobe involvement, with relative preservation of metabolic activity in the primary motor and sensory areas. Chase *et al.* (1984) noted a correlation between focal areas of decreased metabolism and specific neuropsychological deficits, and again reported on the more severe changes noted in the parieto-occipito-temporal area with relative frontal sparing in Alzheimer's disease.

Much interest has been generated by the neuropathological findings of Alzheimer's disease. Macroscopically there may be atrophy, especially in the temporoparietal region, and histo-logically there is loss of neurones, proliferation of astrocytes and the presence of senile plaques and neurofibrillary tangles. Gran-ulovacuolar degeneration, in particular in the hippocampal pyra-midal cells, is also seen. Tangles appear as coils of parallel bundles which stain intensively with silver. On electronmicroscopy they are seen to be made up of paired helical filaments, although their origin is undetermined. The plaques are degenerating nerve termi-nals, astrocytes and microglia with an amyloid centre. The termi-nals also contain paired helical filaments (Tomlinson, 1982). The tangles are in the cell body, usually close to the axon hillock, and the plaques are often located near to blood vessels. This situation of the tangles may lead them to block the normal movement of the macromolecules from the neurones to the terminal. Another established neuronal abnormality of the neurones containing tan-gles is a smaller nucleolus with diminished RNA content (Crapper *et al.*, 1979).

These changes are maximal in the cortex, especially in the temporo-parieto-occipital region, and in limbic-related cortex, hippocampus and amygdala, but also occur in some brainstem nuclei such as the locus coeruleus. Plaques in non-cortical struc-tures are most numerous in the mammillary bodies. Although the molecular biology of the isolated filaments from plaques and tan-gles suggests some link between the two, with some identical protein subunits, as yet their exact relationship has to be clarified. There does seem to be a relationship between the presence of large numbers of these abnormalities and the dementias (Tomlinson, 1982).

Although plaques and tangles are an essential feature of the pathology of Alzheimer's disease, they are not exclusive to that condition. Tangles are found, albeit in smaller numbers, in association with normal aging, and with such pathologies as dementia pugilistica, postencephalitic Parkinson's disease, progressive supranuclear palsy (the Steele–Richardson syndrome), subacute sclerosing panencephalitis and Down's syndrome. This raises the question as to whether or not they represent some non-specific response to a variety of insults. Plaques, too, have been seen in Down's syndrome, Creutzfeld–Jakob's disease and with lead encephalopathy (Cummings and Benson, 1983).

The other line of pathological research has been the discovery of neurochemical defects in Alzheimer's disease. The first to be defined was an abnormality of cholinergic mechanisms. Thus, it is now known that in Alzheimer's disease there is a widespread loss of presynaptic cholinergic activity, notably in the hippocampus, amygdala and neocortex (Bowen and Davison, 1986). The principal abnormality detected is a deficit of the synthesizing enzyme choline acetyl transferase, and a significant relationship exists between the decline in activity and an increasing number of plaques (Perry and Perry, 1980). This contrasts with the presence of normal muscarinic cholinergic receptor activity. It is thought that the loss reflects degeneration of cholinergic neurones from the nucleus basalis, the projections of which are widespread. It has also been shown in fresh biopsy tissue that acetylcholine synthesis in Alzheimer brain tissue is reduced (Francis *et al.*, 1985), and the extent of the reduction correlates with the cognitive impairment. These cortical cholinergic deficits are not found in some other dementias, for example multi-infarct dementia or Huntington's chorea, but do occur in Creutzfeld–Jakob's disease and alcoholic dementia (Bowen and Davison, 1986).

Although some have suggested that Alzheimer's disease is a disorder of cholinergic innervation (Coyle *et al.*, 1983), several other neurotransmitter deficits have now been described (see Table 1). These include diminished noradrenergic and serotonergic innervation to the cortex, with associated neuropathological findings in the locus coeruleus and raphe nuclei (Adolfsson *et al.*, 1979; Mann *et al.*, 1980). Low levels of GABA, dopamine (Adolfsson *et al.*, 1979), dopamine beta hydrolase (Cross *et al.*, 1981b), somatostatin (Francis and Bowen, 1985) and neurotensin with an increase in substance P (Perry and Perry,

1982) have all been reported. A low uptake of serotonin by neocortical biopsy tissue has also been noted (Benton *et al.*, 1982). All these changes may have relevance for the symptomatology of the disease, and are relevant in terms of defining therapies. Not all neurotransmitters are reduced, however, and some peptides such as cholecystokinin and VIP seem normal (Rossor *et al.*, 1980). Bowen and colleagues argue that since cognitive decline can be related to reduced synthesis of acetylcholine, and other monoamine abnormalities have not so clearly been related to the cognitive changes, that these latter changes are not the primary neuropathological events in the disease (Francis *et al.*, 1985).

Of interest recently has been the demonstration of abnormalities of increased binding of glutamate in caudate nucleus preparations and decreased glutamate terminals in cortical and hippocampal areas from Alzheimer's disease brains, suggesting dysfunction of excitatory amino acid release pathways from neocortical neurones (Bowen and Davison, 1986; Hardy *et al.*, 1987). Such data implicate the cortex as a possible site of the primary pathology, loss of descending projections leading to secondary changes in subcortical structures.

CSF studies in general have led to conflicting results, probably due to differing diagnostic criteria of the different authors. In one study of Alzheimer's patients with histological confirmation of the diagnosis, there was a decreased HVA and 5-HIAA levels compared to age-matched controls (Palmer *et al.*, 1984).

Finally, on the basis of clinical and biochemical findings, some have suggested that there are at least two forms of Alzheimer's

Table 1 Summary of some neurotransmitter and receptor changes in Alzheimer's disease

	Transmitter	Receptor
Acetylcholine	↓	N
Noradrenaline	↓	N
Dopamine	↓	N
5-HT	↓	N
Glutamate	↓	↑
Somatostatin	↓	↓
GABA	↓	?

disease. Rossor *et al.* (1984) examined brains of patients and controls, and noted various changes in the former including decreased choline acetyl transferase, GABA, noradrenaline and somatostatin levels. However, older patients, dying in their ninth and tenth decades, had a relatively pure cholinergic deficit with additional decreases in somatostatin, reductions being confined to the temporal cortex. There was no cholinergic loss in the frontal cortex. The younger patients had more widespread changes with regards to acetylcholine and the other neurotransmitters. They suggested that Alzheimer's disease in those under 80 may be a distinct form of the disease. Bondareff *et al.* (1981b) also provided data showing that neuronal dropout in the locus coeruleus characterizes a subgroup with a younger age, more severe disease and earlier death. Mahendra (1984) has developed the concept further. He suggests that one type of Alzheimer's dementia is characterized by earlier onset, signs and symptoms of parietal lobe and language disorders, and cortical and subcortical pathology. In the other, of later onset, the pathology is restricted to subcortical sites, and the presence of the parietal lobe signs is minimal. Some of these differences are shown in Table 2.

In spite of this growing knowledge of the pathology and chemistry of Alzheimer's disease, the aetiology remains obscure. The suggestion that it represents premature aging is not compatible with the evidence (see below) from clinical, radiological and pathological comparisons of elderly people and patients with dementia. The presence of plaques and tangles and possible bichemical links between them may suggest a common genetic defect that leads to their formation, the consequent disruption of neuronal activity then leading to the clinical picture. Others suggest that the plaques are due to degeneration from their cells of origin, in the nucleus basalis, the latter being the crucial site of pathology. Rossor (1981) has proposed that the disease should be conceptualized as a 'disorder of the isodendritic core'. The isodendritic core refers to the fact that cells of the locus coeruleus, substantia nigra, substantia innominata and septal nuclei all share a generalized pattern of dendritic spread, intermingling with other neuronal elements, thus forming a continuous isodendritic core from the spinal cord to the basal forebrain. This idea links Alzheimer's disease and Parkinson's disease, each representing a different region of loss of the core, and may explain the frequent presence of extrapyramidal motor symptoms in Alzheimer's

Table 2 **Summary of some changes in Alzheimer's disease and normal aging**

	Old age	Alzheimer's early onset	Alzheimer's late onset
Plaques in cortex	+	+++	++
Tangles in cortex	–	+++	++
CAT decrease	±	+++	++ (temporal)
↓ cells in locus coeruleus	–	+++	+
↓ cells in nucleus basalis	–	+++	–
Noradrenaline ↓	–	++	+
GABA ↓	+	+++	+
5-HT ↓	+	+++	+
Somatostatin ↓	–	++	+ (temporal only)
Cholecystokinin	–	–	–
VIP	–	–	–

– = no change

disease and the high frequency of cognitive impairment in Parkinson's disease. While tangles are not a regular feature of the latter, profound losses of neurones in the nucleus basalis are seen.

As noted, the cortical/subcortical location of the pathology of Alzheimer's disease has been a matter of much speculation. The early concepts of two types of dementia, one primarily cortical, presenting with focal cortical signs such as aphasia and apraxia, and the other subcortical, with dilapidation of cognition, memory problems and slowing, placed Alzheimer's disease firmly with the cortical dementias. The newer pathological studies have emphasized the subcortical basis for much of the neurochemical change, and the ideas of Rossor (1981) implied a common pathological link between Parkinson's disease, an associated dementia which was classified clinically as subcortical, and Alzheimer's disease. More recently the suggestion of an initial cortical pathology has again arisen with the PET findings of early parietotemporal cortical abnormalities and the glutamic acid studies suggestive of loss of cortical cell bodies projecting down to subcortical structures.

Pathogenic agents discussed have included aluminium intoxication, immunological abnormalities and slow viruses, although no convincing data have supported such ideas. Certainly to date there are no substantial reports of transmission of a similar disease from Alzheimer's disease brain tissue to animals, and the immunological abnormalities reported may well be secondary (Cummings and Benson, 1983). The genetic component needs to be further elaborated but in most cases the condition is sporadic. The link with Down's syndrome is perhaps a promising lead that may bear fruit, especially pursuing the genetic contributions to microtubular pathology. Recently the gene for beta-amyloid protein has been identified on chromosome 21, reinforcing the connection with Down's syndrome (Goldgaber *et al.*, 1987).

Pick's disease

Pick described a form of dementia in 1892 associated with a circumscribed atrophy of the frontal and temporal lobes. It is much less common than Alzheimer's disease and is commoner in females. Inheritance is said to be through a single autosomal dominant gene, although most cases are sporadic.

There are distinguishing features that reflect the underlying pathology and separate it from Alzheimer's disease. Thus abnormalities of behaviour, emotional changes and aphasia are frequently the presenting features. Some have noted elements of the Kluver–Bucy syndrome at one stage or another of the disease (Cummings and Benson, 1983). Interpersonal relationships deteriorate, insight is lost and the jocularity of frontal lobe damage may even suggest a manic picture. The aphasia is reflected in word finding difficulties, empty flat non-fluent speech and paraphasias. With progression the cognitive changes become apparent, which include memory deterioration, but several higher cortical functions are intact, for example the patient continuing to play bridge or even to work at a technical job. Ultimately extrapyramidal signs, incontinence and widespread cognitive decline is seen. Some of the clinical features that distinguish the dementias are shown in Table 3.

The EEG tends to remain normal in this disease, even when the behaviour changes are advanced, and the CT or MRI may provide confirmatory evidence of lobar atrophy (see Figure 1). Likewise the PET picture shows diminished metabolism in the frontal and temporal areas.

Pathologically the brunt of the changes are borne by the frontal and temporal lobes, and are mainly neurone loss with gliosis. The

Table 3 The differential diagnosis of dementia (from Trimble, 1981a, p.118)

	Alzheimer's	Pick's	Creutzfeld–Jacob's	Arteriosclerotic	Hydrocephalic
Early signs	Memory	Behaviour change, aphasia, incontinence	Neurological signs and symptoms	Acute focal deficit	Memory, psychomotor showing, ataxia, incontinence
Focal deficits	+ +	+	+	+ +	– –
Orientation difficulties	Early	Late	–	–	–
Personality change	Late	Early	Early	Late	Early
Extrapyramidal signs	+	+	+	+	±
EEG	Abnormal	Often normal	Always abnormal	Abnormal	Abnormal
Other features	'Mirror sign'	Hyperalgesia	Myoclonus	Pseudobulbar signs	

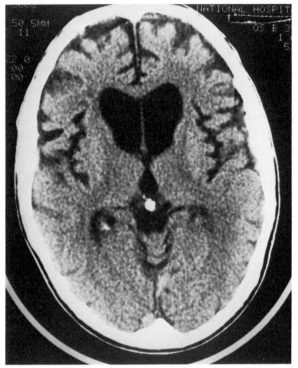

Figure 1. CT scan of a patient with suspected Pick's disease. Note the atrophy of frontal and temporal lobes.

characteristic change is the 'balloon' cell which contains disorganized neurofilaments and neurotubules, and the Pick bodies which are silver staining and are also composed of neurofilaments and tubules. The latter are particularly prominent in the mediotemporal and limbic frontal areas. Plaques and tangles are not a feature of this disease, and the aetiology is unknown.

VASCULAR DEMENTIAS

The concept of vascular dementia has undergone significant changes in recent years, most notably with the recognition that chronic ischaemic changes in the brain are rarely, if ever, responsible for dementia. It is now thought that multiple cerebral infarctions are a common cause of dementia, but that separation of this type of deterioration from Alzheimer's disease is possible on clinical grounds and has therapeutic and prognostic relevance.

The vascular dementias comprise three main groups. Firstly, MID associated predominantly with multiple cortical infarcts; secondly, MID with mainly subcortical infarcts; and thirdly, that type which affects white matter diffusely, Binswanger's disease. In reality the first two types are frequently combined.

The pattern of the presentation relates to the occurrence of multiple infarcts, their site of extracranial origin and their location in the CNS. The most common cause is emboli from the extracranial arteries and the heart, and typically the progression is of a stepwise dementia, often with a history of hypertension and evidence of recurrent strokes. On examination there may be evidence of focal deficits in neurological function, and increased muscular tone, hyperreflexia and Babinski responses may be found. A pseudobulbar state may be apparent, and emotional lability present. Unlike Alzheimer's disease, there is an equal sex preponderance.

The Hachinski score is now an accepted method of helping establish a diagnosis, and is used widely in research (Hachinski *et al.*, 1975). Application of this scale, the features of which are shown in Table 4, leads to a score, the ischaemia score. If over seven, the diagnosis is more likely to be MID, while a score of under 4 suggests parenchymatous dementia. Although there are critisisms of the method and the scale, follow-up studies have been carried out which suggest that four features, namely abrupt onset, stepwise deterioration, focal neurological symptoms and a history of hypertension, are the best discriminators for MID.

In the cortical presentations of MID, the signs and symptoms depend on the site of the lesions. The middle cerebral artery territory is most involved, leading to aphasias, apraxias, visuospatial problems and other signs and symptoms of cortical pathology. In contrast, the subcortical variant affects the basal ganglia, thalamus and internal capsule. It is usually the consequence of infarction of tissue supplied by the lenticulostriate arteries of the middle cerebral artery and other small perforating vessels from the posterior communicating and posterior cerebral arteries.

The pattern of the disorder is progressive, with acute deterioration in the mental and cognitive state of the patient followed by recovery. The latter is rarely to the state prior to the infarct, so a continuous but interrupted decline occurs. Patients often retain insight to their difficulties, and personality is quite preserved

Table 4   The Hachinski scale (from Hachinski *et al.*, 1975)

Abrupt onset	2
Stepwise deterioration	1
Fluctuation	2
Nocturnal confusion	1
Relative preservation of personality	1
Depression	1
Somatic complaints	1
Emotional lability	1
Hypertension	1
History of stroke	2
Focal symptoms	2
Focal signs	2
Other arteriosclerotic signs	1

initially. Affective changes are common, and these must be distinguished from the lability of pseudobulbar palsy. Psychotic episodes with paranoid delusions may be seen, and be the only or initial sign of an infarct. Hypochondriacal complaints may be an early sign. The cognitive state is one of memory impairment, psychomotor slowing and general delapidation of performance. As the condition advances, motor symptoms are clear, including a Parkinsonian syndrome.

The pathology in MID reveals areas of softening and cavitation, and when these are multiple in the basal ganglia the condition is referred to as a lacunar state.

The EEG usually shows severe changes, and focal slow activity is not uncommon. The CT scan reveals multiple infarcts, bilaterally distributed, some of which may be seen in the basal ganglia. Jacoby and Levy (1980b), in their careful study of CT changes in dementia, selected their sample to exclude MID. Nevertheless, they found a significant excess of low attenuation areas affecting 25 per cent of patients, hinting at overlap and a blurring of the boundaries between Alzheimer's disease and MID. The patients with these changes had higher diastolic blood pressures compared with those without them.

Hachinski *et al.* (1975) investigated CBF, using their scale to differentiate those with vascular dementia. They showed widely distributed areas of low flow, greater than that found in non-vascular cases of dementia. With PET, clearer differences between vascular and non-vascular cases have been noted (Frackowiak *et al.*, 1981). In contrast to the frontoparietal degeneration of Alzheimer's disease, MID showed more scattered areas of focal infarction, although in mild dementia the parietal areas were involved in both groups. In general, a low frontal pattern was characteristic of the Alzheimer's disease group. Of importance were the findings that changes in oxygen uptake in the MID patients were coupled to the CBF, the ratio of extracted oxygen (OER) remaining in the normal range. This demonstrates that the pathology is not related to ischaemia (where the OER increases), and raises doubts about the feasibility of using agents that increase blood flow in treatment.

Binswanger's encephalopathy refers to a form of dementia of vascular aetiology with predominantly white matter changes. The cerebral cortex appears well preserved, and patients have a past history of hypertension. The presentation is of a slowly developing dementia, often in the presenium, with a history compatible with multiple small strokes. Neurological signs, pseudobulbar lability and psychopathology are seen. The latter includes affective changes, paranoid delusions and hallucinations.

Pathologically there is loss of myelin and gliosis, and accompanying blood vessels are arteriosclerotic (Janota, 1981). The EEG is usually abnormal, with generalized slowing or focal changes, and the CT scan may reveal decreased white matter attenuation (see Figure 2). The white matter changes are reflected by low oxygen uptake with a PET scan (Frackowiak *et al.*, 1981).

The causes of the vascular occlusions responsible for the vascular dementias are legion (Cummings and Benson, 1983). Included are haematological conditions, inflammatory disorders and infections, and cardiac disease, all of which may lead to emboli, and the prominent role of hypertension has been noted above. This is of utmost relevance for evaluation and treatment. Thus, since vascular dementia is a secondary form of dementia, elicitation of any underlying pathology is of prime importance, especially if the condition is treatable in its own right. This underlines the importance of a full and proper evaluation and investigation of patients with dementia. Ruling out cardiovascular disease, and especially hypertension, may require specialized investigations and repeated estimations of blood pressure. Rarer causes such as systemic lupus erythematosus, giant cell arteritis, atrial myxomas and sarcoid

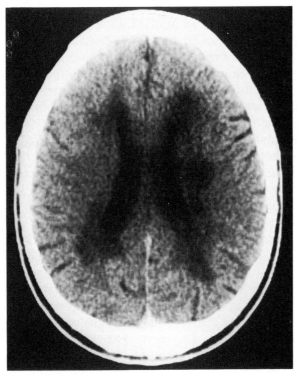

Figure 2. CT scan of a patient with Binswanger's encephalopathy. Note the deep white matter lesions. (Scan kindly supplied by Dr G. Tatler, National Hospitals, Queen Square.)

should be thought of, as well as the commoner diabetes, and emboli from silent myocardial infarctions and atrial fibrillation.

While survival may relate to the underlying condition, it seems that it is longer in Alzheimer's disease (five to ten years) than in MID.

OTHER FORMS OF DEMENTIA

The primary dementias of Alzheimer and Pick can be distinguished from dementia associated with other CNS conditions such as Huntington's chorea and Parkinson's disease, and the secondary dementias such as those due to vascular (for example MID), infective (for example syphilis, AIDS, Creutzfeld–Jacob's disease), traumatic, metabolic, neoplastic and metabolic causes. In addition, one form of dementia, potentially reversible, is now clinically identifiable secondary to hydrocephalus. Some of these conditions are described here (see Table 5).

CNS syphilis

Although rare, this condition is still encountered as a cause of dementia in the Western world, and it is advisable to appropriately test serology in all cases. In its florid form, GPI presents as a progressive deterioration with associated psychopathology. The latter may resemble manic illness, schizophrenia or a depressive illness. The disorder starts insidiously, some ten to fifteen years after the primary infection, but soon loss of judgement and delusions, sometimes with the well-known grandiosity, appear. This may resemble the euphoria of the frontal lobe syndrome, but the grandiosity is quite distinctive from the mood congruent behaviour of mania. On examination, apart from the abnormal mental state, tremor of the lips, tongue and outstretched hands may occur. Dysarthria is common. The typical Argyll–Robertson pupil is seen in about 50 per cent of cases. If associated with tabes dorsalis, neurological features of this, such as loss of vibration and position sense in the limbs, will be found. Convulsions may occur.

Table 5   Some treatable causes of dementia (from Trimble, 1981a, p.125)

Traumatic	Head injury, hydrocephalus after head injury, subdural
Infective	Neurosyphilis, chronic meningitis, parasitic and fungal infections, AIDS
Deficiences	Vitamin B_{12}, folic acid
Neoplasia	Primary or metastatic
Intoxications	Barbiturates, anticonvulsants, alcohol
Metabolic	Hormonal (thyroid, parathyroid, adrenal) Renal failure Hepatic failure Pulmonary or cardiac failure
Dynamic	Hydrocephalus Embolic

Pathologically there is marked atrophy with neuronal loss and gliosis, and iron pigment in the microglia and perivascular spaces is specific for the disease (Catterall, 1977). Treponema pallidum can be seen in the cortex in about 50 per cent of cases.

In the CSF there is elevation of total protein and lymphocyte count, a paretic (first zone) rise in the Lange colloidal gold curve and positive serology. An oligoclonal antibody pattern is also seen. Blood screening with WR or the VDRL is essential, but these give both false positive and negative results. The treponema pallidum immobilization test (TPI) or the fluorescent antibody test (FTA) are much more reliable. After treatment, the VDRL and the WR usually become normal, but this may take several years. The FTA, however, may remain positive, but prior to relapse the clinical manifestations are normally preceded by further CSF changes, notably a rise in cells and protein and increasing antibody titres.

AIDS

This condition has recently assumed great importance for psychiatry, and an AIDS-related encephalopathy may well become as common for this era as CNS syphilis was for earlier generations. This condition is caused by the virus HTLV-111 (HIV—human immunodeficiency virus), which invades T-helper lymphocytes and damages them. Briefly, the T-helper cells promote immunological responses to infection. They have a surface glycoprotein which binds to the envelope glycoprotein of HIV. The HIV is a retrovirus, one which destroys cells it invades by transcribing its own RNA into the DNA of the host cell using the enzyme reverse transcriptase. The depletion of T-helper lymphocytes leads to loss of the infected persons immunological competence, and secondary 'opportunistic' infections develop. Many of these affect the brain, for example toxoplasmosis or cryptococcal meningitis. An alternative expression is the development of certain tumours, for example CNS lymphoma.

It is known that the virus itself is neurotropic and can be isolated from brains and CSF of patients. It may lead to an acute encephalopathy, associated with malaise, mood changes and seizures. However, an insidious dementia may occur with initial features of psychopathology such as lethargy, loss of libido, affective changes and cognitive blunting. Eventually, neurological signs become clear, the EEG changes often showing bilateral slowing and CT may reveal evidence of atrophy. The CSF may show a rise of the cell count and protein. In the final stages, mutism, dementia, incontinence and paraplegia may result. At the present time it is not known what proportion of patients who contact the infection will go on to develop clinical symptoms or survive, but AIDS has a high mortality and there is no cure.

The virus is a blood-borne pathogen, and high-risk patients are intravenous drug abusers, homosexuals and haemophiliacs. It is identified by testing for HIV antibodies.

Creutzfeld–Jakob's disease

Considerable interest in this condition has been aroused by the recognition of its 'viral' aetiology. The original descriptions were of a dementia with pyramidal and extrapyramidal manifestations. It is a rare cause of dementia, males being affected more than females. Rarely, familial cases are described, and autosomal dominant inheritance is suggested (Masters *et al.*, 1979).

Although sudden onset is seen, usually, in the initial phase, there may be only vague somatic complaints followed by mood and personality changes. The progression of the disorder may be fairly rapid, many patients dying within six months of the diagnosis. Soon the dementia is apparent, and localized cortical deficits such as aphasia or apraxia may occur. The accompanying signs are those of extrapyramidal and pyramidal dysfunction, but cerebellar abnormalities and frontal lobe features may also be seen. Muscle wasting, convulsions, particularly myoclonic jerking, delusions and hallucinations form part of the clinical picture. A startle response to sudden loud noises is an interesting sign that may help provide a clue to diagnosis.

Several different forms of the dementia have been described. These include a cerebellar form, an amyotrophic form with marked lower motor neurone signs and the amaurotic variant of Heidenhain. However, some prefer not to split the disorder in this way, regarding the disease as a single entity with various presentations.

The CSF is usually unremarkable, although protein may be elevated. The EEG is always abnormal, with increased slow wave activity and diminution of the alpha rhythm. A pattern of slow sharp-wave discharges is seen, that may be locked to the myoclonic jerks (see Figure 3). Although these may be seen in other conditions such as metabolic encephalopathies, SSPE and some viral

338

encephalitides, their presence with the above clinical picture confirms the diagnosis of Creutzfeld–Jakob's disease. The CT scan may be normal, although mostly shows atrophy and ventricular dilatation, while on PET there are multifocal areas of hypometabolism (Cummings and Benson, 1983).

Of interest has been the transmission of the condition from human brain material to primates. Thus the first degenerative condition of the human CNS to be transmitted to primates was Kuru. This disorder, found among aborigines in New Guinea, causes a pathological state similar to the human disease in the primate brains. In Creutzfeld–Jakob's disease this consists of neuronal loss and gliosis, and status spongiosus—the microscopic appearance of vacuoles leading to a spongiform picture. This has now been transmitted to several species, and there are reports of man-to-man inoculation during neurosurgical procedures (Bernoulli *et al.*, 1977) and more recently from human growth hormone extracts. The pathological agent responsible has yet to be identified, but is thought to be an unconventional slow virus or a protein derivative referred to as a prion.

Hydrocephalic dementias

Although not exactly understood, the dynamics of CSF flow are as follows. The majority is produced by the choroid plexi of the

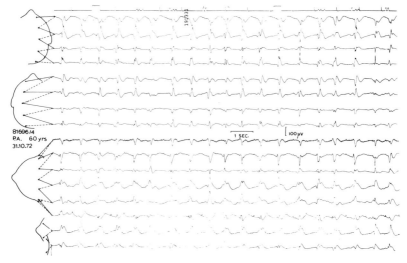

Figure 3. An EEG of a patient with Creutzfeld–Jakob's disease, showing characteristic slow wave complexes.

ventricular system, and flow is from the lateral and third ventricles, through the Sylvian aqueduct to the fourth ventricle, and then out from the interstices of the brain to the subarachnoid space. It then flows either upwards, over the surface of the brain to be absorbed into the saggital sinus, or downwards over the spinal cord. Interference with this flow pattern can lead to hydrocephalus, with accumulation of excess CSF within the ventricular system. Two main varieties of hydrocephalus are recognized, obstructive and non-obstructive (see Table 6).

The non-obstructive conditions have been discussed, and refer to those traumatic, destructive or degenerative states that lead to ventricular enlargement. The obstructive varieties are of two main types. In non-communicating hydrocephalus, the CSF flow is impeded within the ventricular system leading to increased pressure in the ventricles and secondary enlargement. Such states have been long recognized in childhood, but it is now clear that a variety of processes may lead to similar pathology in adulthood, and dementia is one result. Pathologies include tumours, intracranial haemorrhage, colloid cysts of the third ventricle, ectatic basilar artery and periventricular inflammation. The link between stenosis of the aqueduct, a very vulnerable site, and a schizophreniform illness has been noted (see page 224).

In communicating hydrocephalus there is no obstruction of the flow within the ventricular system or its exits, but a failure of absorption of the CSF back into the saggital sinus through blockage. Either the fluid is unable to reach the convexity of the brain or absorption through the arachnoid villi is abnormal. There are several causes of this, including cerebral trauma, previous meningitis, neoplasia or, most commonly, subarachnoid haemorrhage. Normal pressure hydrocephalus was described by Adams *et al.* (1965), and referred to a dementia seen several years after a head

Table 6 Hydrocephalic dementias (after Benson, 1975)

Non-obstructive	Degenerative, e.g. Alzheimer's disease
	Destructive, e.g. arteriosclerotic
Obstructive	Non-communicating with ventricular obstruction
	Communicating—normal pressure hydrocephalus

injury or subarachnoid haemorrhage with characteristic clinical features. These include gait disturbance and incontinence and a normal CSF pressure. The dementia was often of recent onset, and was more related to a psychomotor slowing than to memory and higher cognitive deficits. Patients lost initiative, became apathetic, and in some cases resembled a state of depression.

It is now recognized that the clinical picture can be very varied. Spasticity, especially of the lower limbs, difficulty in initiating movement, frontal lobe signs, and incontinence and ataxia in the presence of dementia should alert to the possibility of this diagnosis, even in the absence of the above associated events in the patient's history, idiopathic cases being well recognized.

The EEG is usually abnormal showing diffuse slowing, and a CT scan reveals large ventricles, often maximally blown in the frontal and temporal regions, in the presence of normal or small cortical sulci. Air encephalography shows air to be present in the enlarged ventricles, but little or no air passing over the cortex. Isotope cisternography will reveal the abnormal pattern of flow.

The possibility of shunting the CSF to either the atrium of the heart or the peritoneal cavity has been tried, but with variable success. Cummings and Benson (1983) conclude: 'Recognised aetiology, short duration before treatment, presence of motor signs, and positive cisternographic findings are the best indicators of possible surgical success. . .' (p.236).

OTHER CAUSES OF DEMENTIA

The causes of dementia are legion, and some of the commoner causes have already been defined. Every physician is looking to exclude a treatable cause, some of which are shown in the table above. Tumours, especially meningiomas, must always be ruled out. Both folic acid and vitamin B_{12} deficiencies can lead to neuro-psychiatric change and dementia, and this can occur in the absence of an anaemia. Nicotinic acid deficiency can lead to a pellagra-like state with dermatological changes, gastroenterological symptoms and dementia. Anticonvulsant drugs, notably phenytoin, in epileptic patients have been implicated with an encephalopathy (Trimble and Reynolds, 1976) and the dementia of chronic alcoholism is recognized (Ron et al., 1979a). Intoxication with psychotropic drugs can lead to cognitive dulling, for example with lithium, and rarely major tranquillizers can provoke or exacerbate a dementia-like syndrome.

Hormone disturbances can lead to dementia, especially hypo-thyroidism, when it is usually accompanied by other signs of myx-oedema. Thyroid function tests will be abnormal, serum cholesterol raised and thyroid antibodies may be present in the serum.

More pervasive causes of dementia include those secondary to such cerebral insults as trauma and anoxia, and the dementia of demyelinating conditions such as multiple sclerosis.

SOME OUTSTANDING ISSUES

Differential diagnosis

It is often suggested that to try and diagnose the cause of dementia in life is a futile exercise. It is asserted that the post-mortem diagnosis is the only valid one, and that clinical diagnosis is often at variance with this. It is further implied that dementia is irreversible and that treatments are ineffective, and hence the diagnosis is purely an academic exercise.

There are several reasons why such views are no longer tenable. Thus, the patterns do differ in their clinical presentation. While the broader issue of cortical and subcortical dementia is discussed below, it seems that there are some forms of dementia that pri-marily present with cortical destruction, with apraxias and aphasias, while others develop gradual cognitive slowing, diffi-culties with planning a future event and impairment of their grasp of complex issues—often initially with minimal memory impair-ment. Alzheimer's and Pick's diseases can be distinguished in many cases, the latter showing behavioural complications in the presence of a relatively well-preserved memory and absence of the parietal signs. EEG and CT data aid this distinction. An important sequel to this is to allow for and expect more florid behavioural problems with Pick's disease, which has consequences not only for management, but also medicolegally.

Both of these forms of dementias must be distinguished from a cortical aphasia syndrome, which may be very difficult in the so-called angular gyrus syndrome, or following an infarct in the dominant hemisphere of a left-handed patient, in whom the clini-cal picture of the aphasia can be misleading. The angular gyrus syndrome is caused by a lesion of the left hemisphere in the region of that gyrus. Patients have combinations of fluent aphasias, apraxias, alexia and parts of the Gerstmann syndrome, comprised of acalculia, right–left disorientation, finger agnosia and agraphia. Such focal syndromes are most likely, particularly if due to a vascular cause, to be non-progressive, thus carrying a very different prognosis to the dementias.

Distinguishing primary parenchymatous dementias from secondary dementias is of utmost importance, especially in view of the number of reversible causes that exist. The separation of the different types of vascular dementias has prognostic and treatment implications. The number of toxic, metabolic and hormonal causes should be remembered, and patients with dementia offered the same medical facilities for investigation as other patients. The exclusion of an acute organic brain syndrome (delirium) from dementia can sometimes be difficult, but the possibility that an established dementia may be exacerbated by such a state must always be thought of, and significant improvements of the mental state can be seen with resolution of the offending cause.

The relevance of careful clinical investigation is apparent with follow-up studies. Marsden and Harrison (1972) in a ten year follow-up, noted 15 out of 106 not to be demented, most having psychiatric conditions of which depression was the commonest. In those with confirmed dementia, eight had an unsuspected tumour, four had hydrocephalic dementia and six were alcoholic. Although this was a selected referral population, and was from an era prior to CT scanning, it reflects the necessity for investigation. Ron *et al.* (1979b) also reported that, in their follow-up study, 31 per cent failed to sustain a diagnosis of dementia, again the commonest missed condition being depression. They gave as the best discriminators of this group a previous history of depressive illness, and affective features on admission. Psychometric tests, with marked verbal/performance discrepancy (but not memory tasks), radiological evidence of cerebral, particularly cortical, atrophy and EEG abnormalities were of maximum value in discriminating those with and without dementia.

The value of investigation is further emphasized from studies at centres where intensive evaluation is carried out, showing that potentially reversible causes are found in from 5 to 15 per cent of cases (Pearce and Miller, 1973; Smith and Kiloh, 1981). In one series of CT scans, the detection of remediable lesions, namely tumour, hydrocephalus or subdural haematoma, was over 10 per cent. Naguib and Levy (1982), in their follow-up study, emphasize the possible importance of the predictive value of CT scanning, those patients with the worst prognosis having lower density values, notably in the right parietal area.

Thus, for some conditions, specific treatments need to be applied. For example, cerebrosyphilis requires antibiotics, usually large doses of penicillin, although steroids are often given in addition to prevent the Herxheimer reaction, an acute febrile state with intensification of symptoms that comes on soon after treatment. A patient with hydrocephalus should be referred to an interested surgeon for consideration of shunting, and tumours will require similar referral. Attempts should be made to correct any endocrine or metabolic causes discovered, and intoxicants, especially any unnecessary drugs, should be removed. It should be remembered that the aging brain, especially one affected by a dementing process, is easily decompensated by such factors, an acute organic brain syndrome thus complicating the underlying deficits. Respiratory and urinary tract infections are notorious offenders, although in patients that have ceased to care for themselves and yet have no one to look after them, nutritional deficiencies may be paramount.

Subtle head injuries may occur, either causing a dementia syndrome, for example with the development of subdural haematomas, or exacerbating an existing condition. Alcohol problems should never be overlooked, many elderly early demented patients taking an excess, with poor food intake, worsening confusion, head injuries and falls.

A diagnosis of MID should lead to a search for the site of origin of any emboli, and any hypertension requires cautious treatment. To prevent further episodes, aspirin, which has an effect on platelet aggregation, is often given on a daily basis, while some advocate even more aggressive anticoagulant treatment—an area of considerable unresolved controversy. In a few selected cases, where the problem relates to carotid artery stenosis, carotid endarterectomy has been tried, although the evidence that this brings lasting benefit is not yet clear.

Many drug therapies are available, but all are symptomatic and most are of little value. Among the most important are the psychotropics. Depression or a depressive component often responds to antidepressants, although choice of drug is difficult. Their anticholinergic properties may increase cognitive problems and lead to urinary retention. Imipramine starting with as small a dose as 10 mg a day has been popular. ECT is not contraindicated.

Of the major tranquillizers, thioridazine seems to provoke minimal extrapyramidal problems and to effectively help two distressing symptoms, namely restlessness and nocturnal wandering. Again small doses are tried initially, but sometimes up to 300 mg or more, with the main loading at night, are of value.

Benzodiazepines should be used with caution, and certainly no patient should be on more than two at the same time. For nocturnal sedation, the shorter acting drugs are preferred, while in the daytime, drugs whose pharmacokinetics are minimally influenced by aging and that have minimal effect on cognition are needed. Oxazepam and clobazam are examples. Chlormethiazole can provide a useful alternative to the benzodiazepines, but barbiturates should be avoided.

Reversible/irreversible

In older definitions of dementia, the criterion that it shall be an irreversible syndrome is often noted. One distinguishing feature between a delirium and a dementia was thus thought to be the acute reversible nature of the former, and the chronic irreversibility of the latter. However, the feature of irreversibility can no longer be accepted. The latter arises from the structural impairment, and if the pathogenesis is functional then the possibility of reversibility can be entertained. There are many examples of a functional dementia noted above, and early treatment may prevent significant morbidity, or prevent structural changes developing.

Dementia/pseudodementia

The presentation of a major affective disorder with a picture resembling dementia has already been discussed (Chapter 9). It has also been noted that follow-up studies indicate that patients who do not deteriorate tend to have an affective disorder in retrospect. Although the term pseudodementia refers to this condition, it is arguably incorrect. Thus if it has the hallmarks of dementia, it should be so diagnosed, recognizing that dementia is the beginning not the end of the diagnostic process. Depression, in addition to several other conditions, becomes a cause of reversible dementia. Others include mania, the depressive 'pseudodementia' of Ganser, hysteria, simulation and neurotic illness. The acknowledgement that these conditions must be considered in the differential diagnosis of dementia hopefully will lead to their presence being sought and the correct diagnosis of a potentially treatable condition made. The evidence from follow-up studies suggests that this is not necessarily the case.

Cortical/subcortical

In this chapter, reference to subcortical dementia has been made. It is suggested that damage to the subcortical nuclei may lead to a dementia syndrome, the presentation of which differs from those disorders that mainly influence cortex. Albert *et al.* (1974) described the features of subcortical dementia as emotional and personality changes, memory disorder, a defective ability to manipulate acquired knowledge and a slowness in the rate of information processing. In contrast to the cortical dementias, aphasias, apraxias and similar symptoms are not seen. This clinical picture may be seen in progressive supranuclear palsy (Steele–Richardson syndrome), Parkinson's disease, Huntington's chorea and Wilson's disease. The dementia of depression also has similar features. They supported this concept by quoting evidence that surgical lesions of the basal ganglia impair performance and prob-lem-solving tasks, and that stimulation of subcortical structures impairs cognitive performance. They also noted the similarity of the symptom complex of subcortical dementia to the behavioural syndrome seen in patients with frontal lobe damage. Pointing to the unique reciprocal connections between the frontal cortex and the limbic system, they also referred to this as frontolimbic dementia.

The concept of the subcortical dementias is most strongly advo-cated by Cummings and Benson (1983). They give as prominent clinical features 'mental slowness, inertia and lack of initiative, forgetfulness, dilapidation of cognition, and mood disturbance' (p.73). The memory changes are more of forgetfulness and diffi-culty of spontaneous recall, and the cognitive state may demon-strate a difficulty with processing of complex problems, 'failing to synthesize the elements properly to achieve the correct answer. . .' (p.10). They also include as causes hydrocephalus and toxic/metabolic disorders that disrupt basal gangia function, and note that many conditions may lead to a combined picture of both cortical and subcortical deficits.

The concept of subcortical dementias has not gained universal acceptance. This stems in part from a traditional reluctance to view some subcortical structures, such as the basal ganglia, as anything but motor in function, and the long-held views that 'higher' cognitive function is the prerogative only of the cortex. Further, the pathological studies viewed above have led to a questioning of the value of the term subcortical in the context of pathology. However, it does emphasize that disruption of cognition can be the result of damage to the deeper nuclear structures of the brain and that dementia has presentations other than the classical one seen in association with Alzheimer's disease.

Senile/presenile dementia

The term senile dementia referred arbitrarily to patients developing dementia over the age of 65. It was referred to, if no other underlying condition was found, as parenchymatous senile dementia, and was thought to present in a similar fashion to the presenile dementia of Alzheimer, but in a milder form. Those who wish to uphold differences between the latter and senile parenchymatous dementia note the genetic difference, and comment clinically on the relative absence of focal cortical signs, extrapyramidal disorder and seizures in the senile group. Further, Sourander and Sjögren (1970) argued there were neuropathological differences, noting the higher density of plaques and tangles in the temporal neocortex, amygdala and hippocampus from brains of Alzheimer patients. The alternative view, that the senile dementia and Alzheimer's disease were the same condition emerged from the early neurochemical studies, in which cholinergic deficits were seen irrespective of age (Bowen et al., 1979).

Recent evidence once again supports the view of two possible types of condition, with differing pathologies. The biochemical changes of younger patients are more severe and pervasive (Rossor et al., 1984; Bondareff et al., 1982b); radiological changes, especially ventricular enlargement, are greater (Jacoby and Levy, 1980b); and patients with the worst survival rates are younger and show marked parietal lobe impairment (McDonald, 1969). The concept of presenile/senile based on arbitrary age limits was poorly conceived, and the question of differing disorders should be based on evidence of the kind now accumulating, particularly of a biochemical nature.

Dementia and aging

A related issue is the extent to which disorders such as Alzheimer's disease merely represent accelerated aging. This view is almost certainly incorrect. It is true that elderly people develop cognitive impairments, notable slowing and memory difficulty, but cognition is often intact in advanced old age, and the other disturbances seen in Alzheimer's disease are not seen. Further, the pattern of psychological subtests seen in dementia is different from aging (Botwinick and Birren, 1951). The genetic evidence argues for a separate condition as does the pathological and radiological data. Thus plaques and tangles are common in the brains of elderly non-demented people, but plaques are usually in smaller numbers and tangles are only rarely found in the cortex. Cell loss is seen, but, unlike Alzheimer's disease, it is less extensive and, where there is a reduction of dendritic arborization, an increase in synaptic contact is noted (Tomlinson, 1982).

Some decline in muscarinic binding sites occurs with aging, but choline acetyltransferase activity is not characteristically diminished and the ability to synthetize acetylcholine is not diminished. The losses of noradrenaline and somatostatin seen in Alzheimer's disease are not a feature of aging (Rossor et al., 1984) (see Table 2). The CSF metabolites in dementia are shown to be reduced, but in normal aging are within the normal range. One interpretation of this is that in spite of some neuronal loss and diminution of biochemical activity with aging, the remaining neurones can cope with the demands on them by increasing their activity, while the neurones in Alzheimer's disease do not possess this reserve capacity (Adolfsson et al., 1979).

In their radiological investigations, Jacoby and Levy (1980a, 1980b) examined age-matched non-demented subjects and could compare CT findings with Alzheimer's disease patients. They showed a trend, noted by others, of an increasing ventricular size with age, and interestingly reported significant negative correlations between a memory and orientation test and sulcal dilatation. Compared to demented patients, the normals had less suggestion of cortical atrophy, although overlap was noted, and cognitive decline in the patients was associated not with cortical atrophy, but with ventricular dilatation.

Mixed types and thresholds

In spite of attempts to clearly distinguish various types of dementia, mixed types are frequently seen. Thus Pick's and Alzheimer's pathology have been seen in the same brain (Smith and Lantos, 1983), and the existence of low attenuation areas on CT scans in patients with presumed Alzheimer's disease is common (Jacoby and Levy, 1980b). The acute onset of Alzheimer's disease following injury or illness is reported (Hollander and Strich, 1970), and several pathogenic influences seem to be linked to the formation of both plaques and tangles. The presence of plaques in normal aging and their correlation broadly with the cognitive performance has led to the suggestion that there are thresholds beyond which dementia occurs. Thus, aging processes provide the nidus upon which other insults operate to increase the changes and eventually throw the brain into 'brain failure', analogous to the development of cardiac failure. The insults could be many, including a vascular episode, minor head injury or anoxia. In spite of the attractiveness of these ideas to explain some of the clinical phenomena, they are not supported by the biochemical evidence accumulated to date.

Replacement therapy

Several drugs are reported to improve blood flow or metabolism, although the evidence that they help dementia is minimal. The futility of merely increasing blood flow in Alzheimer's disease or MID has been demonstrated by the PET studies. Cycladenate and isoxsuprine have been the subject of many poorly designed trials, but the results of use clinically are disappointing and both can precipitate an acute organic brain syndrome. Other drugs in this category include co-dergocrine mesylate, pentifylline and naftidrofuryl. Hydergine, an ergot alkaloid, appears to possess mixed dopamine agonist–antagonist properties, and has been reported in several short-term trials (up to 8 mg daily) to improve behaviour rather than cognition (MacDonald, 1982). Piracetam, thought to enhance acetylcholine release, is another compound for which claims have been made, but its evaluation is as yet incomplete.

The role of other cholinergic agonists to date has been disappointing. It was hoped in Alzheimer's disease, where changes in the choline system can be found, that replacement would be similar to that of Parkinson's disease with L-dopa. This was based on the assumption that the choline deficits were the only or at least the most important of the changes in the brain. However, it is clear that several other transmitter systems are involved and that the acetylcholine abnormalities, while they may link to memory changes, do not necessarily reflect the other behavioural changes so characteristic of dementia. Further, as Kopelman (1985) has shown, even the memory deficits are more pervasive than those provoked by artificial disruption of acetylcholine activity. Treatments have either been with choline precursors such as choline, deanol or lecithin, with anticholinesterases such as physostigmine, or with agonists such as arecholine or the longer acting oxytremorine. At the present time none of these treatments can be recommended, and the only encouraging results have emerged with an oral anticholinesterase drug tetrahydroaminoacridine.

Other therapeutic strategies sometimes employed include giving L-dopa and a decarboxylase inhibitor (sinemet, madopar) to help motor symptoms.

CHAPTER 12

Biological treatments

INTRODUCTION

Physicians for hundreds of years have sought biological therapies for mental disorders. However, the psychopharmacological revolution of the late 1950s and 1960s has had a dramatic effect on the practice of psychiatry and its theoretical orientation. Many patients who would previously have been condemned to long-term institutionalized care have had the course of their illness altered, so much so that some of the florid manifestations of psychopathology that were so apparent in psychiatric hospitals in earlier years are now much less common. The successful use of antipsychotic, antidepressant and more recently anxiolytic drugs has led to an exploration of their biochemical properties, and has accelerated our understanding of the relationship between brain biochemistry and behaviour. The fact that many neurological conditions are treated with a similar range of drugs has helped reinforce the close relationship between psychiatry and neurology, and a common language has developed between various neuroscience disciplines whose common interest is in brain–behaviour relationships.

In spite of this, it is unfortunate that many physicians are still unaware of not only the powerful nature of some of these treatments, but also of the relative specificity of some of them in terms of their effects upon various neurotransmitter systems. Such selectivity means that drug selection for treatment has to be made carefully, but in addition influences the side effect profile of psychotropic drugs, which in itself may determine compliance and therapeutic outcome.

In addition to the psychotropic revolution, it must be recalled that after the First World War a number of other biological treatments became popular, which still have their place today. Amongst these are included electroconvulsive therapy and psychosurgery, both of which will be considered in this chapter.

PHARMACOLOGY: PHARMACOKINETICS AND PHARMACODYNAMICS

Of the several ways that drugs are administered to patients, the oral route is the most common. Following absorption from the gastrointestinal tract, the drug passes to the liver via the portal system, where metabolism may occur, usually by the process of oxidation, reduction, hydrolysis or conjugation. This metabolism is referred to as 'first-pass metabolism', and drugs which are given intramuscularly or intravenously avoid this 'first-pass' effect. The rate of absorption of a drug from the stomach depends upon a number of factors, including the concentration of the active compound, the carrying medium with which they are given, including whether or not they are taken with food, the pH of the gastrointestinal tract, associated disease of the gut, and other active medications which may compete with uptake across the gastrointestinal cell membranes.

Ionization is an important factor determining uptake since only non-ionized drug crosses cell membranes freely, and, unless specific transport mechanisms exist, the rate of movement is proportional to the concentration of the drug across cell membranes. The proportion of ionized to un-ionized drug is dependent on both pH and its dissociation constant. It is immediately apparent how oral ingestion may lead to a wide variation in the amount of drug finally absorbed from the gut, and thus how oral dose does not necessarily relate to serum levels.

Some drugs increase the activity of enzymes responsible for their metabolism or for the metabolism of other drugs within the liver. Barbiturates, phenytoin, carbamazepine and steroids are particularly implicated, although the enzyme-inducing properties of the psychotropic drugs have been relatively little studied. Chlorpromazine is known to induce its own metabolism.

From the bloodstream, drugs become widely distributed throughout the body, initially determined by the relative blood flow of the various organs and the presence of the blood–brain barrier which protects the brain from being affected by many neurotoxic compounds. Further, many drugs are bound to plasma proteins, especially albumin, the presence of the drug in plasma thus being in both bound and unbound (free) forms.

Many psychotropic drugs are secondary or tertiary amines and weak bases and are absorbed better from the duodenum than the stomach. Since lipid solubility is important for passing through the blood–brain barrier, they are highly lipid soluble but are also highly protein bound.

Excretion of drugs is usually via the kidney, although the liver and other organs such as the lung may also be involved.

352

The half-life of a drug refers to the time it takes for its concentration to decrease in the plasma by 50 per cent. The quicker the metabolism and elimination, the shorter the half-life. 'Zero-order' kinetics refers to a situation in which there is an exponential relationship between the dose of a drug and its serum levels (see Figure 1), while in 'first-order' kinetics the relationship is one of equivalence.

Zero-order kinetics arise because the enzymes responsible for drug metabolism and excretion become saturated at levels required for the therapeutic effects. Phenytoin is one drug that follows such kinetics, whereas the majority of psychotropics show first-order kinetics. Knowledge of the half-life of a drug is useful, since it is recommended that the dose interval be equivalent to the half-life. The steady state, namely that in which the serum level of

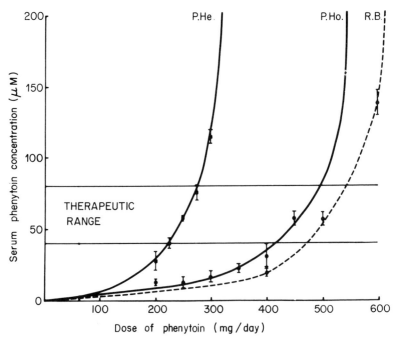

Figure 1. An example of zero-order kinetics. Dose/serum level relationship for phenytoin in three patients in whom steady state concentrations were measured at several doses of the drug. Each point represents the mean ± SD of three to seven separate estimations. The curves were fitted by computer using the Michaelis-Menten equation. The therapeutic range suggested by Buchthal *et al.* (1960) has been drawn in to illustrate the steepness of the relationship within this range. Note: 4 μM = 1 μg/ml. (From Richens, 1976. Reproduced with permission.)

the drug reaches a steady plateau, excretion being in balance with intake, is approximately equivalent to four half-lives.

Since factors which influence drug metabolism include genetics, age, diet, coexistent medications and coexistent disease, careful consideration of pharmacokinetic principles is required, but particularly in certain patients. These include those with diseases of the liver, kidney and heart, but also the young and the elderly. In children, absorption from the stomach is faster than in adults, which may lead to higher peak drug concentrations and thus an increased risk of adverse effects. Plasma protein binding is reduced because of lower albumin and globulin contents of the blood, values comparable to those of adults being reached between the ages of ten and fifteen. The enzyme systems responsible for drug degradation are faster than those of adults in early childhood, and decrease slowly with age, such that adult clearance values develop around puberty. Although the reasons for this are not clear, the increased metabolism of drugs in childhood means dosing requirements need careful adjustment.

In elderly patients, the body composition has altered, with generally a leaner body mass and an increase in adipose tissue. This means that lipid-soluble drugs are more extensively distributed, particularly in elderly females, as the fraction of their total body weight composed of adipose tissue increases more than in males. Alteration of gastrointestinal tract activity, with reduction of gastroparietal cell function and impaired acid secretion with an elevated pH, leads to impaired absorption of certain drugs. Hepatic and renal activity may also be altered. In particular, the hepatic microsomal enzymes responsible for oxidative metabolism, principally hydroxylation and n-dealkylation, may be diminished in this age group, leading to reduced clearance and higher steady state plasma concentrations with multiple drug dosage. Further, reduced hepatic blood flow occurs, on account of reduced cardiac output, with a further decline of clearance. Elderly patients may have diminished plasma albumin with reduced total protein binding, and elimination of drugs by renal clearance is increased since there is a fall of glomerular filtration rate and decreased tubular secretion and absorption capacity of the renal tubules. All of these factors mean alterations in the volume of the drug distribution (the hypothetical volume relating the amount of drug in the body to the plasma concentration at all times after the attainment of distribution equilibrium) and reduced clearance with considerable danger of drug toxicity if dosages employed for younger patients are not modified.

Pharmacodynamics is a term that refers to the biochemical, physiological and behavioural effects of drugs, which in many cases bears no direct relation to pharmacokinetics. With regards to behavioural effects, an important variable is the interaction of a drug with neurotransmitter and receptor mechanisms in the brain, and this is related not only to brain levels but also to the affinity and selectivity of the drug for the various receptor sites. Behavioural toxicity refers to specific side effects of drugs, leading to impaired performance. These problems, frequently encountered in clinical practice, include a whole spectrum from minor mood changes, impairment of psychomotor performance, fatigue and drowsiness, through to severe agitation and psychoses.

Classification

Of the various ways to classify psychotropic drugs, the outline shown in Table 1 has been adopted in this book.

This is based on clinical criteria, including the main illnesses upon which the drugs act. However, it should be made clear that

Table 1   Classification of psychotrophic drugs

Antidepressants	Monoamine oxidase inhibitors (MAOI)
	hydrazines
	non-hydrazines
	Non-MAOI
	tricyclic
	non-tricyclic
Major tranquillizers	Phenothiazines
(neuroleptics)	Butyrophenones, thioxanthines
	Other
Minor tranquillizers	Barbiturates
	Non-barbiturates
Psychostimulants	
Mood stabilizing drugs	Lithium
	Carbamazepine
Others	Beta blockers
	Narcotics and analgesics
	Anticonvulsants

simply because a drug is referred to as an antidepressant, it does not mean that its only property is to relieve depressive illness. Alternative methods of classifying drugs are chemical, electrophysiological and behavioural, the latter referring to their effects in defined biological systems.

Biochemical classifications are assuming importance as more selective compounds are developed, their actions being primarily related to one main biochemical activity. The electrophysiological classifications have depended to a large extent on the effects of various compounds on the EEG. In particular, investigations using power spectra analysis reveal that virtually all psychotropic drugs cause significant changes in the EEG and this has some relationship to their clinical and side effects. In general, neuroleptic compounds increase slow waves (theta and delta activity) and decrease the frequency of alpha and beta frequencies. Minor tranquillizers decrease slow waves and increase fast activity, particularly in the range of 20–40 Hz. Antidepressants increase both slow and fast activities, at the same time decreasing alpha frequencies, while stimulants produce a variable picture (Itil, 1975). However, this tidy scheme is not all it appears, and there are exceptions. For example, the antidepressants do not all conform to the above profile, the less sedative and more alerting compounds (for example MAOI and nomifensine) increasing alpha frequencies (Saletu, 1982). This places some limitations on attempts to use EEG profiles to screen for potential therapeutic drugs.

Psychotropic drugs also influence sleep. Tricyclic antidepressants reliably diminished REM sleep, while having minimal effect on overall sleep duration. Neuroleptics have no consistent effects, while minor tranquillizers increase sleep duration, diminish stage 1 and REM sleep while increasing stage 2 sleep. Stimulants diminish total sleep duration and REM sleep (Speigel and Aebi, 1981).

ANTIDEPRESSANTS

These are divided into two major categories. The monoamine oxidase inhibitors (MAOI) and non-MAOI drugs. The latter are traditionally referred to as tricyclic or non-tricyclic, while the MAOI may be subdivided either by chemical structure into hydrazines and non-hydrazines, or in reference to their enzyme selectivity as MAOA or MAOB inhibitors.

MAOI antidepressants

These compounds, the first of which was isoniazid, were introduced for the treatment of tuberculosis, but were soon recognized to be energizing in their effects. The early forerunners were all hydrazines, and were notable because of their hepatotoxicity and the 'cheese reaction'. The mechanism of the latter is as follows. Monoamine oxidase is widely distributed throughout the body, and together with catechol-O-methyl transferase is responsible for the detoxification of absorbed primary amines. Some symphathomimetic amines, in particular tyramine, exert a hypertensive effect by releasing noradrenaline from tissue. Although the main problem is tyramine, other amines and amine precursors such as tyrosine, histamine and dopamine may also be involved, and such products may derive from protein-containing foods that have undergone degradation or from other drugs.

MAO inhibitors will minimize the degradation of these amines in the gut wall, and thus one explanation for the 'cheese effect' relates to an increased presence of them in the circulation. Alternatively, inhibition of MAO in adrenergic nerve endings will delay the metabolism of tyramine and noradrenaline and thus increase their effects.

It is now known that MAO exists in both A and B forms. The substrates for MAOA include noradrenaline and serotonin, while phenylethylamine is a substrate for MAOB. Tyramine and dopamine are substrates for both forms, but it has been suggested that selective inhibition of only one form of MAO may minimize the chances of a hypertensive reaction.

The symptoms of the reaction include headache, sweating, nausea, vomiting and a rise in blood pressure that can lead to cerebral bleeding. The foods most often involved are outlined in Table 2, although fatalities have almost always been associated with cheese.

Currently marketed hydrazine derivatives include isocarboxide, nialamide and phenelzine, the non-hydrazine groups include tranylcypromine and pargyline. The selective compounds include deprenyl for MAOB and clorgyline, cimoxatone and moclobemide for MAOA.

The place of MAO drugs in the treatment of depression has been evaluated in several recent reviews (Tyrer, 1976; Pare, 1985). Generally they are recommended for patients with 'atypical depressions', although the exact features that respond are often

Table 2 Substances that may interact with MAOI drugs

Cheese—especially matured (not including cottage cheese or cream cheese)

Marmite, Bovril and other protein extracts (not including Bisto)

Pickled herring, liver, game food, broad beans (whole)

Yoghurt

Alcoholic drinks: especially chianti, beer and red wine (excluding spirits)

Drugs: amphetamine, fenfluramine, ephedrine, phenyl-propanolamine, pethidine and other narcotics, antihypertensives, tricylic antidepressants, cocaine, barbiturates and general anaesthetics, antihistamines, L-dopa, insulin and anti-hypoglycaemic drugs

---

less than clearly defined. Tyrer (1976) suggested that the clinical profile most commonly associated with a good response included hypochondriasis, somatic anxiety, irritability, agoraphobia, social phobias and anergia. A poor result is associated with guilt, depressed mood, ideas of reference and nihilistic delusions. Klein and Davis (1969) referred to hysteroid dysphorics with markedly labile mood, vulnerability to interpersonal rejection, with some elements of the hysterical personality, and hyperphagia and hypersomnia. Most workers agree that a patient with typical major affective disorder and endogenous features is the least appropriate for this class of drugs, while additional anxiety or phobic symptoms, or mixed anxiety–depressive states may respond. The presence of somatic symptoms, of the phobic anxiety–depersonalization syndrome and the presence of panic attacks suggest a good response. Following administration there is often a delay before an improvement which may be days or even weeks, although this is less with the non-hydrazine drugs. These compounds suppress REM sleep, and the onset of the clinical improvement coincides with the change in sleep pattern. Dosage is particularly important, and some negative results of earlier trials stemmed from inadequate prescriptions. It is usual to start with doses in the medium range and then increase after one or two weeks, depending on the patient's response. However, doses of up to 90 mg of phenelzine, 20–40 mg of tranylcypromine and 50 mg of isocarboxazid may be necessary. Once treatment has been started it may continue for several years if necessary, and apart from the limitations of interactions with foodstuffs and other drugs, long-term side effects appear to be rare.

The drugs are metabolized by acetylation, and the speed (fast and slow) at which this is carried out is a polygenetically inherited trait. In the United Kingdom, some 40 per cent of the population are fast acetylators, but the clinical relevance of this is unclear.

MAOI drugs may be combined with tricyclic or other antidepressants in certain clinical situations. Although this may lead to unwanted effects, especially hypotension, used carefully such combinations can be useful, particularly with resistant depressions. In general, a patient on a tricyclic antidepressant may be started on an MAOI, while more caution needs to be exercised when patients are already on the latter and need to be given additional tricyclic therapy. Both drugs may be started simultaneously, but it is wise to start each drug at a lower dose than would be used when given as the sole drug. Pare *et al.* (1982) have suggested that a combination of a tricyclic antidepressant and an MAOI might even protect patients from the 'cheese effect' since the tricyclics inhibit the neuronal uptake of tyramine, thus preventing the displacement of noradrenaline and the possible hypertensive consequences. Using the intravenous tyramine test they reported a greater increase in blood pressure in patients on an MAOI alone compared to those on a combination, although it was amitriptyline and not dothiepin or trimipramine which had this protective effect. It has been suggested that clomipramine should not be combined with an MAOI, but some newer antidepressants, such as mianserin, may be safely used.

Apart from the hyper- and hypotensive reactions, other side effects noted include tremor, weakness, dizziness, hyperreflexia, irritability, ataxia, impotence, hypotension, micturition problems, sweating, hyperpyrexia, rashes and, rarely, convulsions. The drugs are contraindicated in liver disease, congestive heart failure and following cerebrovascular accidents. The hypertensive complications respond to alpha adrenergic blocking drugs, such as phentolamine or chlorpromazine.

The newer generation of MAOI drugs currently being investigated are those that show selectivity for one or other of the enzymes. Most work has been carried out with deprenyl, which appears to possess antidepressant properties (Mendlewicz and Youdim, 1983), which can be shown to inhibit platelet MAOB, an effect that may be related to the clinical response. The selectivity for MAOB is probably related to lack of the hypertensive effect with tyramine and lack of postural hypotension as a side effect.

Murphy *et al.* (1983) compared the selective MAOA inhibitor clorgyline to the partially selective MAOB inhibitor pargyline. Clorgyline proved to be significantly more effective as an anti-depressant, associated with effects on noradrenaline metabolism including a decrease in MHPG levels in the plasma and CSF. The changes of MHPG in the CSF were greater than those for 5-HIAA or dopamine metabolites, and a highly significant association was noted between changes in CSF noradrenaline concentration and the reduction of depression and anxiety rating following both clorgyline and pargyline. Pargyline was shown to elevate the urinary excretion of monoamines principally metabolized by MAOB such as phenylethylamine and to produce virtually maximal inhibition of platelet MAOB activity. These authors suggested that inhibition of MAOA is more closely related to the antidepressant effects of these drugs. It has yet to be demonstrated that the antidepressant effect of deprenyl is an MAOB effect, since higher doses are required for the response, and, at such levels, MAOA might well be also inhibited. If it is the case that MAOA inhibition is essential for the antidepressant effect, and this, in addition, is related to hypertensive reactions, the development of selective MAOA compounds with antidepressant effects and minimal side effects may be difficult. Further, there is no direct evidence that inhibition of the MAO activity is directly responsible for the antidepressant effect, since the biochemical inhibition may be demonstrated within a day or two of starting the drug, whereas the clinical effects and some of the side effects do not emerge for up to two weeks or more. Secondary changes must be postulated, included in these being down-regulation of central noradrenergic receptors (Murphy *et al.*, 1983).

Non-MAOI antidepressants

The first of these to be synthesized and used was imipramine, followed shortly by amitriptyline. These two drugs are probably still the most widely used antidepressants. The early members of this group were all variations of the tricyclic nucleus, but more recently drugs have been developed with non-tricyclic structures. Some of these are shown in Figure 2.

An alternative mechanism of classification is shown in Table 3, according to the number of rings in each compound (Richelson,

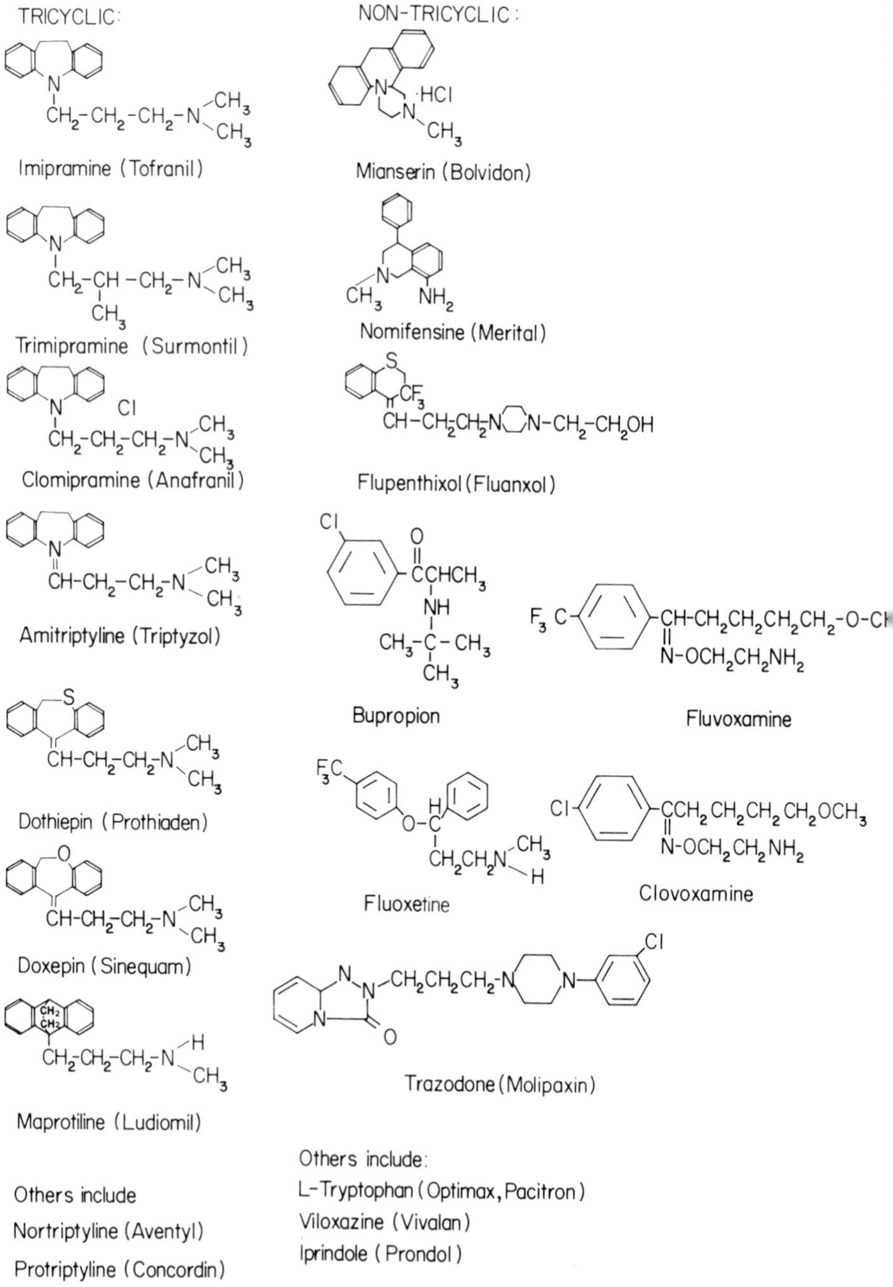

360

Figure 2. Showing the structure of some tricyclic and non-tricyclic antidepressants.

1986). Traditionally, the tricyclic drugs were thought to act by inhibition of monoamine uptake into the presynaptic neurone, thus enhancing the availability of monoamines within the synaptic cleft. Further, it was taught that drugs which are tertiary amines have more of an effect on 5-HT uptake, while the secondary amines are more potent with regards to catecholamine uptake. Some of the non-tricyclic non-MAOI drugs may have an entirely different mode of action however, for example the precursor loading drug L-tryptophan or the neuroleptic drug flupenthixol. The spectrum of action of a group of antidepressants in relationship to biochemical effects in shown in Table 4.

Recently, Richelson (1986), using synaptosomes from rat brain, has shown that desipramine and protriptyline are the most potent at blocking noradrenaline uptake, the least active being trazadone and alprazolam. Many of the other compounds used clinically such as imipramine, dothiepin, amitriptyline and clomipramine also possess the ability to block the reuptake of noradrenaline. More recently, selective 5-HT uptake inhibitors have been developed, which are discussed in more detail below. Anticholinergic effects are noted particularly with amitriptyline, clomipramine and protriptyline, which not only will relate to their side effects, but also to their clinical efficacy if patients find them difficult to take. Antihistaminic effects also vary as shown.

The mode of action of this type of antidepressant has traditionally been related to their ability to inhibit monoamine uptake within neurones of the CNS, and this certainly is a common biological activity they share. However, this effect occurs acutely, while their therapeutic effect may take several weeks to become

Table 3 Classification of newer antidepressants according to the number of rings in the structure

One ring	Two rings	Three rings	Four rings
Bupropion	Fluoxetine	Butriptyline	Alprazolam
Clovoxamine	Viloxazine	Clomipramine	Amoxapine
Fluvoxamine	Zimelidine	Dothiepin	Maprotiline
		Iprindole	Mianserin
		Nomifensine	Oxaprotiline
		Trimipramine	Trazodone

Table 4 Properties for some antidepressant drugs

	Inhibition of uptake			Affinities for receptor	
	5-HT	NA	DA	Muscarinic anticholinergic	Antihistaminic
Amitriptyline	+ +	+ + +	±	+ + +	+ + +
Clomipramine	+ + +	+	–	+ +	±
Imipramine	+ +	+	±	+	+
Maprotiline	–	+ + +	±	±	+
Desipramine	+	+ + +	–	+	–
Nortriptyline	+	+ + +	±	+	+
Bupropion	–	–	+ +	–	–
L-tryptophan	–	–	–	–	–
Mianserin	–	+	+	–	+ +
Viloxazine	–	+	+	–	–
Citalopram	+ + +	–	–	–	–
Fluoxetine	+ + +	–	–	–	–
Trazadone	+	–	–	–	±
Iprindole	–	–	±	–	–
Fluvoxamine	+ +	–	–	–	–
Dothiepin	+	+	±	±	+ + +
Protriptyline	+	+ + +	±	+ + +	±

+ + + = maximum
–　　 = minimum or zero

apparent. In addition, compounds such as mianserin and iprindole minimally inhibit amine uptake in vivo. More recently, attention has been paid to the chronic effects of these and other antidepressant treatments on the sensitivity of catecholamine receptors, in particular, down-regulation of beta receptor activity. This leads to a decrease in glycogenolysis in the postsynaptic cell, small changes at the receptor being magnified through the coupler, effector and amplifier system of the postsynaptic cell membrane into larger dynamic changes. It is known that an intact 5-HT system is required for the beta receptor changes to occur. These data have led to hypotheses that relate depressive illness to a supersensitivity at these receptor sites, itself related to decreased intrasynaptic levels of neurotransmitters, such as 5-HT. The mechanism of the down-regulation and subsensitivity of noradrenergic receptors by antidepressants is unclear, but it could be related to a change of affinity, a reduction of density or interference with cyclic AMP coupling or activity.

Some of the newer antidepressants, such as mianserin, zimelidine and fluoxetine fail to change the density of beta receptors, but still cause down-regulation of the system, implying that density changes alone are not sufficient. Attention has also been paid to the alpha-2 adrenergic receptor since long-term but not short-term antidepressant treatment reduced the sensitivity of the alpha-2 autoreceptor (Crews and Smith, 1978). The functional effect of this is to increase noradrenergic impulse flow and turnover with behavioural activation. Charney *et al.* (1983) examined alpha receptor function in nine patients with major depressive illness before and following a four to six weeks course of treatment with amitriptyline. Alpha-2 autoreceptor sensitivity was estimated by measuring changes of plasma-free MHPG and patient-related sedation in response to clonidine, while postsynaptic alpha-2 function was determined by the release of growth hormone, also following clonidine. They demonstrated that the antidepressant treatment reduced the autoreceptor sensitivity but had no effect on the postsynaptic receptor. Although some other antidepressants, for example desipramine and imipramine, have also been shown to reduce alpha-2 autoreceptor sensitivity, at the present time information on other drugs, particularly in patient studies, is very limited. Nonetheless, these findings are in keeping with a hypothesis that hypersensitivity of the presynaptic receptors in depression would be associated with decreased release of neurotransmitters and up-regulation of the postsynaptic beta receptor. Antidepressants thus regulate the presynaptic receptor and normalize the postsynaptic receptor. The association of these findings to the decreased postsynaptic alpha-2 activity in depressed patients (Siever and Uhde, 1984) is unclear. It is of interest that mianserin is an alpha-2 presynaptic receptor antagonist, an action which may be relevant to its antidepressant action.

Most antidepressants decrease the receptor density of 5-HT$_2$ receptors in the frontal cortex, an effect which distinguishes them from ECT which increases 5-HT$_2$ receptors. As a generalization therefore, antidepressants and ECT down-regulate alpha-2, beta and 5-HT$_1$ receptors, and increase GABA-B receptors. Their action on the 5-HT$_2$ receptor differs.

Some newer antidepressant compounds

In recent years a number of drugs, most of which differ from classical tricyclic drugs, have been developed. These will be briefly described. Some of them are not yet available for clinical use, but show promise. Other compounds, such as zimelidine and nomifensine, which have been introduced clinically but withdrawn on account of side effects, are not discussed.

364

Mianserin

This is a tetracyclic compound, whose main mode of action appears to be as an antagonist at the presynaptic alpha adrenoceptor. It has antihistaminic but only minimal anticholinergic and serotonergic activity. It was originally identified by its EEG profile, which was similar to that of amitriptyline. Its biochemistry confers certain advantages, for example minimal anticholinergic side effects and cardiotoxicity, although it is epileptogenic. Unlike tricyclic antidepressants, it does not significantly decrease the antihypertensive action of drugs such as bethanidine, debrisoquine or guanethidine.

It is rapidly absorbed following oral administration, peak plasma concentrations occurring in two to three hours. Its half-life is ten to seventeen hours. It is highly protein bound, and the majority is metabolized by hydroxylation, N-oxidation or N-demethylation. It has been shown in several trials to possess antidepressant activity at doses between 30 and 120 mg daily, and it is customary to prescribe it as a single night-time dose.

Recently blood dyscrasias have been noted, including agranulocytosis, which are usually reversible. It appears relatively safe if taken in overdose, a marked advantage over tricyclic drugs (Crome and Newman, 1977).

Maprotiline

Although often referred to as a tetracyclic drug, this is tricyclic in nature. It is thought to be relatively selective for blocking noradrenergic reuptake. It is low in anticholinergic effects, and may even have cardiac antiarrhythmic properties. It is well absorbed after oral administration, peak plasma levels being reached between six and nineteen hours, the half-life being around 30 hours. This makes it ideal for single daily administration.

It appears to have antidepressants effects, equivalent to tricyclic drugs, but seizures are a specific problem which have emerged with its clinical use, particularly at higher doses (Trimble, 1980).

Trazadone

This is a triazolopyridine with an added phenylpiprazine group. It has no anticholinergic properties and again is free from cardiovascular side effects, but is a 5-HT$_2$ antagonist, a 5-HT uptake inhibitor and an alpha-2 adrenoceptor antagonist. It is thus both alpha adrenergic and serotoninergic. It is rapidly and completely absorbed following oral administration and its metabolites are inactive. The half-life is about four hours, and its clinical dosage is approximately twice that of tricyclic drugs, going to a maximum of 600 mg per day. It has similar efficacy to tricyclic antidepressants, but is sedative, and like mianserin is relatively safe when taken in overdose. It is reported to provoke priapism in males (Scher *et al.*, 1983) but may increase libido in females (Gartrell, 1986).

Viloxazine

This drug has been available for some time, and also has minimal anticholinergic properties. It is rapidly absorbed after oral administration, with maximal blood levels between one and four hours and a half-life of two to five hours. In animal models it is stimulant, and is a weak inhibitor of noradrenergic uptake. Its main disadvantages are nausea and vomiting, but, of the antidepressants, it has minimal convulsant potential (Trimble, 1978b). However, its use in epilepsy is inhibited because of its adverse pharmacokinetic interaction with carbamazepine (Pisani *et al.*, 1984). It has limited antihistaminic and anticholinergic properties, but is mildly sympathomimetic.

Flupenthixol

This is a neuroleptic compound, discussed further below, which has been used in small doses as an antidepressant. It is a dopamine receptor antagonist, which in small doses appears to have some alerting properties. It is well absorbed after oral administration. It may be superior for patients with mixed anxiety depressive states but its antagonism at the dopamine receptor raises the possibility of extrapyramidal side effects. It is one of a number of major tranquillizers that have been used in the treatment of depression, including thioridazine, chlorpromazine, perphenazine, fluphenazine and the substituted benzamides (see below) such as sulpiride. There is an extensive literature on the use of thioxanthine drugs in depression (Robertson and Trimble, 1982), flupenthixol belonging to this chemical group. The onset of action tends to be rapid (Trimble and Robertson, 1983) and its clinical value may be more in patients with non-endogenous dysthymic disorder.

Amoxapine

This is a demethylated metabolite of the antipsychotic drug loxapine. It is rapidly absorbed following oral administration. It has minimal anticholinergic properties, but does block dopamine receptors, which contribute to its side effect profile. This includes extrapyramidal reactions and hyperprolactinaemia, but in addition, seizures may be a problem.

L-tryptophan

Some of the literature that relates to the antidepressant properties of tryptophan is discussed in Chapter 9. It is an essential amino acid, and its antidepressant effects, potentiated in particular by MOAI drugs, form part of the evidence for implication of 5-HT mechanisms in depression. It possesses no anticholinergic, anti-adrenergic or dopaminergic properties, with a half-life of around four hours. It may, in addition, be usefully combined with tricyclic drugs, in particular amityriptyline and clomipramine. It has few side effects, other than drowsiness.

Selective 5-HT uptake inhibitors

A new generation of selective 5-HT uptake inhibitor drugs has been developed, fluoxetine being one of the first. Zimelidine, a compound with similar biochemical effects, has been withdrawn from clinical use on account of neurotoxic side effects, in particular the Guillain-Barre syndrome and seizures. Other drugs at present being developed include fluvoxamine, femoxatine, citalopram, indalpine and paroxetine. In general, they block the reuptake of 5-HT although this action is rapid in animal models occurring within a matter of hours. This is associated with reduced activity in serotonin neurones, which slowly recovers over a period of fourteen days (Montigney and Blier, 1985). With some drugs, for example zimelidine, there is an associated down-regulation of the $5-HT_2$ receptor, but this is not seen with citalopram or fluoxetine, an effect less constant therefore than the down-regulation of beta receptors already discussed, although interesting in view of the increased number of $5-HT_2$ receptors noted in post-mortem studies of some depressed patients (Stanley and Mann, 1983). It is not clear what these alteration 5-HT receptor functions mean in terms of antidepressant action, or how they relate to other receptor changes associated with antidepressant treatment.

Fluoxetine is a bicyclic drug with high selectivity for inhibition of 5-HT uptake and virtually no effect on catecholamine neurones. It has a half-life of 6–14 days. It reduces REM sleep and increases REM latency although its effect on the seizure threshold, as with other drugs in this group, has yet to be evaluated. Several of these selective 5-HT uptake inhibitors have minimal sedative effects, and do not impair psychomotor performance. Fluvoxamine is a single ringed compound with no anticholinergic properties, which is rapidly absorbed after oral administration and has a half-life of approximately fifteen hours. It is extensively metabolized and its metabolites also have no effect on the catecholamine uptake process. Gastrointestinal side effects appear to be a particular problem, although it has minimal effects on the EEG profile (Saletu et al., 1983). It has a half-life of approximately fifteen hours, and can therefore be given on a once daily basis.

Some other novel or new antidepressants

Iprindole is a weak inhibitor of both noradrenaline and 5-HT uptake, with relatively weak antidepressant action. Like mianserin, its lack of effect on traditional monoamine systems has been one piece of evidence which has led to questioning of the classical neurotransmitter hypothesis of affective disorder. Clovoxamine inhibits both noradrenaline and 5-HT uptake, and appears from its EEG profile to have some activating properties (Saletu et al., 1983). Another compound with alerting properties is bupropion, a drug with a single ring novel structure that has no effect on 5-HT or noradrenaline uptake, and does not inhibit monoamine oxidase. Although it may block dopamine reuptake and has a chemical structure which resembles amphetamine, at higher doses it provokes seizures and may thus not become clinically acceptable. Lofepramine is a newly developed tricyclic antidepressant with similar properties and profile of clinical effect to the other tricyclic drugs, but an apparent excellent safety profile. S-adenosyl-methionine is a CNS methyl donor at present being investigated for its antidepressant properties, its main disadvantage being that it has to be given intramuscularly or intravenously. The rationale for its use stems from the link between folate metabolism and mood as discussed in Chapter 9.

Some general principals of treatment

Although many of the newer drugs seem to have equivalent clinical efficacy with the established tricyclic drugs, their main benefit may lie in having less side effects, particularly those related to anti-cholinergic activity. Many of them, for example mianserin, are much safer in overdose, although these benefits must be seen alongside the known long-term safety profile of the tricyclics, and the enthusiasm for some of the newer compounds has been lessened by the withdrawal of such drugs as zimelidine. Some 15 per cent of all fatal poisonings are due to tricylic drugs, and 3.3 per cent of tricylic overdoses have a fatal outcome. Amitriptyline and related tricyclics are responsible for approximately 1.66 deaths by suicide per 10 000 patients prescribed the drug whereas the comparable figure for mianserin is around 0.13. There are also major differences between the drugs in regard to their sedative properties, some of which are related to their antihistaminic action. The more sedative compounds include amitriptyline, trimipramine, dothiepin, clomipramine and mianserin, while less sedative are protriptyline, flupenthixol and some of the newer selective 5-HT uptake inhibitors. The clinical implications of this are that patients with depression that require sedation, either because of anxiety, agitation or insomnia, may do better on the more sedative compounds, whereas those with psychomotor retardation require the least sedation. If insomnia is prominent, then the whole of the prescribed dose should be given at night-time, so that maximum sedation is obtained without the need for additional hypnotic drugs. Some patients, especially the elderly or those with heart or urinary problems, will be unable to tolerate the anticholinergic properties of some of the drugs, and those with minimal anti-cholinergic activity will be required.

Much attention in the past has been paid to some specific side effects, in particular cardiac and neurological problems. Tricyclic drugs increase the atrioventricular conduction time (Burrows *et al.*, 1976) and can convert a partial to a complete heart block. In overdose they provoke a variety of arrhythmias, these being the commonest cause of death from overdose. The antidepressants with minimal anticholinergic effects, including the newer selective uptake inhibitors, are safer in this regard. In one study, a comparison between fluoxetine and amitriptyline, an increased heart rate, prolongation of the P–R interval and QRS complex were noted with the tricyclic drug, but not with fluoxetine (Fisch, 1985).

Nearly all the non-MAOI antidepressants lower the seizure threshold and may precipitate seizures with the possible exception of viloxazine and nomifensine (Trimble, 1978b). The mechanism of this side effect is not understood, although it may be related to interference with monoamine or GABA activity. Nonetheless, patients with organic neurological disease, who may have a lowered seizure threshold, should be prescribed tricyclic drugs with caution. The management of epileptic patients is discussed further below.

Impairment of cognitive function and performance on psychological tests probably occurs with most of the non-MAOI drugs, although this has not been well evaluated. Most studies are single dose or short term in volunteers, and while patient data tends to show improvement of cognitive function on antidepressant therapy, this may well be due to the relief of the cognitive effects of the depression rather than being related to the antidepressant per se. Evidence from healthy volunteers suggests differences between drugs, for example, imipramine, amitriptyline and mianserin giving the most detrimental effects, nomifensine and viloxazine being associated with least problems (Thompson and Trimble, 1982b). As noted, some of the newer selective 5-HT uptake inhibitors may also be more beneficial in this regard.

Choice of antidepressant needs therefore to take into account the clinical pattern of the depression, the age of the patient and additional medical diagnoses. It is helpful to take a drug history from the patient and to find out if any close relative has had a depressive illness and, if so, to which drug they have responded. If a patient has been reliably treated before on a particular compound and has suffered few side effects from it, it is logical to start on the same preparation, unless there are no other contraindications. Potential suicide risk may be one of these, and drugs which are safe in overdose have obvious advantages. It is wise, especially if the patient has previously experienced side effects or has some associated medical problem such as a seizure disorder, to start on low doses and build up the prescription over the ensuing one or two weeks. If a rapid early response is required, flupenthixol seems to be helpful, and may be used initially. Polypharmacy should be avoided, however, and no patient should require an additional hypnotic to an antidepressant if a sedative antidepressant can be given as a single night-time dose. Useful combinations, apart from those with MAOI drugs, include L-tryptophan and clomipramine, or clomipramine and lithium in intractable cases. Some preparations are still available that combine antidepressants and phenothiazines, for example motival, which is fluphenazine and nortriptyline. If possible, these should be avoided. In unresponsive patients, higher than usual doses may be given, the increments being given until side effects occur or a clinical response is obtained. Once started, an antidepressant should be continued, if successful, for six to twelve months.

Pharmacology

Serum level monitoring of antidepressant drugs can be undertaken. It is usually carried out using gas–liquid chromatography, although radioimmunoassay and mass spectrometry are also used. With regards to the tricyclic drugs, following absorption, they are metabolized by methylation and hydroxylation in the liver, before passing into the circulation, where they are strongly protein bound. Tertiary tricyclics, for example imipramine and amitriptyline, are demethylated to secondary amines, which themselves possess antidepressant properties. They are absorbed well and rapidly, peak plasma concentration occurring in two to six hours, although marked variation between patients is noted in terms of the serum levels for identical doses of medication. The half-lives are very variable, from 8 hours for imipramine to over 80 hours for protriptyline. They are highly bound to plasma protein, with about 10 per cent circulating as free drug. Most of the studies that have examined the relationship between clinical response and serum levels have measured total rather than free levels. Further, since the presence of metabolites has to be taken into account, it is hardly surprising that the results obtained are difficult to interpret. Some authors have claimed that a therapeutic window exists, such that levels below or above this lead to poor results. This has mainly been noted with nortriptyline (Sorensen *et al.*, 1978). In contrast, for imipramine, the relationship is linear, levels below 150 ng/ml (540 nmol/l) being less effective (Glassmann *et al.*, 1977). In general it may be said that high levels of drugs are more likely to lead to side effects, while patients with low levels respond poorly. In practice, measurement of serum levels is helpful in patients not responding as expected on good clinical doses of the drug, or in a patient apparently experiencing side effects on small doses. It may also be useful in monitoring compliance where this is suspect. Interactions between tricyclic drugs and others show that barbiturates and some other anticonvulsants lower, while major tranquillizers raise the serum levels of antidepressants, these effects mainly occurring by alteration of activity of metabolizing enzymes in the liver.

A list of side effects with these drugs is shown in Table 5.

Table 5   Some side effects of non-MAOI antidepressant drugs

Sedation	Tremor
Dry mouth	Dyskinesia
Palpitations and tachycardia, changes on the ECG	Myopathy, neuropathy
	Convulsions
Visual difficulties	Ataxia
Postural difficulties	Delirium
Postural hypotension	Agitation
Nausea, vomiting, heartburn	Transient hypomania
Constipation	Depersonalization
Glaucoma	Aggression
Urinary retention, impotence, delayed ejaculation	Jaundice (cholestatic)
	Weight gain
Paralytic ileus	Impairment of cognitive function
Galactorrhoea	
Sweating	Rashes
Fever	

Some of these occur frequently but may be tolerable, for example dry mouth, while others are rarer and can be very discomforting, such as dyskinesias or seizures. Some may be used therapeutically, for example the hypnotic effect.

'Flu-like reactions have been described with several compounds including zimelidine and nomifensine, with headaches, joint pains and elevation of liver enzymes. Weight gain is a particularly difficult problem for patients and this is not solely attributable to an increase in appetite. Recently a withdrawal syndrome on stopping antidepressants after long-term treatment has been suggested. Symptoms include anxiety, panic, abdominal cramping, vomiting and diarrhoea. In addition, insomnia with nightmares, some restlessness, and occasionally hypomanic, manic or even psychotic pictures have been described. These, like withdrawal syndromes generally, tend to occur in patients who have been on higher doses for long periods of time, who stop their drugs suddenly. They can be avoided by careful reduction of dosage and warning to the patient at the time of initial prescription not to suddenly stop taking their medication.

MAJOR TRANQUILLIZERS

These drugs naturally fall into four groups: phenothiazines, butyrophenones, thioxanthines and others. The phenothiazines have a tricyclic nucleus in which different configurations of the side chain lead to alteration of their properties (see Figure 3). Three subgroups are recognized, one with an aliphatic side chain, such as chlorpromazine, one with a piperidine side chain, such as thioridazine, and one with piperazine side chains, such as trifluoperazine. The thioxanthines have a structure similar to the phenothiazines and include clopenthixol, flupenthixol, thiothixine and related drugs.

The butyrophenones, such as haloperidol, and related diphenylbutylpiperidines, such as pimozide, fluspiriline and penfluridol, have a different chemical structure, and some drugs, for example fluspiriline and penfluridol, are long-acting oral preparations. Other major tranquillizers include molindone, reserpine, tetrabenazine, oxypertine, loxapine and the substituted benzamides, such as sulpiride.

The distinguishing property of all these drugs is their ability to block dopamine receptors, and clinically they are antipsychotic. In addition they may evoke extrapyramidal symptoms of various types. They all inhibit apomorphine-induced stereotypy and agitation; provoke an acute increase in dopamine turnover with raised HVA levels in areas such as the corpus striatum, nucleus accumbens, olfactory tubercle and frontal cortex; block the stimulation of dopamine-sensitive adenylate cyclase; and displace receptor binding with H_3 dopamine or H_3 spiroperidol at postsynaptic dopamine receptor sites. The relative receptor binding profiles for some of these drugs is shown in Table 6.

The most potent dopamine receptor antagonist used clinically is benperidol, while pimozide is the most specific. With few exceptions, the ability of these drugs to block the receptor correlates with their clinical antipsychotic action. Since the majority readily provoke extrapyramidal effects, it has been suggested that the antipsychotic potential is due to antagonism of dopamine receptors in the mesolimbic or mesocortical areas of the brain, while the motor effects relate to the nigrostriatal system. There are a few drugs that appear to possess minimal potential to evoke extrapyramidal effects, namely sulpiride, clozapine and thioridazine. One explanation for this has been the anticholinergic potential of these drugs which may counteract the tendency to provoke extrapyramidal symptoms. Alternatively, it has been suggested that

Nucleus:

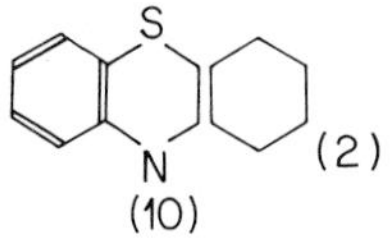

(2)

(10)

Aliphatic side-chain: e.g. chlorpromazine (Largactil)

$$(10) \ -CH_2-CH_2-CH_2-N(CH_3)_2$$
$$(2) \ -Cl$$

Piperidine side-chain: e.g. thioridazine (Melleril)

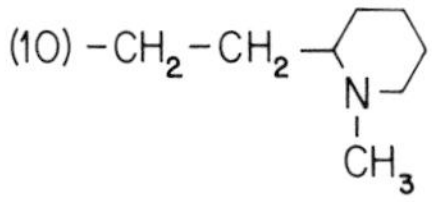

$$(2) \ -S-CH_3$$

Other examples: Pericyazine (Neulactil)

Piperazine side-chain e.g. trifluoperazine (Stelazine)

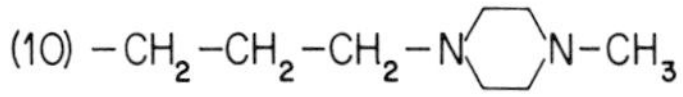

Other examples: Perphenazine (Fentazin)

Fluphenazine (Moditen)

Thiopropazate (Dartalan)

(a) Structures of the phenothiazine compounds

Haloperidol (Haldol)

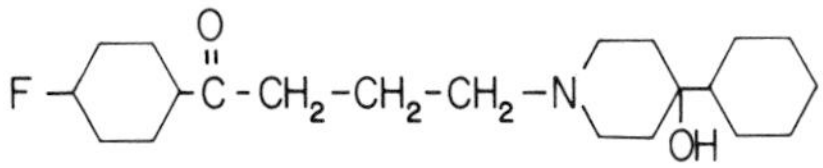

Related drugs: Pimozide (Orap)

Penfluridol

Fluspiriline (Redeptin)

(b) Structure of the butyrophenones

Figure 3. Showing the structure of some phenothiazines and butyrophenones.

Table 6   Receptor binding properties of neuroleptics

	DA	5-HT	Alpha adrenergic	Histamine	ACh
Benperidol	+++++	±	±	–	–
Droperidol	+++++	+	+	–	–
Haloperidol	+++++	–	±	–	–
Pimozide	+++++	–	–	–	–
Bromperidol	+++++	–	±	–	–
Fluspiriline	+++++	+	–	–	–
Thiothixine	++++	+	±	+	–
Trifluoperazine	++++	±	±	±	–
Perphenazine	++++	+	–	+	–
Flupenthixol	++++	+	+	±	–
Fluphenazine	+++	+	+	+	–
Penfluridol	+++	–	–	–	–
Chlorprothixine	+++	++	++	++	++
Thioridazine	++	+	++	+	++
Chlorpromazine	++	++	+++	+++	++
Sulpiride	+	–	–	–	–
Promazine	±	+	+++	+++	+++

they preferentially act on dopamine receptors in mesolimbic areas, rather than at the striatum. Although studies examining dopamine metabolites do not confirm a preferential increase in levels when comparing mesolimbic to striatal structures for various neuroleptics, those examining the disappearance or release of dopamine from selective sites do support a suggestion of a more preferential action in mesolimbic areas for these compounds (Leysen and Niemegeers, 1985; Scatton and Zivkovic, 1984). Since sulpiride does not have anticholinergic properties it would seem that the most likely explanation for these differing clinical effects of some of the neuroleptics relates to differential blockade of dopamine receptors in limbic as opposed to striatal areas.

When neuroleptics are given chronically, it is shown in animal models that tolerance occurs, and in patients initially elevated HVA levels in the CSF tend to decrease after a few weeks of drug administration (Post and Goodwin, 1975). However, it seems that this tolerance is observed in the striatum but not in mesolimbic and mesocortical dopaminergic systems (Scatton and Zivkovic, 1984), possibly explaining the clinically effective antipsychotic action of these drugs which persists over time.

It should be noted that of the various subclasses of dopamine receptors described, it is antagonism of the D2 receptor which is thought to have the most clinical potential. Table 7 shows a comparison of the antagonism at D1 and D2 receptors for some neuroleptic drugs.

In general, the rank order of the potency of the drugs for interaction with the D1 receptor is unrelated to any of the behavioural tests of measuring dopaminergic activity, and as yet the relationship of this receptor to CNS function is undetermined. However, the D2 receptor binding does correlate with effects on behavioural tests of dopaminergic function, and probably relates to their antipsychotic function. Following treatment with these drugs, it has been shown in animal models that the number of D2 receptor binding sites increases, which, on drug withdrawal, slowly reverts to pretreatment values (Leysen and Niemegeers, 1985). Other effects mediated by the D2 receptor are dopamine-activated locomotion, prolactin release, dopamine-induced vomiting and impaired learning noted following administration of dopamine antagonists. The alpha-1 adrenergic blockade is related to cardiovascular problems including hypotension, tachycardia and sedative effects—the latter may be enhanced by any antihistaminic effect.

There has recently been a growing interest in the substituted benzamide drugs, such as sulpiride, raclopride, remoxepride and tiapride. These, derived from metaclopramide, act as dopamine receptor antagonists, but while tiapride seems to be preferential for the striatum, sulpiride has more effect on the mesolimbic system and is a selective D2 antagonist. They have no effects on

Table 7 D1 and D2 receptor site antagonism

	D1	D2
Pimozide	+	+ + + +
Butaclamol	+ + + +	+ + + +
Chlorpromazine	+ +	+ + +
Thioridazine	+ +	+ + +
Flupenthixol	+ + + +	+ + +
Haloperidol	+ +	+ + + +
Sulpiride	–	+ + +
Clozapine	+ +	+ +
Fluphenazine	+ + +	+ + +

other receptor systems, and sulpiride is without effect on GABA binding. At low doses, it is antiemetic (150–600 mg per day), while at medium doses it is disinhibitory, having some form of antidepressant activity. However, in higher doses (above 800 mg per day) it is antipsychotic. It has a powerful effect on prolactin release and unlike traditional neuroleptics does not readily provoke catalepsy or inhibit apomorphine-induced circling and stereotypical behaviour in rodents. These latter findings suggest it may have less powerful an effect on motor systems and thus have a low incidence of extrapyramidal side effects.

Following oral administration, chlorpromazine is easily absorbed and metabolized by the liver with peak plasma level occurring in one to three hours. Its half-life is 17 hours. Some metabolites, such as the sulfoxide, have little pharmacological activity, while others, for example the hydroxy derivatives, are more potent. It is strongly protein bound, and preferentially accumulates in the brain with a brain–plasma ratio of about 5:1. After termination of treatment, excretion of the drug or one of its metabolites may continue for several months.

Haloperidol is less rapidly absorbed, maximal concentrations occurring around five hours, with a half-life of 13–20 hours. It is 90 per cent protein bound, and does not induce its own metabolism. Pimozide has a half-life of over 50 hours, and it is possible to give the drug on less than a daily basis. Once weekly treatment has been tried successfully in maintenance therapy for psychotic patients. The half-life of sulpiride is eight hours.

The dose of major tranquillizers prescribed needs to be titrated for individual patients against their symptoms, but in some cases large doses are necessary. With drugs that are alpha adrenergic blockers, for example chlorpromazine, such doses may lower blood pressure and monitoring of the latter may be necessary. It is usual in clinical practice to start patients on oral medications, and often once daily prescription is possible. Following control of psychotic symptoms with oral therapy, especially if the patient has schizophrenia, a change to intramuscular preparations may be preferred.

Esterified drugs, mostly dissolved in oil, are given intramuscularly, and released over a varying period of time, up to about four weeks. They include the decanoate preparations of haloperidol, fluphenazine, flupenthixol, clopenthixol and fluspiriline. The latter is held in aqueous solution as opposed to a vegetable oil base, and may be given on a once weekly regime.

These drugs provoke the same incidence of extrapyramidal problems as do oral preparations, although the onset may be more rapid (Ayd, 1974). Trials comparing groups of patients on injectable preparations or oral pimozide suggest little difference in relapse rate (McCreadie *et al.*, 1980), although some studies have reported oral therapy to be superior with regards to several aspects of social adjustment (Falloon *et al.*, 1978).

In schizophrenia, once treatment has been started, it probably needs to be continued indefinitely. Discontinuation of therapy leads to relapse in approximately 20 per cent of patients in six months and 45 per cent of patients at one year (Curson *et al.*, 1985). It is estimated that some 60–65 per cent of patients will relapse over a 24 month period if not taking drugs, comparable data for those in maintenance therapy being 35 per cent. Poor response to treatment relates to younger age of onset of illness, prominent initial negative symptoms, impairment of cognitive performance and an enlarged ventricular–brain ratio on the CT scan.

A relationship between clinical response to serum levels of neuroleptics or plasma prolactin has not been demonstrated in schizophrenia (Kolakowska *et al.*, 1985a). In contrast, some authors have reported a relationship between extrapyramidal symptoms and elevations of prolactin (Rao *et al.*, 1980) and in acute mania, improvement in clinical symptoms parallels the prolactin rise. Recently, the suggestion that maintenance should be with low dose neuroleptics (for example 5 mg of fluphenazine decanoate every two weeks) has been made, which may reduce the long-term incidence of side effects. Low doses of neuroleptic medication have been used in other conditions, for example depressive illness, borderline personalities and anxiety neurosis. The preferential response of monosymptomatic psychoses to pimozide has been reported (Riding and Munroe, 1975), and for aggression, in particular in patients with brain damage, clopenthixol may have special value.

Major tranquillizers are also used in the management of manic depressive illness and in patients with acute or chronic organic brain syndromes. They may be used in alcohol withdrawal states, although their potential to lower seizure threshold is a problem in this setting.

In some cases it is necessary to tranquillize patients rapidly, and intramuscular or intravenous doses may be given. For example a regime may include haloperidol 10–20 mg every 30–60 minutes, following an initial loading dose of 10–30 mg intramuscularly. In these situations, changeover to oral therapy should be carried out as soon as possible. Side effects, such as acute dystonias, seem to be rare. With haloperidol, the chances of severe side effects such as hypotension or a seizure are minimized.

Side effects

The side effects of major tranquillizers are similar to those listed for antidepressants (Table 5). Of particular interest, however, are the extrapyramidal syndromes, which include dystonias, akinesia, akathisia, Parkinsonism and tardive syndromes.

In general, these disorders fall into two groups, as shown in Table 8. In practice, some admixture of symptoms is seen, and the division may not be so clear. The acute disorders include acute dystonias, akathisia, akinesia and Parkinsonism. The chronic ones are mainly tardive dystonia and tardive dyskinesia. Acute dystonia is one of the earliest extrapyramidal side effects and usually occurs within the first two or three days of treatment. Typically, the movements are uncoordinated and spasmodic, and may involve the body, the limbs, the head and the neck. The jaws may be tightly clenched together, the tongue may be forcibly protruded and facial grimaces occur. Retrocollis, torticollis, antecollis, oculogyric crises or opisthotonos may all be seen. Males are preferentially affected and some suggest that up to 50 per cent of patients may develop some form of reaction following treatment with high potency neuroleptics (Winslow *et al.*, 1986). There are repeated spasms of muscles with hypertonicity between attacks, and the condition can be distressing and painful. Dystonia is usually treated by intramuscular or intravenous administration of an anticholinergic drug such as benztropine or orphenadrine, although benzodiazepines are also effective. It is thought to be due to increased dopamine turnover that occurs following acute administration of dopamine antagonists, stimulating dopamine receptors not blocked by the action of the drugs and thus provoking the movement disorder.

Much more common is akinesia, which is usually seen within 24 hours of starting the drugs. Patients have diminished spontaneous movements, reduced facial expression and may complain of fatigue. Muscle tone is not increased, and the clinical picture may be mistaken for an increasing apathy of depression or schizophrenia. It is usually helped by lowering the dose of the major tranquillizer or adding an anticholinergic drug.

Table 8   Extrapyramidal effects of psychotrophic drugs

Acute	Chronic
Dystonia	Tardive dyskinesia
Akathisia	Tardive dystonia
Akinesia	
Parkinsonism	
Rabbit syndrome	

Akathisia is sometimes less acute, but occurs very frequently, affecting over 50 per cent of patients. It is characterized by a subjective sense of restlessness and presents as motor hyperactivity, with shifting posture and inability to sit or stay still for more than a few moments. It thus resembles agitation, and may lead to a mistaken diagnosis of agitated depression, or a deterioration of the psychosis if unrecognized. Gibb and Lees (1986) have pointed out that a group of patients exist who also have orofacial dyskinesia, recognizing the frequent occurrence of the two disorders in the same patient. They also note that, particularly in those with late onset and persistent akathisia, the subjective restlessness is often not manifest, although patients still demonstrate motor restlessness. Akathisia usually responds to a reduction of dose or to the administration of anticholinergic or benzodiazepine drugs. Since similar clinical pictures have been reported in patients following L-dopa therapy in Parkinson's disease, it is thought that it somehow relates to abnormalities of dopamine transmission within the basal ganglia.

The classical picture of Parkinsonism, with increased muscle tone, rigidity, increased salivation, gait and posture disturbances, may be seen in patients prescribed neuroleptic drugs, and over 60 per cent of patients may have mild symptoms. In contrast to idiopathic Parkinson's disease, tremor tends to occur late in the picture and is less common than rigidity and akinesia. Akathisia may also be associated with the Parkinsonian picture. The Parkinsonism tends to come on gradually, and may be preceded by complaints of weakness or limb pains. Females are more affected than males. A variant is the so-called 'rabbit syndrome' in which rapid chewing-like movements of the lips occur that resemble a rabbit eating. This is to be distinguished from tardive dyskinesia.

It has been suggested that the incidence of Parkinsonism, and indeed some of the other extrapyramidal syndromes, may be diminished by the administration of routine prophylactic anticholinergic drugs. However, it may be argued that since anticholinergic drugs may exacerbate some motor disorders, for example tardive dyskinesia, may provoke a toxic psychosis, may delay gastric emptying and by neurochemical antagonism of the dopamine blocking potential of the antipsychotic drugs may diminish their therapeutic potential, such routine prescription should be avoided.

As noted, some antipsychotic drugs provoke less in the way of Parkinsonian and other extrapyramidal side effects, sulpiride and thioridazine being the two which are in clinical use. Again, treatment is either by reducing the dose of the neuroleptic drug or by changing to one of these alternative prescriptions. Administration of long-term anticholinergic drugs is probably best avoided.

Other conditions seen after varying time intervals of introducing neuroleptic drugs include the blepharospasm–oromandibular–dystonia syndrome (Meige's or Bruegel's syndrome), catatonic reactions and the neuroleptic malignant syndrome. The blepharospasm–oromandibular–dystonia syndrome is characterized by prolonged spasms of the jaw and mouth, usually in association with blepharospasm, which is seen both as an idiopathic form and also following neuroleptic treatment. Females are more affected than males, and the onset is usually in the sixth decade. The dystonia can be extremely painful, the teeth being forced together and sometimes damaged, or alternatively tongue biting occurring. The mouth may be forced into an open position for varying periods, which if severe may lead to difficulties with speaking, eating and sometimes jaw dislocation. Tongue protrusion, lip pouting and occasionally dystonic posturing in other parts of the body may also be noted. The pathogenesis is unknown, but again it is thought to be related to abnormalities of dopamine activity within the basal ganglia. It is one of a group of newly recognized tardive dystonias, which include other forms of dystonic posturing, spasmodic dysphonia, and abnormal vocalizations which sometimes are in association with tics, a tardive form of the Gilles de la Tourette syndrome.

Catatonic reactions involve posturing, waxy flexibility, withdrawal, mutism and associated Parkinsonism, which may be severe and life threatening and misinterpreted as an exacerbation of the underlying psychosis.

The neuroleptic malignant syndrome is one of the most serious of the extrapyramidal complications, presenting as hyperpyrexia and rigidity. It may emerge from a catatonic reaction and be associated with a variety of other abnormal involuntary movements. Autonomic disturbances including cardiovascular and respiratory difficulties, perspiration, salivation and incontinence may be seen, and death may occur from respiratory, cardiac, hepatic or renal failure. It can develop quite suddenly and has been described following a single injection of a neuroleptic. Its appearance may be facilitated by the combined administration of lithium. Its pathogenesis is not understood, but presumably relates to dopamine receptor blockade in the basal ganglia and hypothalamus. In view of its high mortality (20–30 per cent), attention to the patient's medical state is extremely important. Leucocytosis and elevated creatine kinase levels in the presence of abnormal liver function tests are often found. Treatment with bromocryptine, dantrolene and amantadine have all been tried.

Tardive dyskinesia

This condition is a chronic disorder secondary to the administration of major tranquillizers, although idiopathic forms with an identical clinical picture are noted. In addition, it has been associated with the taking of antihistamines, anticholinergic drugs, anticonvulsants, particularly phenytoin, and the tricyclic antidepressants. It usually comes on after about three months of therapy, and its appearance is gradual. In some patients, the first movements are noted following reduction of drug dosage. This withdrawal dyskinesia is frequently seen in patients who have been on neuroleptic medication for a long period of time.

The characteristic features of tardive dyskinesia are persistent abnormal muscular movements, predominantly affecting the tongue and perioral region, but, in addition, choreiform and athetoid movements in the limbs, and occasionally the trunk. There is smacking of the lips with masticatory jaw movements and protrusion of the tongue, often in combination. Sometimes the only clinical manifestation is increasing writhing movements of the lips. In other patients, blepharospasm, blinking, tics, abdominal movements and laryngeal spasms may also be noted. More rarely, particularly in younger patients, a to-and-fro clonic-type movement of the spine is seen. Although it is sometimes stated that the condition does not cause much stress, and it is true that patients often lightly dismiss the dyskinesia, putting their problems down to 'denture difficulties', it nevertheless in some patients is very uncomfortable and may be socially quite disabling.

Tardive dyskinesia is found more frequently in patients receiving neuroleptics than in control populations, is commoner in females and is found with increasing frequency with age. Younger patients tend to have involvement of the extremities and trunk, occasionally with bizarre postures and ballistic movements with gait abnormalities and rocking, while in the elderly a perioral distribution with associated limb movements is the more frequent picture. Kidger *et al.* (1980), using a principal components analysis of the symptoms, suggested three components to the overall syndrome, which were an orofacial factor, a trunk and limb movement factor and a Parkinsonian factor.

In some cases the dyskinesia is persistent, although a withdrawal dykinesia will tend to disappear over weeks to months, following cessation of the neuroleptic. Present estimates suggest that about 50 per cent of patients with tardive dykinesia will remain unchanged at follow-up. No convincing association between duration, dose or type of antipsychotic drug treatment has emerged, although there is a suggestion that patients who develop tardive dyskinesia are more likely to show impairments on psychological testing (Wegner *et al.*, 1985; Struve and Willner, 1983), and an increased incidence of CT scan changes including ventricular dilatation (Owens *et al.*, 1985).

The pathogenesis of tardive dyskinesia has yet to be clarified. The facts that it is commonly related to drugs whose principal action is dopamine antagonism and that it is a tardive disorder has led to the suggestion that it is related to the development of postsynaptic dopamine receptor supersensitivity. This is supported by observations that similar movements may be seen following L-dopa therapy for Parkinson's disease and that L-dopa itself may exacerbate the movements of tardive dykinesia. However, there are serious shortcomings to the concept that the condition is simply related to some form of receptor disuse supersensitivity. These include the discrepancies between the development of the clinical syndrome and the time of the increase in dopamine receptors following the beginning of treatment, which can be shown to occur rapidly in animal models. Further, all animals given neuroleptics develop supersensitivity, whereas only some 20 per cent of patients develop the persisting dyskinesia. In addition, in animal models where increased receptor sensitivity is shown, no equivalent of tardive dyskinesia has been seen. The receptor changes tend to revert to normal after withdrawal, but again, in patients, persistence of the syndrome can continue for many years. Finally, in patient post-mortem studies, no difference in binding has been shown with respect to either D1 or D2 receptors in the brain when patients with schizophrenia with or without movement disorders are compared (Waddington, 1985).

An alternative hypothesis relates to an alteration of GABA, since significant reductions in GAD activity have been shown in the globus pallidus, subthalamus and substantia nigra of primates receiving long-term neuroleptic therapy (Gunne et al., 1984). This deficit appeared related to abnormal orofacial movements in the animals. The hypothesis receives some support from early suggestions that GABA agonists may improve some of the symptoms of tardive dyskinesia in patients (Casey et al., 1980). These data have recently been replicated using gamma-vinyl GABA, in studies in which dyskinetic schizophrenic patients were reported to show lower CSF GABA levels than those without dyskinesias (Thaker et al., 1987). Although no consistent abnormalities or neuropathological changes at post-mortem have been described, there are several reports of microscopic changes in some basal ganglia areas, including the substantia nigra in patients receiving long-term neuroleptics (Christensen et al., 1970), perhaps suggesting that the clinical picture arises from the combination of some form of intrinsic neuronal damage in these crucial regions of the brain and long-term dopamine receptor blockade.

A large number of drugs have been tried in the treatment of tardive dyskinesia, but success has been very limited. Most of the studies have been continued for a few weeks only, and the majority are not double-blind. Neuroleptic drugs themselves are the most effective method of suppressing the symptoms, although in the long term it seems hardly logical to use them. Anticholinergic drugs exacerbate the symptoms, and withdrawal should be undertaken if they are concurrently prescribed in a patient with the syndrome (Burnett et al., 1980).

Other side effects

Agranulocytosis, due to a direct toxic effect of phenothiazines on the bone marrow, may occur and depression of the white cell count is often encountered. Photosensitivity may be a problem with chlorpromazine, and may lead to skin eruptions on exposure to sunlight or a pattern of contact dermatitis. Retinal pigmentation has been described with thioridazine. Combinations of lithium and haloperidol may lead to an organic psycho-syndrome. A withdrawal syndrome has been seen after long-term treatment, with insomnia, anxiety, restlessness and the already mentioned movement disorders. A depressive illness has been reported to occur in some patients treated with neuroleptics, although the exact relationship between the medication and the depression is unclear, since postpsychotic depression is a well-recognized clinical entity. One suggestion is that suppression of the psychotic symptoms permits the expression of preexistent affective symptoms.

MINOR TRANQUILLIZERS

Three main groups are included: barbiturates, benzodiazepines and others. As such, they are the most widely used drugs in psychiatry, and possess sedative and anticonvulsant properties in addition to being anxiolytic. The main differences between the barbiturates and the benzodiazepines reside in the lack of suicide potential with the latter and the greater tendency to addiction with the former.

Barbiturates include phenobarbitone, butobarbitone and amylobarbitone. They are rapidly absorbed from the GI tract and are powerful hepatic enzyme inducers. Their duration of action is around eight hours, but their generalized effect on the brain leads to respiratory depression, which may cause death in overdose. Since the introduction of the benzodiazepines, they are used far less frequently, although occasional patients still benefit from the prescription of an hypnotic barbiturate in very selected circumstances. Although phenobarbitone at one time was an important drug in the management of epilepsy, its use these days is not encouraged.

The benzodiazepines have a common structure, but differ with respect to their metabolites (see Figure 4).

Ultimately, they are conjugated with glucuronic acid, and a number of the metabolic products themselves are active compounds. However, some of the benzodiazepines (particularly the short-acting ones) tend not to have active intermediaries. Many of the longer-acting ones have desmethyldiazepam as their active metabolite, which has a half-life of some 50 hours. However, benzodiazepines differ both with regards to their half-life and with their potential for anxiolytic, anticonvulsant, muscle relaxant,

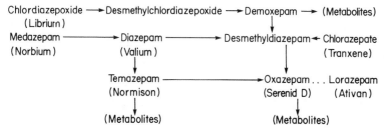

Figure 4. Showing the pathway of benzodiazepine metabolism.

sedative and amnesic effects. Some of these differences are shown in Tables 9 and 10.

On the basis of their half-lives, they may be divided into long, intermediate and short duration of action. Some of these pharmacokinetic differences are shown in Table 11.

In general, those with a long duration of action tend to be prescribed as anxiolytics, while those in the short-acting class are hypnotics. The clearance of many of these drugs is increased with age, although oxazepam, lorazepam and temazepam show only minor differences in their kinetics with advancing years. The metabolism of lorazepam and oxazepam are little influenced by liver disease.

The discovery of the benzodiazepine receptor has led to a clearer understanding of their mode of action (Braestrup and

Table 9   Half-life of different benzodiazepines

	Hours
Temazepam	8
Oxazepam	8
Lorazepam	12
Medazepam	6–20
Flurazepam	10–20
Chlordiazepoxide	24
Diazepam	30
Chlorazepate	30–60
Nitrazepam	48
Triazolam	2
Clonazepam	53
Clobazam	18

Table 10   Differential effect of different benzodiazepines

Drug	Anxiolytic	Anticonvulsant	Muscle relaxing	Sedative	Amnesic
Lorazepam	+ +	+ + +	+	+	+ + +
Diazepam	+ +	+	+ + +	+ +	+
Temazepam	+	±	+	+ + +	±
Clonazepam	±	+ + +	+ +	+	±
Nitrazepam	+	+ +	+	+ + +	±
Clobazam	+ +	+ + +	+	±	±

Nielsen, 1982). The benzodiazepine binding site, thought to represent part of the GABA–receptor chloride ionophor complex, is in some way related to the behavioural actions of these drugs, although it does not explain all of their effects. For example, meprobamate and alcohol, both effective anxiolytics, do not bind to the receptor. This is one element of the argument which has led Gray (1982) to suggest that at least the anxiolytic effect of the benzodiazepines is related to enhancement of GABA transmission, probably at selective sites within the CNS, but that interaction with other neurotransmitter systems, in particular the ascending monoamines, is also involved (Iversen, 1983). Benzodiazepine antagonists counteract some of the effects of benzodiazepines, and provoke anxiety in humans (Dorow *et al.*, 1983). Respiratory depression does not appear to be a complication of benzodiazepine therapy, and after overdose, if taken alone, benzodiazepines rarely result in death.

The differing profile of benzodiazepines is reflected in two recently introduced compounds, namely clobazam and

Table 11   Pharmacokinetic differences among benzodiazepines

Long	Intermediate	Short
Chlordiazepoxide	Alprazolam	Brotizolam
Clorazepate	Bromazepam	Midazolam
Clobazam	Flunitrazepam	Triazolam
Diazepam	Lorazepam	
Flurazepam	Lormetazepam	
Ketazolam	Nitrazepam	
Medazepam	Oxazepam	
Prazepam	Temazepam	

alprazolam. Clobazam is a 1,5-benzodiazepine, in which the nitrogen on the heterocyclic ring is moved from the 4 to the 5 position. This appears to confer a better therapeutic potential of the drug with regards to its anticonvulsant effect, the drug possessing minimal sedative, myorelaxant and cognitive side effects (Trimble, 1986d). Alprazolam is a triazolobenzodiazepine, which in addition to its anxiolytic properties is reported to be effective in the control of panic disorder and may possess antidepressant properties (Judd et al., 1986). It appears that most benzodiazepines are ineffective for panic attacks, while tricyclic antidepressants, MAOI drugs and alprazolam are therapeutically useful. Alprazolam is antidepressant for patients with reactive or neurotic depression (Imlah, 1985) and mania has been reported as a side effect (Arana et al., 1985).

Recently, concern has been expressed about benzodiazepine dependence. This has been reported after as short a time as six weeks of treatment, although tends to occur in patients who have been on high doses for prolonged periods. Withdrawal symptoms may occur, particularly if the dose of the drug is withdrawn at an inappropriate rate. The withdrawal syndrome in many cases represents a return of earlier anxiety, although some authors have suggested that perceptual distortions and feelings of depersonalization are characteristic (Ashton, 1984). Withdrawal seizures are certainly one manifestation, although again, in the clinical setting, probably reflect too rapid a decrease in dose. The presence of the withdrawal syndrome suggests how effective these compounds are biologically, and thus how they should be used judiciously in clinical practice. It has been reported that premorbid personality characteristics may be important in predicting those patients who will show withdrawal reactions, those with passive and dependent personality traits being more susceptible than those showing premorbid conscientiousness, rigidity or even premorbid anxiety proneness (Tyrer et al., 1983).

Benzodiazepine withdrawal symptoms occur somewhat later than those due to barbiturates, and they do not appear to correlate with serum levels of benzodiazepines or their metabolites. Treatment with propranolol, clonidine, tricyclic antidepressants and oxypertine have all been suggested.

Other side effects include oversedation, problems with concentration and memory, and in the elderly, ataxia and confusion, particularly with the longer-acting and more sedative compounds. Depression has been reported, but it is also seen following long-term benzodiazepine withdrawal (Olajide and Lader, 1984).

Release of aggression has also been noted in both animals and humans.

Other minor tranquillizers include meprobamate, which is absorbed rapidly, induces its own metabolism and has a half-life of about twelve hours. It is approximately halfway between the barbiturates and the benzodiazepines in terms of producing tolerence, sedation and cortical depression. Other hypnotics include chloral hydrate, dichloralphenazone, glutethamide, paraldehyde and chlormethiazole. The latter may be particularly useful in the management of alcohol withdrawal syndromes.

Buspirone is a cyclopyrrolone, which is well absorbed and widely distributed throughout the body. It has a half-life of approximately two to three hours, and although a dopamine antagonist does not appear to be antipsychotic. It has anxiolytic properties, possibly related to an action at the dopamine receptor, but lacks sedative, muscle relaxant and anticonvulsant effects. It does not appear to interact with benzodiazepine or GABA receptors, and thus has a relatively unique profile for an anxiolytic compound. Zopiclone is also a cyclopyrrolone, which has a short half-life and is effective as an hypnotic.

When using minor tranquillizers, doses of drugs have to be based on clinical judgement, and for tranquillization once daily or twice daily regimes can be used. Although some patients develop tolerance to these drugs, requiring increasing doses over time, this is not usual and many patients continue to get clinical benefit on small doses. However, it is important that they should not be given for longer than is necessary, and that when withdrawal is undertaken, it should be done slowly and with care.

BETA-ADRENERGIC BLOCKERS

Beta-adrenergic blockers, such as propranolol, are widely used in the management of cardiovascular disorders, and clinically decrease the heart rate, lower the blood pressure and may cause bronchial constriction. Their use in the management of anxiety disorders has been advocated, one suggestion being that they influence the somatic symptoms such as palpitations, sweating and diarrhoea as opposed to psychic symptoms (Tyrer and Lader, 1974). However, improvement of psychic symptoms has also been reported (Kathol et al., 1980), and the suggestion that their effect is primarily on peripheral receptors may need revision. Some beta blockers such as practolol, with little ability to cross the blood–

brain barrier, also appear to be effective anxiolytics. They are of little value in agoraphobia and panic attacks and do not influence lactate-induced panic (Gorman *et al.*, 1983). There has been interest in their use in schizophrenia, but the results of various trials are contradictory. If they are of value, it is only in high doses, over 600 mg per day, and at least part of their clinical efficacy may be related to their interaction with neuroleptics, significantly elevating serum chlorpromazine levels (Peet, 1981). They are contraindicated in patients with respiratory and cardiac disorders, where beta blockade may lead to deterioration of the clinical state, and are poorly tolerated by some people who develop a severe malaise and lethargy which, if unrecognized, may be taken for further symptoms of the underlying psychiatric disturbance. A withdrawal syndrome has been described with abrupt termination of treatment. Their use as single doses (40 mg of oxprenolol) to quell stage fright and other brief-lived episodes of stress-induced anxiety may be helpful, but generally in the management of patients with anxiety, benzodiazepines are preferred, particularly by patients (Tyrer and Lader, 1974).

LITHIUM

Lithium carbonate was first introduced for the treatment of manic depressive illness in 1949 and has in recent years become the drug of choice for prophylactic management of manic depressive psychosis. Following ingestion, it is absorbed rapidly, peak concentrations occurring in one to two hours, with a half-life of approximately 24 hours. It is mainly excreted in the urine, and thus patients with renal disease readily become intoxicated. Since it is reabsorbed with sodium into the proximal renal tubules, any drug that leads to a negative sodium balance, such as a diuretic, will lead to increased retention of lithium. This also occurs with alteration of the diet, heavy sweating and diseases that reduce sodium intake. For a hypertensive patient, a beta blocker or clonidine is preferred, and thiazide diuretics should be avoided.

Its mode of action is still unknown in spite of its widespread use, but it does reduce sodium content of the brain, increase central 5-HT synthesis and noradrenaline turnover, increase platelet 5-HT uptake (Coppen *et al.*, 1980) and reduce urinary noradrenaline, MHPG, VMA and whole body noradrenaline turnover (Linnoila *et al.*, 1983a). Rangel-Guerra *et al.* (1983) reported that using MRI, T_1 proton relaxation time was reduced from elevated levels in 20 patients with bipolar affective disorder following lithium therapy of 900 mg per day for ten days.

The main indication for lithium is in bipolar manic depressive illness, although it is now known to be useful in the management of recurrent unipolar affective disorder. It may also be used in the acute treatment of affective disorder, especially mania, when it is usually started in combination with a major tranquillizer. Other uses of lithium include recurrent aggressive disorders, migraine, cluster headaches, cycloid psychoses and organic mental disorders with secondary affective symptoms. In one trial (Coppen et al., 1978), lithium was found to be superior to mianserin in the long-term maintenance treatment of depressive illness.

It has a number of toxic effects, which are shown in Table 12. Although these are minimized by regular monitoring of serum lithium levels, with a suggested non-toxic range of 0.6–1.5 μmol/l, severe toxicity has been described at lower levels, and coexistent medication such as phenytoin, carbamazepine and haloperidol may be related to this. Ibuprofen, indomethacin, mefenamic acid, diclofenac and piroxicam inhibit lithium excretion, and diuretics cause lithium retention, which may increase serum levels. Patients with cardiac or renal disease, or in other situations that may interfere with the clearance of lithium, will obviously need regular monitoring and, prior to starting therapy, it is customary to assess renal and hepatic function. Thyroid function is also checked since hypothyroidism, sometimes associated with goitre or even advanced myxoedema, has been observed. Lithium therapy may decrease thyroxine and T_3 and increase TSH levels which may lead to abnormalities of thyroid function tests even in the absence of clinical signs of hypothyroidism. If lithium maintenance therapy is essential, then supplementary thyroxine treatment will be required if the patient develops myxoedema.

Although a teratogenic affect of lithium in humans has not been demonstrated, there are reports of a high incidence of congenital malformations in babies born to mothers who take lithium, and it should probably be discontinued if possible during pregnancy. One of the commonest side effects relates to altered renal function, with polyuria and polydipsia. Urinary concentrating ability is impaired, which may be exacerbated by combination with neuroleptics. The polyuria may result in compensatory increases in antidiuretic hormone secretion, although occasionally a picture of nephrogenic diabetes insipidus is seen. In spite of these findings,

Table 12   Toxic effects of lithium

Neuropsychiatric	Drowsiness
	Confusion
	Psychomotor retardation
	Restlessness
	Stupor
	Headache
	Weakness
	Tremor
	Ataxia
	Myasthenia gravis syndrome
	Peripheral neuropathy
	Choreoathetoid movements
	Dysarthria
	Dysgeusia
	Blurred vision
	Seizures
	Dizziness, vertigo
	Impaired short-term memory and concentration
Gastrointestinal	Anorexia, nausea, vomiting
	Diarrhoea
	Dry mouth, metallic taste
	Weight gain
Renal	Microtubular lesions
	Impairment of renal concentrating capacity
Cardiovascular	Low blood pressure
	ECG changes
Endocrine	Myxoedema
	Hyperthyroidism
	Hyperparathyroidism
Other	Polyuria and polydipsia
	Glycosuria
	Hypercalciuria
	Rashes

long-term follow-up does not suggest that serious renal damage occurs with prolonged therapy.

Severe intoxication may lead to a clear organic brain syndrome with hyperactive reflexes, seizures and tremor. On occasions, unilateral neurological abnormalities have been reported, which may be interpreted as an alternative neurological diagnosis. If toxicity results in coma, dialysis should be considered, especially if clearance is in any way delayed. On stopping the drug, the serum concentration usually falls by about half each day, and after routine therapy withdrawal symptoms including irritability and emotional lability have been described (King and Hullin, 1983).

ANTICONVULSANT TREATMENT

Some of the anticonvulsant drugs presently in use are shown in Table 13. The older barbiturate related compounds and phenytoin are gradually being replaced by newer drugs such as carbamazepine and sodium valproate. One problem has been the growing recognition of chronic toxic side effects that occur with the long-term administration that the treatment of epilepsy requires.

Phenytoin is highly plasma bound and cleared from the plasma by hepatic metabolism. Varying serum levels may be noted amongst different patients on the same dose, and small increments in prescription can lead to rapidly escalating serum levels on account of its zero-order pharmacokinetics (Figure 1). In spite of its long use, its mechanism of action is still unclear although there are suggestions that it may interact with sodium or calcium channels in excitable neurones, thus limiting the potential for high frequency neuronal discharges. It is a membrane stabilizer and also possesses some benzodiazepine binding and thus has some influence at the GABA receptor, particularly at higher concentrations.

Primidone is partially converted to phenobarbitone, although the primidone component itself probably exerts independent anticonvulsant activity. Phenobarbitone also influences the transcellular transport of sodium, calcium and potassium ions influencing the neurotransmitter release of GABA, glutamate and aspartate. Further, it enhances GABA postsynaptic inhibition interacting at the benzodiazepine–GABA receptor.

Carbamazepine is structurally related to the tricyclic antidepressants, and has a mode of action different from phenytoin and phenobarbitone. Its biochemical actions include partial agonism of adenosine receptors; it acutely increases the firing of the locus

Table 13   Some anticonvulsant drugs in current use

Name	Half-life (h)	Recommended serum level (μmol/l)	Indications
Carbamazepine (Tegretol)	8–45	16–50	Generalized seizures; simple or complex partial seizures; secondary generalized seizures
Clobazam (Frisium)	22	—	
Clonazepam (Rivotril)	20–40	—	Myoclonic epilepsy
Ethosuximide (Zarontin)	30–100	300–700	Generalized absence seizures
Phenobarbitone	36 (children)	60–180	Generalized or simple partial seizures
Phenytoin (Epanutin)	—	40–100	Generalized seizures: simple or complex partial seizures
Primidone (Mysoline)	3–12	—	Generalized: complex or simple partial seizures
Sodium valproate (Epilim)	10–15	—	Generalized absence seizures: myoclonic epilepsy; simple or complex partial seizures
Sulthiane (Ospolot)	—	—	Complex partial seizures

coeruleus, and decreases CSF somatostatin and HVA accumulation after probenacid (Post and Uhde, 1986; Post *et al.*, 1986). Further, in animal models, carbamazepine is shown to be relatively more effective than other anticonvulsants in inhibiting the seizures developed from amygdala kindling, suggesting some limbic system selectivity for the drug (Albright and Burnham, 1980). Ever since its introduction for the management of epilepsy it has been reported to have some psychotropic properties, and its recent use as a mood stabilizer in manic depressive illness has been widely investigated and reviewed (Post and Uhde, 1986). It appears to be as effective as conventional neuroleptics in the acute management of mania, and to be equivalent to lithium in the long-term prophylaxis of bipolar affective disorder. Although some trials have been carried out on patients who are lithium resistant, neither this nor the presence of EEG abnormalities are related to a beneficial clinical response. Some patients respond well to a combination of carbamazepine and lithium, while not responding to each individual drug alone. Although its main use is in the control of complex partial seizures, for which it is now the drug of choice, it is also used in schizoaffective disorders, in the management of aggression and episodic dyscontrol and in some schizophrenic patients. Trials in the latter condition are sparse and the indications for its use have yet to be evaluated.

Sodium valproate is thought to be a GABA agonist, although the mechanism of its anticonvulsant action is unknown at the present time. It also reduces sodium and potassium conductance, reducing the excitability of nerve membranes. As with carbamazepine, it has been suggested as having some mood stabilizing properties, although the case is less secure.

The role of benzodiazepines in the management of epilepsy has been largely restricted to acute use in status epilepticus. However, clonazepam and clobazam have been used for oral therapy. Clonazepam finds more use in childhood, but is markedly sedative, in contrast to clobazam, a non-sedative 1,5-benzodiazepine. Clobazam has effective antiepileptic properties in a subgroup of patients who are non-responsive to other drugs, and is used as adjunctive therapy.

The side effects of anticonvulsants are many. While acute toxic effects have been recognized for a long time, the chronic ones, especially subtle changes of cognition and behaviour, have only recently become widely discussed (see Table 14).

Neuropsychiatric side effects, in particular of phenytoin, include an encephalopathy and deterioration of intellectual function, while apathy, depression, dysphoria, irritability and occasionally hyperactivity are seen in association with the barbiturates and polytherapy. Chronic dyskinesias are occasionally seen, while an acute dystonic reaction has been noted with carbamazepine. Sodium valproate has been associated with liver failure in a small number of young patients, and also produces a reversible alopecia and weight gain. Carbamazepine may be associated with water intoxication, although the mechanism of this is not clear. This is in contrast to the polyuria provoked by lithium, and emphasizes the different pharmacological profiles of lithium and carbamazepine, even though both have mood stabilizing effects.

Interactions between anticonvulsants and other drugs, or between anticonvulsants themselves, may present problems in management. Of particular importance are the drugs that elevate phenytoin levels and may lead to phenytoin toxicity (see Table 15), and interactions with psychotropic drugs. There is some

Table 14   Chronic toxic effects of some anticonvulsant drugs (from Reynolds, 1975)

Nervous system	Cerebellar atrophy (?)
	Peripheral neuropathy
	Encephalopathy
	Other mental symptoms
Haemopoietic system	Folic acid deficiency
	Neonatal coagulation defects
Skeletal system	Metabolic bone disease
	Vitamin D deficiency
Connective tissue	Gum hypertrophy
	Facial skin changes
	Wound healing
	Dupytren's contracture
Skin	Hirsutism
	Pigmentation
	Acne
Liver	Enzyme induction
Endocrine system	Pituitary–adrenal
	Thyroid–parathyroid
	Hyperglycaemia (diabetogenic)
Other metabolic disorders	Vitamin B_6 deficiency (?)
	Heavy metals
Immunological disorders	Lymphotoxicity
	Lymphadenopathy
	Systemic lupus erythaematosus
	Antinuclear antibodies
	Immunoglobulin changes (?)
	Immunosuppression

evidence that patients on phenytoin, because of induced hepatic enzymes, will have lower serum levels of antidepressants, and thus prescription of the usual dose may be subtherapeutic. Serum levels of neuroleptics may likewise be significantly lower in patients treated with anticonvulsants than in controls. Viloxazine has been shown to provoke carbamazepine intoxication (Pisani *et al.*, 1984).

It is generally accepted that newly diagnosed patients should be treated by the prescription of only one anticonvulsant drug if

Table 15 Some interactions between anticonvulsants and between anticonvulsants and other drugs

	Effect on phenytoin levels
Sulthiame	↑
Diazepam, clonazepam	↓
Carbamazepine[a]	↓
Phenobarbitone	↓
Valproate[b]	↑ (free levels)

Effect of these compounds reduced	May induce anticonvulsant toxicity
Warfarin and coumarin anticonvulsants	Isoniazid
Cortisol, dexamethasone and prednisolone	Dicoumarol
Contraceptive pill	Disulfiram
Vitamin D	Chloramphenicol
Phenylbutazone	Imipramine
Antidepressants	Chlorpromazine
Chlorpromazine	Chlorpheniramine
Digoxin	Methyl phenidate
Diazepam	

[a] Carbamazepine reduces the serum concentration of phenytoin and vice versa.
[b] Sodium valproate displaces phenytoin from its protein binding sites, increasing the unbound fraction of phenytoin.

possible. It has recently been shown that upwards of 80 per cent of new patients with appropriate serum level monitoring and adequate serum levels will be satisfactorily controlled on monotherapy. It is not clear that addition of a second drug will lead to better management of seizures in those who continue to have attacks, with rare exceptions. Recent research has suggested that patients who have further seizures are likely to do so within a year of presentation with the first attack, and it is thus to some extent predictable who is likely to become the patient with chronic uncontrolled seizures. It is this group in particular that are liable to receive polytherapy, and, in the long term, who may suffer neuropsychiatric complications.

The question of which anticonvulsant drug to use for which type of seizure is often a matter of clinical choice, but some guidelines are clear. In some instances, for example, the use of steroids or ACTH for infantile spasms and the almost exclusive use of ethosuximide for generalized absence seizures, there is high specificity. However, for the majority of seizures, there is more overlap, as noted in Table 13. There is some recent evidence that carbamazepine has superiority over the other drugs for the management of complex partial seizures, but aside from this, the choice of prescription relates to side effects and patients' tolerability. Phenytoin is particularly unsuitable for a number of patients because of its side effects, including cognitive dulling, hirsutes, gum hypertrophy and acne with coarsening of the facial features. Teratogenic effects also occur with anticonvulsant drugs, although again carbamazepine would appear to bring with it the minimal risk. During pregnancy, serum levels of anticonvulsants may fall, and they thus need to be carefully monitored if control of the epilepsy proves difficult.

Dosage of the drugs will vary with each individual, although generally it is wise to start with a small dose and increase gradually until satisfactory serum levels are achieved. Many anticonvulsants can be given on a once daily or twice daily regime and compliance may be enhanced by this prescription.

CONVULSIVE THERAPY

Although the original observations of von Meduna led to the introduction of convulsive therapy with camphor, electroconvulsive therapy (ECT) was introduced by Cerletti and Bini for the treatment of schizophrenia. However, it was clear that it gave better results in depressive illness, the main indication for its use today. Although it was eclipsed by the successful introduction of antidepressants in the 1960s, more recently there has been an upsurge of interest. This has stemmed partly from the realization that antidepressant drugs may be ineffective in severe affective disorder, and further from the troublesome side effects of psychotropic drugs which may be seen with long-term treatment, sometimes required in psychotic patients, for example the extrapyramidal complications of neuroleptic drugs. Its current place in therapy has been extensively reviewed (Fink, 1986a; Malitz and Sackheim, 1986). The conclusions of an NIH consensus development conference stated: 'ECT is demonstrably effective for a narrow range of severe psychiatric disorders in a limited number of diagnostic categories; delusional and severe endogenous depression and manic and certain schizophrenic syndromes' (Consensus Development Conference Statement, 1986).

Fink (1986a) refers to the changes in behaviour that occur consequent on ECT, dividing them into those which are seizure dependent (see Table 16) and those which are subject dependent (see Table 17).

The seizure dependent effects are a direct result of the seizure or the seizure induction method and include neurophysiological and hormonal consequences, the majority of which are usually transient, returning to pretreatment levels within days or a few weeks of the seizures. The subject dependent effects are related to the state of the patient at the time of administration of the seizure, one of the most persistently observed consequences being elevation of mood in severely depressed patients, an effect being particularly noted in patients who are suicidal or psychotic.

Table 16 Seizure dependent effects

Organic mental syndrome
    Memory difficulty
    Amnesia
    Disorientation, confusion
    Aphasia
    Dementia

Interseizure EEG
    Delta/theta slowing
    Amplitude increase
    Burst patterns

Rise in brain seizure threshold

Rise in plasma prolactin

Increased permeability of the blood–brain barrier

Headache

Table 17   Subject dependent effects

Behavioural consequences vary with clinical syndrome	
Major depression	Relief of depression
Psychosis	Normalized thought patterns
Excitement, mania	Reduced hypermotility
Stupor	Alerting; normal behaviour
Parkinsonism	Reduced rigidity
Pseudodementia	Relief of dementia
Neuroleptic malignant syndrome	Syndrome relieved
Characterological issues	
Hypochondriasis	Symptoms worsened
Hysterical character	Increased complaints
Denial personality	Increased use of denial

Stimulus parameters have received considerable attention, as has the issue of unilateral or bilateral electrode placement. Waveform, either sine wave or brief pulse stimuli (short current bursts with lower energy content), have been compared, as have different stimulus intensities. At present there is no evidence of a difference in therapeutic outcome between high and low energy stimuli, although the latter provokes less acute cognitive and electrophysiological abnormalities (Weiner, 1986). Supra threshold stimuli do not produce additional therapeutic benefits (Ottosson, 1960).

The issue of whether unilateral ECT is as effective as bilateral ECT has been the subject of considerable investigation. The consensus seems to be that no differences in outcome are demonstrated between the two forms of electrode placement, although some studies demonstrate a therapeutic advantage for bilateral ECT, especially if a fixed number of treatments are compared. Memory disruption is considerably greater with bilateral electrode placement, as are other side effects such as post-seizure confusion and headache. Unilateral non-dominant hemisphere seizure discharge seems to be associated with less intracerebral current and less postictal suppression of the contralateral hemisphere.

Although its use has been established for many years, recently several double-blind controlled trials of ECT have been carried out (see Crow and Johnstone, 1986b). The majority of these have been in affective disorder, and demonstrate a significant benefit for electroconvulsive therapy. A consistent predictor of response has been the presence of delusions, although clinically 'endogenicity' has been a valuable guide. Several authors have looked at ECT response in relationship to outcome (Fink, 1986b). Generally, while the prognosis seems unrelated to the pretreatment DST status, normalization of an abnormal DST suggests a good clinical outcome and failure to normalize should be cause for concern. Prolactin has been shown to rise following the seizure (Trimble, 1978), elevations being greater for bilateral as opposed to unilateral electrode placement. Abrams and Schwartz (1985) have reported an inverse relationship between the prolactin release at fifteen minutes of the first four treatments and clinical outcome. Those with good response showed lower peak prolactin elevations than poor responders.

Trials against simulated ECT have also been reported for schizophrenia (Taylor and Fleminger, 1980), demonstrating the benefit of the seizure, and successful use of non-dominant hemisphere unilateral ECT in manic episodes has been shown (Small *et al.*, 1986). Other situations where ECT has occasionally been helpful have been in the management of Parkinson's disease, organic mental disorders, particularly associated with severe affective disorder, in delirium and in epilepsia partialis continua in order to bring the seizure to an end.

The mechanism of action of ECT is not known. Changes of brain function evolve over time, reflected in the usual clinical practice of administering therapy two or three times a week. The antidepressant effect seems directly related to the seizure activity (Ottosson, 1960), cumulative seizure duration being an important variable. Maletsky (1978) estimated that if total seizure time was less than 201 seconds, no response was noted, while most patients respond after 1000 seconds, beyond this little additional improvement being noted. In animal models a consistent effect is down-regulation of beta adrenergic receptor sites, and enhanced behavioural responses to 5-HT, possibly related to increased numbers of 5-HT_2 receptors, have been noted. Dopamine related behaviours are also shown to be enhanced by repeated seizures (Green, 1986).

In man, Slade and Checkley (1980) examined growth hormone responses to clonidine and methylamphetamine in patients with affective disorder before and after a course of ECT. No significant changes were noted. The effects of ECT on neuroendocrine responses to apomorphine have also been reported but are variable. CBF is reduced following treatment, as is glucose metabolism (Silfverskiöld *et al.*, 1986).

Contraindications to the use of ECT are few, but include the presence of intracranial tumours and a recent cerebrovascular accident. Since an increase in CSF pressure occurs during the seizure discharge, ECT is best avoided in conditions where raised intracranial pressure is suspected. It carries with it minimal risk of mortality, and the morbidity is more related to complications of the accompanying anaesthetic than to the therapy itself.

PSYCHOSURGERY

The early experiments of Fulton and Jacobsen (1935) demonstrated that primates with destruction of the frontal lobes became more placid and less anxious. Moniz (1936) became the first to sever connections between the frontal lobes and other areas of the limbic system in psychiatric patients, which led Freeman and Watts (1947) to develop a standardized leucotomy technique. The early operations were radical frontal leucotomies in which a large section of white matter was severed between the frontal lobes and the rest of the brain, although since that time the operation has been remarkably refined. Thus, restricted frontal leucotomy was followed by orbital undercutting in which only the medial situated frontothalamic fibres were destroyed. Other selective lesions include cingulectomy, in which the anterior 4 cm of the cingulum are removed, and subcaudate tractotomy, in which lesions are placed beneath the head of the caudate nucleus. Stereotactic techniques have been used to place lesions with greater accuracy, and during some surgical procedures stimulation is carried out. This provokes subjective experiences in patients, but also is used to evaluate autonomic changes such as alteration of heart rate, blood pressure and forearm blood flow in order to locate sites for surgical destruction. In one procedure, multifocal leucocoagulation, patients have lesions made through chronically implanted electrodes after various intervals of time, the change in symptoms being continuously observed. When clinical status improves, further lesions are withheld.

The main frontolimbic connections which are severed pass from the lower medial quadrant of the frontal lobe to the septal and nucleus accumbens regions, thalamus and hypothalamus. Additional target areas are the frontocingular connections passing to the cingulate gyrus and hippocampus. The subcaudate pathway interrupts frontal and temporal connections, in addition to the ascending monoamine projections from the ventral tegmental area to the frontal cortex and vice versa.

In the United Kingdom, two main procedures are used at the present time. These are subcaudate tractotomy and limbic leucotomy, in which small lesions are placed in the lower medial quadrant of the frontal lobe and in the anterior cingulate gyrus.

Although the very early techniques had a mortality of around 6 per cent and a high morbidity, the modified and restricted operations can be carried out safely. Mitchell-Heggs *et al.* (1976) presented data on 66 patients who had a limbic leucotomy; 73 per cent were improved at six weeks and 76 per cent at sixteen months. The best results were in obsessional neurosis, anxiety and depression, although six of seven schizophrenic patients also responded, particularly if the schizophrenic symptoms were accompanied by anxiety, depression or obsessional states. In this follow-up, no intellectual deterioration was noted, and adverse personality changes were reported as minimal. Clinical improvements occurred gradually, for up to a period of a year. Patients with good premorbid personalities did better than those with poor preoperative adjustment. Patients with obsessional illness seemed to do particularly well with stereotactic limbic leucotomy.

Postoperatively, marked frontal lobe oedema can be seen on the MRI scan and a characteristic frontal slow wave activity is seen on the EEG. The amount of this shortly after the operation correlates with a beneficial clinical outcome one year later (Evans *et al.*, 1981).

The indications for psychosurgery have been clarified. Patients should have had a severe psychiatric illness, be potentially suicidal and have been ill for an average of ten years. Further, they must have been shown to have failed to respond to all alternative forms of therapy, including a good trial with available psychotropic medications. The best responses are seen in patients suffering from depression and obsessional neurosis, with good premorbid personalities, and from a stable home environment. Some schizophrenic patients do well, showing a reduction in the number of their psychotic episodes and a reduced need for phenothiazine medication. Psychopathy is an absolute contraindication, and patients who are addicted to drugs or alcohol are not suitable. Complications include cerebral haemorrhage, postoperative suicide, postoperative seizures, personality changes, urinary and faecal incontinence, increased weight, sleep disturbance and diabetes insipidus.

Other neurosurgical procedures used to ameliorate psychopathology include unilateral or bilateral amygdalotomy in patients with aggression, especially lesions of the medial amygdala in the relief of aggressive behaviour disturbances associated with epilepsy (Narabayashi, 1971). Thalamotomy has been used for obsessional illness, while placing lesions in the hypothalamus and stria terminalis have been tried for aggression.

References

Abdulla, Y.H., and Hamadah, K. (1970). 3,5 cyclic adenosine monophosphate in depression and mania, *Lancet*, **i**, 378–81.

Aberg Wistedt, A., and Wistedt, B. (1985). Higher CSF levels of HVA and 5HIAA in delusional compared to non-delusional depression, *Archives of General Psychiatry*, **42**, 925–6.

Abrahams, R., and Schwartz, C.M. (1985). ECT and prolactin release: relation to treatment response in melancholia, *Convulsive Therapy*, **1**, 38–42.

Abrams, R., and Taylor, M.A. (1979). Differential EEG patterns in affective disorder and schizophrenia, *Archives of General Psychiatry*, **36**, 1355–58.

Ackenheil, M., Albus, M., Muller, F., *et al.* (1979). Catecholamine response to short time stress in schizophrenic and depressive patients. In E. Usdin (Ed.), *Catecholamines: Basic and Clinical Frontiers*, Vol. 2, Pergamon Press, New York, pp. 1937–9.

Ackerknecht, E.H. (1973). Contributions of Gall and the phrenologists to knowledge of brain function. In *The Brain and Its Functions*, B.M. Israel, Amsterdam, pp. 149–53.

Adamec, R.E., and Stark-Adamec, C. (1983). Limbic kindling and animal behaviour, *Biological Psychiatry*, **18**, 269–93.

Adams, F. (1939), *The Genuine Works of Hippocrates*, Williams and Wilkins, Baltimore.

Adams, R.D., Fisher, C.M., Hakim, S., Ojemann, R., and Sweet, W.H. (1965). Symptomatic occult hydrocephalus with normal CSF pressure. A treatable syndrome, *New England Journal of Medicine*, **243**, 117–26.

Adolfsson, R., Gottfries, C-G., Oreland, L., Roos, B., Wiberg, A., and Winblad, B. (1978). Monoamine oxidase activity and serotonergic turnover in human brain, *Progress in Neuropsychopharmacology*, **2**, 225–30.

Adolfsson, R., Gottfries, C-G., Roos, B.E., and Winblad, B. (1979). Changes in brain catecholamines in patients with dementia of the Alzheimer type, *British Journal of Psychiatry*, **135**, 216–23.

Akiskal, H.S., Bitar, A.H., Puzantian, V.R., Rosenthal, T.L., and Walker, P.W. (1978). The nosological status of neurotic depression, *Archives of General Psychiatry*, **35**, 756–66.

Albert, M.L., Feldman, R.G., and Willis, A.L. (1974). The 'subcortical dementia' of progressive nuclear palsy, *Journal of Neurology, Neurosurgery and Psychiatry*, **37**, 121–30.

Albrecht, P., Boone, E., Fuller Torrey, E., Hicks, J.T., and Daniel, N. (1980). Raised cytomegalovirus–antibody levels in CSF of schizophrenic patients, *Lancet*, **ii**, 769–71.

Albright, P.S., and Burnham, W.I. (1980). Development of a new pharmcological seizure model: effects of anticonvulsants on cortical and amygdala-kindled seizures in the rat, *Epilepsia*, **21**, 681–9.

Albus, M., Ackenheil, M., Munch, U., and Naber, D. (1984). Ceruletide: a new drug for the treatment of schizophrenic patients, *Archives of General Psychiatry*, **41**, 528.

Alexopoulos, G.S., Inturrisi, C.E., and Lipman, R., *et al.* (1983). Plasma immunoreactive beta–endorphin levels in depression, *Archives of General Psychiatry*, **40**, 181–3.

Alzheimer, A. (1907). Uber eine eigenartige Erkrankung der Hirrinde. *Allegemeine Zeitschrift fur Psychiatrie*, **64**, 146–8.

American Psychiatric Association (1980). *Diagnostic and Statistical Manual of Mental Disorders*, 3rd edition, APA, Washington.

Anden, N.E. (1975). Animal models of brain dopamine function. In W. Birkmayer and O. Hornykiewicz (Eds.), *Advances in Parkinsonism*, Roche, Basle, pp. 169–77.

Anden, N.E., Dahlstrom, A., Fuxe, K., Larsson, K., Olson, L., and Ungerstedt, U. (1966). Ascending monoamine neurones to the telencephalon and diencephalon, *Acta Physiologica Scandinavica*, **67**, 313–26.

Andermann, E. (1980). Genetic aspects of epilepsy. In P. Robb (ed.), *Epilepsy Updated: Causes and Treatment*, Medical Year Book, Chicago, pp. 11–24.

Andreasen, N.C., and Olsen, S. (1982). Negative and positive schizophrenia, *Archives of General Psychiatry*, **39**, 789–94.

Andreasen, N.C., and Winokur, G. (1979). Newer experimental methods for classification of depression, *Archives of General Psychiatry*, **36**, 447–52.

Andreasen, N., Nasrallah, H.A., Van Dunn, V., *et al.* (1986). Structural abnormalities in the frontal system in schizophrenia, *Archives of General Psychiatry*, **43**, 136–44.

Angelini, L., Mazzacchi, A., Picciotto, F., Nardocci, N., and Broggi, G. (1980). Focal lesions of the right cingulum: a case report in a child, *Journal of Neurology, Neurosurgery and Psychiatry*, **43**, 355–7.

Angst, J., Felder, W., and Lohmeyer, B. (1979). Schizoaffective disorders: results of a genetic investigation, *Journal of Affective Disorders*, **1**, 139–53.

Appell, J., Kertesz, A., and Fishman, M. (1982). A study of language functioning in Alzheimer's patients. *Brain and Language*, **17**, 73–91.

Arana, G.W., and Baldessarini, R.J. (1985). The dexamethasone suppression test for diagnosis and prognosis in psychiatry, *Archives of General Psychiatry*, **42**, 1193–204.

Arana, G.W., Pearlman, C., and Shader, R.I. (1985). Alprazolam induced mania, *American Journal of Psychiatry*, **142**, 368–3.

Ardrey, R. (1966). *The Territorial Imperative*, Atheneum, London.

Ariel, R.N., Golden, C.J., Berg, R.A., Quaife, M.A., Dirksen, J.W., Forsell, T., Wilson, J., and Graber, E. (1983). rCBF in schizophrenics, *Archives of General Psychiatry*, **40**, 258–63.

Arregui, A., Mackay, A.V.P., Spokes, E.G., and Iversen, L.L. (1980). Reduced activity of angiotensin converting enzyme in basal ganglia in early onset schizophrenia, *Psychological Medicine*, **10**, 307–13.

Åsberg, M., Träskman, L. and Thoren, P. (1976). 5-HIAA in the CSF: a biochemical suicide predictor, *Archives of General Psychiatry*, **33**, 1193–7.

Ashton, H. (1984). Benzodiazepine withdrawal: an unfinished story, *British Medical Journal*, **288**, 1135–40.

Ayd, F.J. (1974). Side effects of depot fluphenazines, *Comprehensive Psychiatry*, **15**, 277–84.

Bach, Y., Rita, G., Lion, J.R., Climent, C.E., and Ervin, F.R. (1971). Episodic dyscontrol: a study of 130 violent patients, *American Journal of Psychiatry*, **127**, 1473–8.

Baker, H.F., Ridley, R.M., Crow, T.J., Bloxham, C.A., Parry, R.P., and Tyrrell, D.A.J. (1983). An investigation of the effects of intracerebral injection in the marmoset of cytopathic CSF from patients with schizophrenia or neurological disease, *Psychological Medicine*, **13**, 499–511.

Ballenger, J.C., Goodwin, F.K., Major, L.F., *et al.* (1979). Alcohol and central serotonin metabolism in man, *Archives of General Psychiatry*, **36**, 224–7.

Banki, C.M., Vojnick, M. and Molnar, G. (1981). CSF amine metabolites, tryptophan and clinical parameters in depression, *Journal of Affective Disorders*, **3**, 81–9.

Banki, C.M., Arato, M., and Papp, Z. (1983). CSF Biochemical examinations, *Biological Psychiatry*, **18**, 1033–44.

Bannon, M.J., Reinhard, J.F., Bunney, E.B., and Roth, R.H. (1982). Unique response to antipsychotic drugs is due to absence of terminal autoreceptors in mesocortical dopamine neurones, *Nature*, **296**, 444–6.

Baron, M., Levitt, M., and Perlman, R. (1980). Low platelet MAO activity: a possible biochemical correlate of borderline schizophrenia, *Psychiatry Research*, **3**, 329–35.

Baron, M., Levitt, M., Greuen, R., Kane, J., and Asnis, L. (1984). Platelet MAO activity and genetic vulnerability to schizophrenia, *American Journal of Psychiatry*, **141**, 836–42.

Barraclough, B. (1981). Suicide and epilepsy. In E.H Reynolds and M.R. Trimble (Eds.), *Epilepsy and Psychiatry*, Churchill Livingstone, Edinburgh, pp. 72–6.

Baumgartner, A., Gräf, K.J., and Kurten, I. (1985). The dexamethasone suppression test in depression, in schizophrenia and during experimental stress, *Biological Psychiatry*, **20**, 675–9.

Baxter, L.R., Phelps, M.E., Mazziotta, J.C., *et al.* (1985). Cerebral metabolic rates for glucose in mood disorders, *Archives of General Psychiatry*, **42**, 441–7.

Baxter, L.R., Phelps, M.E., Mazziotta, J.C., Guze, B.H., Schwartz, B.H., and Selin, C.E. (1987). Local cerebral metabolic rates in obsessive–compulsive disorder, *Archives of General Psychiatry*, **44**, 211–18.

Bear, D. (1986a). Hemispheric asymmetries in emotional function: a reflection of lateral specialisation in cortical–limbic connections. In B.K. Doane and K.E. Livingston (Eds.), *The Limbic System: Functional Organization and Clinical Disorders*, Raven Press, New York, pp. 29–42.

Bear, D. (1986b). Behavioural changes in TLE. Conflict, confusion, challenge. In M.R Trimble and T. Bolwig (Eds.), *Aspects of Epilepsy and Psychiatry*, John Wiley and Sons, Chichester, pp. 19–30.

Bear, D., and Fedio, P. (1977). Quantitative analysis of interictal behaviour in temporal lobe epilepsy, *Archives of Neurology*, **34**, 454–67.

Beckmann, H., Saavedra, J.M., and Gattaz, W.F. (1984). Low angiotensin converting enzyme activity in CSF of schizophrenics, *Biological Psychiatry*, **19**, 679–84.

Behar, D., Rapoport, J.L., and Berg, C.J., *et al.* (1984). CAT and neuropsychological test measures in adolescents with obsessive–compulsive disorder, *American Journal of Psychiatry*, **141**, 363–9.

Ben-Ari, Y. (1981). Transmitters and modulators in the amygdaloid complex: a review. In Y. Ben-Ari (Ed.), *The Amygdaloid Complex*, Elsevier, North Holland, pp. 163–74.

Benes, F.M., Davidson, J., and Bird, E.D. (1986). Quantitative cytoarchitectural studies of the cerebral cortex of schizophrenics, *Archives of General Psychiatry*, **43**, 31–5.

Bennett, G.W., and Whitehead, G.A. (1983), *Mammalian Neuroendocrinology*, Croom Helm.

Bennett, J.P., Enna, S.J., Sylund, D.B., Gillin, J.C., Wyatt, R.J., and Snyder, S.H. (1979). Neurotransmitter receptors in frontal lobe cortex of schizophrenics, *Archives of General Psychiatry*, **36**, 927–34.

Benson, D.F. (1975). The hydrocephalic dementias. In D.F Benson and D. Blumer (Eds.), *Psychiatric Aspects of Neurologic Disease*, Grune and Stratton, New York, pp. 83–97.

Benson, D.F. (1979). *Aphasia, Alexia and Agraphia*, Churchill Livingstone, Edinburgh.

Benton, J.S., Bowen, D.M, and Allen, S.J., *et al.* (1982). Alzheimer's disease as a disorder of isodendritic core, *Lancet*, **i**, 456.

Berger, P.A., Faull, K.F., Kilkowski, J., *et al.* (1980a). CSF monoamine metabolites in depression and schizophrenia, *American Journal of Psychiatry*, **137**, 174–80.

Berger, P.A., Watson, S.J., Akil, H., *et al.* (1980b). Beta endorphin and schizophrenia, *Archives of General Psychiatry*, **37**, 635–40.

Berman, K.F., Zec, R.F., and Weinberger, D.R. (1986). Physiologic dysfunction of dorsolateral prefrontal cortex in schizophrenia, *Archives of General Psychiatry*, **43**, 126–35.

Bernoulli, C., Siegfried, J., Baumgartner, G., *et al.* (1977). Danger of accidental person-to-person transmission of Creutzfeld–Jakob disease by surgery, *Lancet*, **i**, 478–79.

Berrettini, W.H., Nurnberger, J.I., Hare, T.A., Alling, S.S., Gershon, E.S., and Post, R.M. (1983). Reduced plasma and

CSF GABA in affective illness: effect of lithium carbonate, *Biological Psychiatry*, **18**, 185–94.

Berrettini, W.H., and Post, R.M. (1984). GABA in affective illness. In R.M Post and J.C. Ballenger (Eds.), *Neurobiology of Mood Disorders*, Williams and Wilkins, Baltimore, pp. 673–85.

Bertelsen, A., Harvald, B., and Hauge, M. (1977). A Danish twin study of manic depressive disorders, *British Journal of Psychiatry*, **130**, 330–51.

Besson, J.A.O., Corrigan, F.M., Foreman, E.I., Eastwood, L.M., Smith, F.W., and Ashcroft, G.W. (1985). NMR II. Imaging in dementia, *British Journal of Psychiatry*, **146**, 31–5.

Besson, J.A.O., Corrigan, F.M., Cherryman, G.R., and Smith, F.W. (1987). NMR in chronic schizophrenia, *British Journal of Psychiatry*, **150**, 161–3.

Betts, T.A. (1974). A follow-up study of a cohort of patients with epilepsy admitted to psychiatric care in an English city. In P. Harris and C. Mawdsley (Eds.), *Epilepsy — Proceedings of the Hans Berger Centenary Symposium*, Churchill Livingstone, Edinburgh, pp. 326–38.

Biedermann, J., Rimon, R., Ebstein, R., Belmaker, R.H., and Davidson, J.T. (1977). Cyclic AMP in the CSF of patients with schizophrenia, *British Journal of Psychiatry*, **130**, 64–7.

Bigelow, L.B., Nasrallah, H.A., and Rauscher, F.P. (1983). Corpus callosum thickness in chronic schizphrenia, *British Journal of Psychiatry*, **142**, 284–7.

Bingley, T. (1958). Mental symptoms in temporal lobe epilepsy and temporal lobe gliomas, *Acta Psychiatrica et Neurologica Scandinavica*, Suppl. 120, pp. 1–151.

Bird, E.D., Spokes, E.G.S., and Iversen, L.L. (1979). Increased dopamine concentration in limbic areas of brain from patients dying with schizoprenia, *Brain*, **102**, 347–60.

Bird, J.M., Levy, R., and Jacoby, R.J. (1986). Computed tomography with the elderly: changes over time in a normal population, *British Journal of Psychiatry*, **148**, 80–5.

Birkmeyer, W., Jellinger, K., and Riederer, P. (1977). Striatal and extrastriatal dopaminergic functions. In A.R. Cools *et al.* (Eds.), *Psychobiology of the Striatum*, Elsevier, North Holland, pp. 141–52.

Bleuler, E. (1911). *Dementia Praecox or the Group of Schizophrenics* (Translated by J. Zenkin, 1950), New York International University Press.

Bleuler, E. (1924). *Textbook of Psychiatry* (Translated by A.A. Brill, 1924), Dover Publications.

Blumer, D. (1984). The psychiatric dimension of epilepsy. In D. Blumer (Ed.), *Psychiatric Aspects of Epilepsy*, APA, Washington, pp. 1–65.

Blumer, D., and Benson, D.F. (1975). Personality changes with frontal and temporal lobe lesions. In D.F Benson and D. Blumer (Eds.), *Psychiatric Aspects of Neurologic Disease*, Grune & Stratton, New York, pp. 151–69.

Bogerts, B., Hantsch, J., and Herzer, M. (1983). A morphometric study of the dopamine-containing cell groups in the mesencephalon of normals, Parkinson patients and schizophrenics, *Biological Psychiatry*, **18**, 951–70.

Bogerts, B., Meertz, E., and Schonfeldt-Bausch, R. (1985). Basal ganglia and limbic system pathology in schizophrenia, *Archives of General Psychiatry*, **42**, 784–91.

Bondareff, W., Baldy, R., and Levy, R. (1981a). Quantitative computed tomography in senile dementia, *Archives of General Psychiatry*, **38**, 1365–8.

Bondareff, W., Mountjoy, C.Q., and Roth, M. (1981b). Selective loss of neurones of origin of adrenergic projection to cerebral cortex in senile dementia, *Lancet*, **i**, 783–4.

Bondy, B., Ackenheil, M., Birzle, W., Elbers, R., and Frohler, M. (1984). Catecholamines and their receptors in blood, *Biological Psychiatry*, **19**, 1377–93.

Botwinick, J., and Birren, J.E. (1951). Differential decline in the Wechsler–Bellevue Subtests in the senile psychoses, *Journal of Gerontology*, **6**, 365–8.

Bouman, K.H. (1929). Central nervous system in schizophrenia, *Psychiatrie en Neurologie*, **32**, 517–39.

Bourne, H.R., Bunney, W.E., Colburn, R.W., Davis, J.M., Davis, J.N., Shaw, D.M., and Coppen, A.J. (1968). Noradrenaline, 5-HT and 5-HIAA in hindbrains in suicidal patients, *Lancet*, **ii**, 805–8.

Bowen, D.M., Spillane, J.A., Curzon, G., *et al.* (1979). Accelerated ageing or selective neuronal loss as an important cause of dementia, *Lancet*, **i**, 11–13.

Bowers, M.B. (1973). 5-HIAA and HVA following probenecid in acute psychotic patients treated with phenothiazines, *Psychopharmacology*, **28**, 309–18.

Bowers, M.B. (1974). Central dopamine turnover in schizophrenic syndromes, *Archives of General Psychiatry*, **31**, 50–4.

Bowery, N.G., Price, G.W., Hudson, A.L., Hill, D.R., Wilkin, G.P., and Turnbull, M.J. (1984). GABA receptor multiplicity, *Neuropharmacology*, **23**(2B), 219–31.

Bowlby, J. (1975). *Attachment and Loss*, Penguin Books, London.

Braddock, L. (1986). The dexamethasone suppression test: fact and artefact, *British Journal of Psychiatry*, **148**, 363–74.

Braestrup, C., and Nielsen, M. (1982). Anxiety, *Lancet*, **ii**, 1030–4.

Brambilla, F., Smeraldi, E., Sacchetti, E., *et al.* (1978). Deranged anterior pituitary responsiveness to hypothalamic hormones in depressed patients, *Archives of General Psychiatry*, **35**, 1231–8.

Breggin, P.B. (1964). The psychophysiology of anxiety, *Journal of Nervous and Mental Diseases*, **139**, 558–68.

Bridges, P.K., Bartlett, J.R., Sepping, P., Kantamaneni, B.D., and Curzon, G. (1976). Precursors and metabolites of 5-HT and dopamine in the ventricular CSF of psychiatric patients, *Psychological Medicine*, **6**, 399–405

Briley, M.S., Langer, S.Z., Raisman, R., Sechter, D., and Zarifian, E. (1980). Tritiated imipramine binding sites are decreased in platelets of untreated depressed patients, *Science*, **209**, 303–5.

Briquet, P. (1859), *Traite Clinique et Therapeutique de L'hysterie*, Balliere, Paris.

Broadhurst, P.L. (1975). The Maudsley reactive and non-reactive strain of rats, *Behaviour and Genetics*, **5**, 299–319.

Broca, P. (1878). Anatomie comparee des circonvolutions cerebrals: le grand lobe limbique et la scissure limbique dans la serie des mammiferes, *Revue Anthrapologie*, Serie 2, **1**, 385–498.

Brodal, A. (1969), *Neurological Anatomy in Relation to Clinical Medicine*, Oxford University Press, Oxford.

Brooks, D.N., and McKinlay, W. (1983). Personality and behaviour change after severe blunt head injury — a relative's view, *Journal of Neurology, Neurosurgery and Psychiatry*, **46**, 336–44.

Brown, G.L., Ballanger, J.C., Minichello, M.D., and Goodwin, F.K. (1979). Human aggression and its relationship to CSF 5HIAA, 3MHPG and HVA. In M. Sandler (Ed.), *Psychopharmacology of Aggression*, Raven Press, New York, pp. 131–48.

Brown, G.L., Ebert, M.H., Goyer, P.F., Jimerson, D.C., Klein, W.J., Bunney, W.E., and Godwin, F.T. (1982). Aggression, suicide and serotonin: relationship to CSF amine metabolism, *American Journal of Psychiatry*, **139**, 741–6.

412

Brown, R., Colter, N., Corsellis, N., Crow, T.J., *et al.* (1986). Post-mortem evidence of structural brain changes in schizophrenia, *Archives of General Psychiatry*, **43**, 36–42.

Brown, R.G., Marsden, C.D., Quinn, N., and Wyke, M.A. (1984). Alterations in cognitive performance and affect–arousal state during fluctuations in motor function in Parkinson's disease, *Journal of Neurology, Neurosurgery and Psychiatry*, **47**, 454–65.

Brown, W.A., and Laughren, T.P. (1981). Tolerance to the prolactin-elevating effect of neuroleptics, *Psychiatry Research*, **5**, 317–22.

Brusov, O.G., Fomenko, A.M., and Katasonov, A.B. (1985). Human plasma inhibitors of platelet serotonin uptake and imipramine receptor binding: extraction and heterogeneity, *Biological Psychiatry*, **20**, 235–44.

Buchanan, F.H., Parton, R.V., Warren, J.W., and Baker, E.P. (1975). Double blind trial of L-dopa in chronic schizophrenia, *Australian and New Zealand Journal of Psychiatry*, **9**, 269–71.

Buchsbaum, M.S, Goodwin, F., Murphy, D., and Borge, G. (1971). AER in affective disorders, *American Journal of Psychiatry*, **128**, 19–25.

Buchsbaum, M.S., Coursey, R.D., and Murphy, D.L. (1976). The biochemical high risk paradigm: behavioural and familial correlates of low platelet MAO activity, *Science*, **194**, 339–41.

Buchsbaum, M.S., Wu, J., DeLisi, L.E., *et al.* (1986). Frontal cortex and basal ganglia metabolic rates assessed by PET with 18–(F)2–deoxyglucose in affective illness, *Journal of Affective Disorders*, **10**, 137–52.

Buchthal, F., Svensmark, O., and Schiller, P.J. (1960). Clinical and EEG correlations with serum levels of diphenylhydentoin, *Archives of Neurology*, **3**, 624–30.

Burnett, G.B., Prange, A.J., Wilson, I.C., Jolliff, L.A., Creese, I.C., and Snyder, S.H. (1980). Adverse effects of anticholinergic antiparkinsonian drugs in tardive dyskinesia, *Neuropsychobiology*, **6**, 109–20.

Burrows, G.D., Vohra, J., Hunt, D., Sloman, J.G., Scoggins, B.A., and Davies B. (1976). Cardiac affects of different tricyclic antidepressant drugs, *British Journal of Psychiatry*, **129**, 335–41.

Bustany, P., Henry, J.F., De Rotrou, J., *et al.* (1985). Correlations between clinical state and PET measurements of local brain protein synthesis in Alzheimer's dementia, Parkinson's disease, schizophrenia and gliomas. In T. Greit *et al.* (Eds.), *The Metabolism of the Human Brain Studied with PET*, Raven Press, New York, pp. 241–9.

Butler, P.W.P., and Besser, G.M. (1968). Pituitary–adrenal function in severe depressive illness, *Lancet,* **i**, 1234–6.

Caine, E. (1981). Pseudodementia: current concepts and future directions, *Archives of General Psychiatry*, **38**, 1359–64.

Calloway, S.P., Dolan, R.J., Fonagy, P., De Souza, V.F.A., and Wakeling, A. (1984). Endocrine changes and clinical profiles in depression. The TRH test, *Psychological Medicine,* **14**, 759–65.

Cameron, O.G., Smith, C.B., Hollingsworth, P.J., Nesse, R.M., and Curtis, G.C. (1984). Plasma alpha-2 adrenergic receptor binding and plasma catecholamines. *Archives of General Psychiatry,* **41**, 1144–8.

Cannon, W.B. (1927). The James–Lange theory of emotion; a critical examination and an alternative theory, *American Journal of Psychology,* **39**, 106–24.

Cantello, R., Gilli, M., Riccio A., and Bermamasco, B. (1986). Mood changes associated 'end of dose' deterioration in Parkinson's disease: a controlled study, *Journal of Neurology, Neurosurgery and Psychiatry,* **49**, 1182–90.

Capstick, N., and Seldrup, J. (1977). Obsessional states, *Acta Psychiatrica Scandinavica,* **56**, 427–31.

Carey, G., and Gottesman, I.I. (1981). Twin and family studies of anxiety, phobic and obsessional disorders. In D.F Klein and J. Rabkin (Eds.), *Anxiety: New Research and Changing Concepts*, Raven Press, New York, pp. 117–35.

Carlsson, A. (1977). The influence of antidepressants on central monoamine systems. In H. van Praag and J. Bruinvels (Eds.), *Neurotransmission and Disturbed Behaviour*, Bohn Scheltema & Holkena, Utrecht, pp. 19–33.

Carney, M.W.P., Roth, M., and Garside, R.F. (1965). The diagnosis of depressive syndromes and the prediction of ECT response, *British Journal of Psychiatry,* **111**. 659–74.

Carroll, B.J., Greden, J.F., Haskett, R.F., *et al.* (1980). Neurotransmitter studies of neuroendocrine pathology in depression, *Acta Psychiatrica Scandinavica,* **61**, Suppl. 280, 183–200.

Carroll, B.J., Feinberg, M., Greden, J.F., *et al.* (1981). A specific laboratory test for the diagnosis of melancholia, *Archives of General Psychiatry,* **38**, 15–22.

Casey, D., Gerlach, J., Magelund, G., and Christensen, T.R. (1980). Gamma acetylenic GABA in tardive dyskinesia, *Archives of General Psychiatry*, **37**, 1376–9.

Castellani, S., Ziegler, M.G., van Kammen, D.P., *et al.* (1982). Plasma norepinephrine and dopamine beta hydrolase activity in schizophrenia, *Archives of General Psychiatry*, **39**, 1145–9.

Catterall, R.D. (1977). Neurosyphilis, *British Journal of Hospital Medicine*, **17**, 585–604.

Chalmers, R.J., and Bennie, E.H. (1978). The effect of fluphenazine on basal prolactin concentrations, *Psychological Medicine*, **8**, 483–6.

Chapman, A., Meldrum, B., and Mendes, E. (1983). Acute anticonvulsant activity of structural analogues of valproic acid and changes in brain GABA and aspartate content, *Life Sciences*, **32**, 2023–31.

Charcot, J.M. (1877). *Lectures on the Diseases of the Nervous System* (Translated by G. Sigerson), New Sydenham Society, London.

Charney, D.S., Heninger, G.R., Sternberg, D.E., *et al.* (1981). Presynaptic adrenergic receptor sensitivity in depression, *Archives of General Psychiatry*, **38**, 1334–40.

Charney, D.S., Heninger, G.R., and Sternberg, D.E. (1983). Alpha-2 adrenergic receptor sensitivity and the mechanism of action of antidepressant therapy, *British Journal of Psychiatry*, **142**, 265–75.

Charney, D.S., Henninger, G.R., and Breier, A. (1984a). Noradrenergic function in panic anxiety, *Archives of General Psychiatry*, **41**, 751–63.

Charney, D.S., Henninger, G.R., and Sternberg, D.E. (1984b). The effect of mianserin on alpha-2 adrenergic receptor function in depressed patients, *British Journal of Psychiatry*, **144**, 407–16.

Chase, T.N., Foster, N.L., Fedio, P., Brooks, R., Mansi, L., and Di Chiro, G. (1984). Regional cortical dysfunction in Alzheimer's diasease as determined by PET, *Annals of Neurology*, **15s**, 170–4.

Checkley, S.A. (1979). Corticosteroid and growth hormone responses to methyl amphetamine in depressive illness, *Psychological Medicine*, **9**, 107–15.

Checkley, S. A. (1985). Biological markers in depression. In Granville–Grossman (Ed.), *Recent Advances in Clinical Psychiatry*, Churchill Livingstone, Edinburgh, pp. 201–24.

Chomsky, N. (1980). On cognitive structures and their development: a reply to Piaget. In M. Piatelli-Palmarini (Ed.), *Language and Learning*, Routledge and Kegan Paul, London, pp. 23–54.

Christensen, E., Møller, J.E., and Faurbye, A. (1970). A neuropathological investigation of 28 brains from patients with dyskinesia, *Acta Psychiatrica Scandinavica*, **46**, 14–23.

Christensen, N.J., Vestergarrd, P., Sorensen, T., and Rafaelsen, O.J. (1980). CSF adrenaline and noradrenaline in depressed patients, *Acta Psychiatrica Scandinavica*, **61**, 178–82.

Christiansen, K.O. (1974). The genesis of aggressive criminality. In J. De Wit and W.W. Hastings (Eds.), *Determinants and Origins of Aggressive Behaviour*, Mouton, The Hague, pp. 233–53.

Ciesielski, K.T., Beech, H.R., and Gordon, P.K. (1981). Some electrophysiological observations in obsessional states, *British Journal of Psychiatry*, **138**, 479–84.

Clark, C.M., Kessler, R., Buchsbaum, M.S., Margolin, R.A., and Holcomb, H.H. (1984). Correlational methods for determining regional coupling of cerebral glucose metabolism: a pilot study, *Biological Psychiatry*, **19**, 663–78.

Claude, H., and Bourguignon, G. (1927). Signe de Babinski transitoire dans un cas démence précoce, *Revue Neurologique*, **T1**(6), 1078–81.

Cleobury, J.R., Skinner, G.R.B., Thouless, M.E., and Wildy, P. (1971). Association between psychopathic disorder and serum antibody to herpes simplex virus, type 1, *British Medical Journal*, **i**, 438–9.

Clow, A., Jenner, P., Theodorou, A., and Marsden, C.D. (1979). Neuroleptic drugs and the dopamine hypothesis, *Lancet*, **i**, 934.

Cobb, W.A. (1975). In L.S. Illis (Ed.), *Viral Diseases of the CNS*, Balliere Tindall, London, pp. 76–89.

Coffman, J.A., Andreasen, N.C., and Nasrallah, H.A. (1984). Left hemisphere density deficits in chronic schizophrenia, *Biological Psychiatry*, **19**, 1237–48.

Cohen, S.I. (1980). Cushing's syndrome: a psychiatric study of 29 patients, *British Journal of Psychiatry*, **136**, 120–4.

Consensus Development Conference Statement (1986). *Electroconvulsive Therapy*, **5**(11), NIH.

Cools, A.R. (1981). The puzzling 'cascade' of multiple receptors for dopamine, *Trends in the Pharmacological Sciences*, July **1981**, 171–83.

Cooper, S.J., Kelly, J.G., and King, D.J. (1985). Adrenergic receptors in depression, *British Journal of Psychiatry*, **147**, 23–9.

Coppen, A.J., and Shaw, D.M. (1963). Mineral metabolism in melancholia, *British Medical Journal*, **ii**, 1439–44.

Coppen, A., Shaw, D.M., and Farrell, M.B. (1963). Potentiation of the antidepressive effect of a MAOI by tryptophan, *Lancet*, **ii**, 79–81.

Coppen, A.J., Malleson, A., and Shaw, D.M. (1965). Effects of lithium carbonate on electrolyte distribution in man, *Lancet*, **i**, 682–3.

Coppen, A., Prange, A.J., Whybrow, P.C., and Noguera, R. (1972). Abnormalities of indoleamines in affective disorders, *Archives of General Psychiatry*, **26**, 474–8.

Coppen, A., Ghose, K., Rao, R., Bailey, J., and Peet, M. (1978). Mianserin and lithium in the prophylaxis of depression, *British Journal of Psychiatry*, **133**, 206–10.

Coppen, A., and Wood, K. (1978). Tryptophan and depressive illness, *Psychological Medicine*, **8**, 49–57.

Coppen, A., Swade, S., and Wood, K. (1980). Lithium restores abnormal platelet 5-HT transport in patients with affective disorders, *British Journal of Psychiatry*, **136**, 235–8.

Coppen, A., Abou–Saleh, M., Milln, P., Metcalfe, M., Harwood, J., and Bailey, J. (1983). DST in depression and other psychiatric illness, *British Journal of Psychiatry*, **142**, 498–504.

Coppen, A., Milln, P., Harwood, J., and Wood, K. (1985), Does the DST predict antidepressant treatment success?, *British Journal of Psychiatry*, **146**, 294–6.

Corsellis, J.A.N., Goldberg, G.J., and Norton, A.R. (1968). 'Limbic encephalitis' and its association with carcinoma, *Brain*, **91**, 481–96.

Coursey, R.D., Buchsbaum, M.S., and Murphy, D.L. (1982). Two year follow up of subjects and their families defined as at risk for psychopathology on the bases of platelet MAO activities, *Neuropsychobiology*, **8**, 51–6.

Cowdry, R.W., Pickar, D., and Davies, R. (1986). Symptoms and EEG findings in the borderline syndrome, *International Journal of Psychiatry and Medicine*, **15**, 201–11.

Cox, S.M., and Ludwig, A.M. (1979). Neurological soft signs and psychopathology. *Journal of Nervous and Mental Diseases*, **167**, 161–5.

Coyle, J., Prince, D.L., and DeLong, M.R. (1983). Alzheimer's disease: a disorder of cholinergic innervation, *Science,* **219**, 1184–90.

Craig Risch, S., and Janowsky, D.S. (1984). Cholinergic–adrenergic balance in affective illness. In R. M. Post and J. Ballenger (Eds.), *Neurobiology of Mood Disorders,* Williams & Wilkins, Baltimore, pp. 652–63.

Crapper, D.R., Quittkat, S., and De Boni, U. (1979). Altered chromatin conformation in Alzhemier's disease, *Brain,* **102**, 483–95.

Crawley, J.C.W., Crow, T.J., Johnstone, E.C., *et al.* (1986). Dopamine D2 receptors in schizophrenia studied in vivo, *Lancet,* **ii**, 224.

Crayton, J.W., and Meltzer, H.Y. (1976). Motor endplate alterations in schizophrenic patients, *Nature,* **264**, 658–9.

Creese, I. (1982). Dopamine receptors explained, *Trends in the Neurosciences,* **5**, 40–3.

Crews, F.T., and Smith, C.B. (1978) Presynaptic alpha–receptor sensitivity after long term antidepressant treatment, *Science,* **202**, 322–4.

Crome, P., and Newman, B. (1977). Poisoning with maprotiline and mianserin, *British Medical Journal,* **2**, 260.

Cross, A.J., Crow, T.J., and Owen, F. (1979). GABA in the brain in schizophrenia, *Lancet,* **i**, 560–1.

Cross, A.J., Crow, T.J., and Owen, F. (1981a). 3H–flupenthixol binding in post mortem brains of schizophrenics: evidence for a selective increase in dopamine D2 receptors, *Psychopharmacology,* **74**, 122–4.

Cross, A.J., Crow, T.J., Perry, E.K., Perry, R.H., Blessed, G., and Tomlinson, B.E. (1981b). Reduced dopamine beta hydrolase activity in Alzheimer's disease, *British Medical Journal,* **1**, 93–4.

Crow, T.J. (1980). Molecular pathology of schizophrenia: more than one disease process, *British Medical Journal,* **i**, 66–8.

Crow, T.J. (1984). A re–evaluation of the viral hypothesis, *British Journal of Psychiatry,* **145**, 243–53.

Crow, T.J., and Johnstone, E.C. (1986a). Schizophrenia – the nature of the disease process and its biological correlates. In F. Plum (Ed.), *Handbook of Physiology: Higher Functions of the Nervous System,* American Physiological Society (in press).

Crow, T.J., and Johnstone, E.C. (1986b). Controlled trials of ECT. In S. Malitz and H.A. Sackheim (Eds.), *ECT*, Annals of the New York Academy of Sciences, Vol. 462, pp. 12–29.

Crow T.J., Johnstone, E.C., and Owen, F. (1979a). Research on schizophrenia. In *Recent Advances in Clinical Psychiatry*, Churchill Livingstone, Edinburgh. pp. 1–36.

Crow, T.J., Baker, H.F., Cross, A.J., *et al.* (1979b). Monoamine mechanisms in chronic schizophrenia: post-mortem neuro-chemical findings, *British Journal of Psychiatry*, **134**, 249–56.

Cullen, W. (1800). *Nosology*, Creech, Edinburgh.

Cummings, J.L. (1985). *Clinical Neuropsychiatry*, Grune & Stratton, New York.

Cummings, J.L., and Benson, D.F. (1983). *Dementia; A Clinical Approach*, Butterworths, London.

Cummings, J.L., Benson, F., Hill, M.A., and Read, S. (1985). Aphasia in dementia of the Alzheimer type, *Neurology*, **35**, 394–7.

Curson, D.A., Barnes, T.R.E., Bamber, R.W., Platt, S.D., Hirsch, S.R., and Duffy, J.C. (1985). Long term depot maintenance of chronic schizophrenic out patients, *British Journal of Psychiatry*, **146**, 464–80.

Dalby, J.T., and Williams, R. (1986). Preserved reading and spelling ability in psychotic disorders, *Psychological Medicine*, **16**, 171–5.

Damascio, A.R., and van Hoesen, G.W. (1985). The limbic system and the localization of herpes simplex encephalitis, *Journal of Neurology, Neurosurgery and Psychiatry*, **48**, 297–301.

Darwin, C. (1889). *The Expression of Emotion in Man and Animals*, 2nd edition (Edited by F. Darwin, 1904), John Murray, London.

Davis, P. (1941). Electroencephalograms of manic-depressive patients, *American Journal of Psychiatry*, **98**, 430–3.

Davison, K. (1966). Schizophrenia-like psychoses associated with organic brain disease. Preliminary observations on fifty patients, *Newcastle Medical Journal*, **29**, 67–73.

Davison, K., and Bagley, C.R. (1969). Schizophrenia-like psychoses associated with organic disorders of the central nervous system. In R.N. Herrington (Ed.), *Current Problems in Neuropsychiatry*, Headley Brothers, Kent, pp. 113–84.

del Castillo, J., and Katz, B. (1954). The effects of magnesium on the activity of motor nerve endings, *Journal of Physiology*, **124**, 553–9.

Delgado, J.M.R. (1966). Aggressive behaviour evoked by radio stimulation in monkey colonies, *American Zoologist*, **6**, 669–81.

Delgado-Escueta, A., Mattson, R.H., King, L., *et al.* (1981). The nature of aggression during epileptic seizures, *New England Journal of Medicine*, **305**, 711–16.

De Lisi, L.E. (1984). Is immune dysfunction associated with schizophrenia? A review of the data, *Psychopharmacology Bulletin*, **20**, 509–13.

De Lisi, L.E., Neckers, L.M., Weinberger, D.R., and Wyatt, R.J. (1981). Increased whole blood serotonin concentrations in chronic schizophrenic patients, *Archives of General Psychiatry*, **38**, 647–50.

De Lisi, L., Wise, C.O., Bridge, T., *et al.* (1982). Monoamine oxidase and schizophrenia. In E. Usdin and I. Hanin (Eds.), *Biological Markers in Psychiatry and Neurology*, Pergamon Press, New York, pp. 79–96.

De Lisi, L.E., and Buchsbaum, M.S. (1986). PETT of cerebral glucose use in psychiatric patients. In M.R. Trimble (Ed.), *New Brain Imaging Techniques in Psychopharmacology*, Oxford Unversity Press, Oxford, pp. 48–62.

De Lisi, L., Goldin, L.R., Hamovit, J.R., Maxwell, E., Kurtz, D., and Gershon, E.S. (1986). A family study of the association of increased ventricular size with schizophrenia, *Archives of General Psychiatry*, **43**, 148–53.

Denny-Brown, D., and Russell, W.R. (1941). Experimental cerebral concussion, *Brain*, **64**, 93–164.

Dewan, M.J., Pandurangi, A.K., Lee, S.H., *et al.* (1983). Central brain morphology in chronic schizophrenic patients: a controlled CT study, *Biological Psychiatry*, **18**, 1133–9.

de Weid, D. (1974). Pituitary–adrenal system hormones and behaviour. In F.O. Schmidt and G.F. Worden (Eds.), *The Neurosciences: 3rd Study Program*, MIT Press, Cambridge, Mass., pp. 653–66.

Dewhurst, K. (1980). *Willis' Oxford Lectures*, Sandford Publications, Oxford.

Dewhurst, K. (1982a). Thomas Willis and the foundations of British neurology. In F. Clifford Rose and W.F. Bynum (Eds.), *Historical Aspects of the Neurosciences*, Raven Press, New York, pp. 327–46.

Dewhurst, K. (1982b). *Hughlings Jackson on Psychiatry*, Sandford Publications, Oxford.

420

Dolan, R.J., Calloway, S.P., Fonagy, P., DeSouza, F.V.A., and Wakeling, A. (1985a). Life events, depression and hypothalamic pituitary–adrenal axis function, *British Journal of Psychiatry*, **147**, 429–34.

Dolan, R.J., Calloway, S.P., and Mann, A.H. (1985b). Cerebral ventricular size in depressed subjects, *Psychological Medicine*, **15**, 873–8.

Doran, A.R., Rubinow, D.R., Roy, A., and Pickar, D. (1986). CSF somatostatin and abnormal response to dexamethasone administration in schizophrenic and depressed patients, *Archives of General Psychiatry*, **43**, 365–9.

Dorrow, R., Horowski, R., Paschelke, G., Amin, M., and Braestrup, C. (1983). Severe anxiety induced by FG 7142, *Lancet*, **ii**, 98–9.

Dorus, E. (1980). Variability in the Y chromosome and variability in human behaviour, *Archives of General Psychiatry*, **37**, 587–94.

Dworkin, R.H., and Lenzenweger, M.F. (1984). Symptoms and the genetics of schizophrenia implications for diagnosis, *American Journal of Psychiatry*, **141**, 1541–6.

Eccles, J.C. (1964). *The Physiology of Synapses*, Springer, Berlin.

Edeh, J., and Toone, B.K. (1985). Antiepileptic therapy, folate deficiency, and psychiatric morbidity: a general practice survey, *Epilepsia*, **26**, 434–40.

Eeg-Olofsson, O., Petersen, I., and Sellden, U. (1971). The development of the EEG in normal children from the age of 1 through 15 years, *Neuropaediatrie*, **2**, 375–404.

Egland, J.A., Gerhard, D.S., Pauls, D.L., *et al.* (1987). Bipolar affective disorders linked to DNA markets on chromosome 11, *Nature*, **325**, 783–7.

Egrise, D., Rubinstein, M., Schoutens, A., Cantraine, F., and Mendelwicz, J. (1986). Seasonal variation of platelet serotonin binding in normal and depressed subjects, *Biological Psychiatry*, **21**, 283–92.

Eichelmann, B. (1979). Role of biogenic amines in aggressive behaviour. In M. Sandler (Ed.), *Psychopharmology of Aggression*, Raven Press, New York, pp. 61–93

Ellis, W.G., McCulloch, J.R., and Corley, C.L. (1974). Presenile dementia in Down's syndrome: ultrastructural identity with Alzheimer's disease, *Neurology*, **24**, 101–6.

Emrich, H.M., Dose, M., and von Zerssen, D. (1984). Action of sodium valproate and of oxycarbazepine in patients with affective disorders. In H.M. Emrich *et al.* (Eds.), *Anticonvulsants in Affective Disorders*, Excerpta Medica, Oxford, pp. 45–55.

Esler, M., Turbott, J., Schwartz, R., Leonard, P., Bobik, A., Skews, H., and Jackman, G. (1982). The peripheral kinetics of norepinephrine in depressive illness, *Archives of General Psychiatry*, **39**, 295–300.

Evans, B.M., Bridges, P.K., Bartlett, J.R. (1981). EEG changes as prognostic indicators after psychosurgery, *Journal of Neurology, Neurosurgery and Psychiatry*, **44**. 444–7.

Evans, P. (1972). Henri Ey's concept of the organisation of consciousness and its disorganisation: an extension of Jacksonian theory, *Brain*, **95**, 413–40.

Extein, I., Tallman, J., Smith, C.C., and Goodwin, F.K. (1979). Changes in lymphocyte beta adrenergic receptors in depression and mania, *Psychiatric Research*, **1**, 191–7.

Extein, I., Pottash, A.L.C., and Gold, M.S. (1981). Relation of TRH test and DST abnormalities in unipolar depression, *Psychiatry Research*, **4**, 49–53.

Extein, I., Pottash, A.L.C., Gold, M.S., and Silver, J.M. (1982). TSH response to TRH in unipolar depression before and after clinical improvement, *Psychiatry Research*, **6**, 161–9.

Ey, H. (1978). Hughlings Jackson's fundamental principles applied to psychiatry. In H. Riese (Ed.), *Historical Explorations in Medicine and Psychiatry*, Springer, New York, pp. 204–19.

Falloon, I., Watt, D.C., and Shepherd, M. (1978). The social outcome of patients in a trial of long term continuation therapy in schizophrenia: primozide vs fluphenazine, *Psychological Medicine*, **8**, 265–74.

Farley, I.J., Price, K.S., and Hornykiewicz, O. (1977). Dopamine in the limbic regions of the human brain, *Advances in Biochemical Psychopharmacology*, **16**, 57–64.

Farmer, A., McGuffin, P., Jackson, R., and Storey, P. (1985). Classifying schizophrenia, *Lancet*, **i**, 1333.

Feighner, J.P., Robins, E., Guze, S.B., Woodruff, R.A., Winokur, G., and Munoz, R. (1972). Diagnostic criteria for use in psychiatric research, *Archives of General Psychiatry*, **26**, 57–63.

Fenton, G.W. (1972). Epilepsy and automatism, *British Journal of Hospital Medicine*, **7**, 57–64.

Fenton, G.W., Fenwick, P.B.C., Dollimore, J., Dunn, T.L., and Hirsch, S.R. (1980). EEG spectral analysis in schizophrenia, *British Journal of Psychiatry*, **136**, 445–55.

Fenwick, P. (1981). Precipitation and inhibition of seizures. In E.H. Reynolds and M.R. Trimble (Eds.), *Epilepsy and Psychiatry*, Churchill Livingstone, Edinburgh, pp. 242–63.

Fenwick, P. (1986). Aggression and epilepsy. In M.R. Trimble and T. Bolwig (Eds.), *Aspects of Epilepsy and Psychiatry*, John Wiley and Sons, Chichester, pp. 31–60.

Ferrier, I.N., Cotes, P.M., Crow, T.J., and Johnstone, E.C. (1982). Gonadotrophin secretion abnormalities in chronic schizophrenia, *Psychological Medicine*, **12**, 263–73.

Ferrier, I.N., Johnstone, E.C., Crow, T.J., and Rincon-Rodriguez, I. (1983). Anterior pituitary hormone secretion in chronic schizophrenia, *Archives of General Psychiatry*, **40**, 755–61.

Ferrier, I.N., Crow, T.J., Roberts, G.W., *et al.* (1984a). Alterations in neuropeptides in the limbic lobe in schizophrenia. In M.R. Trimble and E. Zarifian (Eds.), *Psychopharmacology of the Limbic System*, Oxford University Press, Oxford, pp. 244–54.

Ferrier, I.N., Johnstone, E.C., and Crow, T.J. (1984b). Clinical effects of apomorphine in schizophrenia, *British Journal of Psychiatry*, **144**, 341–8.

Ferrier, N., Johnstone, E.C., Crow, T.J., and Rodriguez, I.R. (1986). Anterior pituitary hormone secretion in chronic schizophrenics, *Archives of General Psychiatry*, **40**, 755–61.

Fink, M. (1984). Meduna and the origins of convulsive therapy, *American Journal of Psychiatry*, **141**, 1034–41.

Fink, M. (1986a). Convulsive therapy and epilepsy research. In M.R. Trimble and E.H. Reynolds (Eds.), *What is Epilepsy?* Churchill Livingstone, Edinburgh, pp. 217–28.

Fink, M. (1986b). Neuroendocrine predictors of ECT outcome. In S. Malitz and H.A. Sackeim (Eds.), *ECT,* Annals of the New York Academy of Sciences, Vol. 462, pp. 30–6.

Finley, G.W., and Campbell, C.M. (1941). Electroencephalography in schizophrenia, *American Journal of Psychiatry*, **98**, 374–84.

Fisch, C. (1985). Effect of fluoxetine on the electrocardiogram, *Journal of Clinical Psychiatry*, **46**, 42–4.

Fischer, M. (1973). Genetic and environmental factors in schizophrenia, *Acta Psychiatrica Scandinavica*, Suppl. 238.

Floderus-Myrhed, B., Pedersen, N., and Rasmuson, I. (1980). Assessment of heritability for personality, *Behaviour Genetics*, **10**, 153–62.

Flor-Henry, P. (1969). Psychosis and temporal lobe epilepsy, *Epilepsia*, **10**, 363–95.

Flor-Henry, P. (1983). *Cerebral Basis of Psychopathology*, John Wright, Bristol.

Folstein, M.F., Maiberger, R., and McHugh, P.R. (1977). Mood disorder as a specific complication of stroke, *Journal of Neurology, Neurosurgery and Psychiatry*, **40**, 1018–20.

Foster, G.M., and Anderson, B.G. (1978). *Medical Anthropology*, John Wiley and Sons, Chichester.

Fowler, C.J., von Knorring, L., and Oreland, L. (1980). Platelet MAO in sensation seekers, *Psychiatry Research*, **1980**, 273–9.

Fox, J.H., Topel, J.L., and Huckman, M.S. (1975). Use of computerized axial tomography in senile dementia, *Journal of Neurology, Neurosurgery and Psychiatry*, **38**, 948–53.

Frackowiak, R.S.J., Lenzi, G.L., Jones, T., and Heather, J.D. (1980). Quantitative measurements of regional CBF and oxygen metabolism in man using 15 O and PET: theory, procedure and normal values, *Journal of Computer Assisted Tomography*, **4**, 727–36.

Frackowiak, R.S.J., Pozzilli, C., Legg, N.J., *et al.* (1981). Regional cerebal oxygen supply and utilisation in dementia, *Brain*, **104**, 753–8.

Francis, P.T., and Bowen, D.M. (1985). Relevance of reduced concentrations of somatostatin in Alzheimer's disease, *Biochemical Society Transactions*, **13**, 170–1.

Francis, P.T., Palmer, A.M., Sims, N.R., and Bowen, D.M., *et al.* (1985). Neurochemical studies of early onset Alzheimer's disease, *New England Journal of Medicine*, **313**, 7–11.

Frank, K., and Fuortes, M.G.F. (1957). Presynaptic and postsynaptic inhibition of monosynaptic reflexes, *Federation Proceedings*, **16**, 39–40.

Franzen, G., and Ingvar, D.H. (1975). Absence of activation in frontal structures during psychological testing of chronic schizophrenics, *Journal of Neurology, Neurosurgery and Psychiatry*, **38**, 1027–32.

Freeman, W., and Watts, J.W. (1947). Psychosurgery during 1936–46, *Archives of Neurology and Psychiatry*, **58**, 417–25.

Freud, S. (1953). *On Aphasia* (Translated by E. Stengel), Imago Publishing Co., London.

Friedman, M.J., Stolk, J.M., Harris, P.Q., and Cooper, T.B. (1984). Serum dopamine–beta-hydrolase activity in depression and anxiety, *Biological Psychiatry,* **19**, 557–70.

Frolich, E.D., Tarazi, R.C., and Dunstan, H.P. (1969). Hyperdynamic beta-adrenergic circulatory state, *Archives of Internal Medicine,* **123**, 1–7.

Fuller Torrey, E. (1980). Neurological abnormalities in schizophrenic patients, *Biological Psychiatry,* **15**, 381–8.

Fuller Torrey, E.F., and Peterson, M.R. (1973). Slow and latent viruses in schizophrenia, *Lancet,* **ii**, 22–4.

Fuller Torrey, E., Torrey, B.B., and Peterson, M.R. (1977). Seasonality of schizophrenic births in the United States, *Archives of General Psychiatry,* **34**, 1065–70.

Fulton, J.F., and Jacobsen, C.G. (1935). The functions of the frontal lobes, a comparative study in monkeys, chimpanzees and men, *Advances in Modern Biology,* **4**, 113–23.

Fuster, J.M. (1980). *The Pre-frontal Cortex,* Raven Press, New York.

Gainotti, G. (1969). Reactions, 'catastrophiques' et manifestations d'indifference au cours des oteintes cerebrales, *Neuropsychology,* **7**, 195–204.

Gainotti, G. (1972). Emotional behaviour and hemispheric side of the lesion, *Cortex,* **8**, 41–55.

Galin, D., Diamond, R., and Braff, D. (1977). Lateralization of conversion symptoms: more frequent on the left, *American Journal of Psychiatry,* **134**, 578–80.

Garcia-Sevilla, J.A., Athanasios, P.Z., Hollingsworth, P.J., Greden, J.F., and Smith, C.B. (1981). Platelet alpha 2 adrenergic receptors in major depressive disorder, *Archives of General Psychiatry,* **38**, 1327–33.

Garcia-Sevilla, J.A., Guimon, J., Garcia-Valleto, P., and Fuster, M.J. (1986). Biochemical and functional evidence of supersensitive platelet alpha-2 adrenoceptors in major affective disorder, *Archives of General Psychiatry,* **43**, 51–7.

Gartrell, N. (1986). Increased libido in women receiving trazadone. *American Journal of Psychiatry,* **143**, 781–2.

Gattaz, W.F., Cramer, H., and Beckmann, H. (1983a). Low CSF concentrations of cyclic GMP in schizophrenia, *British Journal of Psychiatry,* **142**, 288–91.

Gattaz, W.F., Riederer, P., Reynolds, G.P., Gattaz, D., and Beckmann, H. (1983b). Dopamine and noradrenaline in the CSF of schizophrenic patients, *Psychiatric Research,* **8**, 243–50.

Gentsch, C., Lichtsteiner, M., and Freer, H. (1981). 3-H diazepan binding sites in Roman high- and low-avoidance rats, *Experientia*, **37**, 1315–16.

George, A.J., de Leon, M.J., Ferris, S.H., and Kricheff, I.I. (1981). Parenchymal CT correlates of senile dementia, *American Journal of Neuroradiology*, **2**, 205–10.

Gerlach, J., and Luhdorf, K. (1975). The effect of L-dopa on young patients with simple schizophrenia treated with neuroleptic drugs, *Psychopharmacologia*, **44**, 105–10.

Gerner, R.H., Fairbanks, L., Anderson, G.M., *et al.* (1984). CSF neurochemistry in depressed, manic and schizophrenic patients compared with that of normal controls, *American Journal of Psychiatry*, **141**, 1533–40.

Gershon, E. (1983). The genetics of affective disorders. In L. Grinspoon (Ed.), *Psychiatry Update*, Vol. 2, APA, Washington, pp. 434–56.

Geschwind, N. (1979). Behavioural changes in TLE, *Psychological Medicine*, **9**, 217–19.

Geschwind, N., and Levitsky, W. (1968). Human brain: left–right asymmetries in temporal speech region, *Science*, **161**, 186–9.

Ghose, K., Turner, P., and Coppen, A. (1975). Intravenous tyramine pressor response in depression, *Lancet*, **i**, 1317–18.

Gibb, W.R.G., and Lees, A.J. (1986). The clinical phenomenon of akathisia, *Journal of Neurology, Neurosurgery and Psychiatry*, **49**, 861–6.

Gibbs, F.A. (1951). Ictal and non-ictal psychiatric disorders in T.L.E., *Journal of Nervous and Mental Diseases*, **113**, 522–8.

Gillin, J.C., Sitaram, N., Wehr, T. *et al.* (1985). Sleep and affective illness. In R.M. Post and J.C. Ballenger (Eds.), *Neurobiology of Mood Disorders*, Williams and Wilkins, Baltimore, pp. 157–89.

Gjessing, R. (1947). Biological investigations in endogenous psychoses, *Acta Psychiatrica Neurologica Scandanavica*, Suppl. 47.

Glaser, G.H., and Pincus, J.H. (1969). Limbic encephalitis, *Journal of Nervous and Mental Diseases*, **149**, 59–68.

Glass, I.B., Checkley, S.A., Shur, E., and Dawling, S. (1982). Effect of desipramine upon central adrenergic function in depressed patients, *British Journal of Psychiatry*, **141**, 372–6.

Glassman, A.H., Perel, J.M., Shostak, M., *et al.* (1977). Clinical implications of imipramine plasma levels for depressive illness, *Archives of General Psychiatry*, **34**, 197–204.

426

Glaus, A. (1931). Ueber Kombinationen von Schizophrenie und Epilepsie, *Zeitschrift für die Gesamte Neurologie und Psychiatrie*, **135**, 450–500.

Glen, A.I.M., Ongley, G.C., and Robinson, K. (1968). Diminished membrane transport in manic-depressive psychosis and recurrent depression, *Lancet*, **i**, 241–3.

Gloor, P., Olivier, A., Quesney, L.F., Andermann, F., and Horowitz, S. (1982). The role of the limbic system in experiental phenomena of TLE, *Annals of Neurology*, **12**, 129–44.

Glowinski, J., Tassin, J.P., and Thierry, A.M. (1984). The meso-cortico–prefrontal dopaminergic neurones, *Trends in Neurosciences*, **7**, 415–18.

Goldgaber, D., Lerman, M.I., McBride, O.W., Saffiotti, U., and Gajdusek, D.C. (1987). Characterisation and chromosomal localisation of a CDNA encoding brain amyloid of Alzheimer's disease, *Science*, **235**, 837–80.

Golden, C.J., Graber, B., Coffman, J., Berg, R.A., Newlin, D.B., and Bloch, S. (1980). Brain density deficits in chronic schizophrenia, *Psychiatry Research*, **3**, 179–84.

Goldstein, G., and Halperin, K.M. (1977). Neuropsychological differences among subtypes of schizophrenia, *Journal of Abnormal Psychology*, **86**, 34–40.

Gomes, U.C.R., Potgieter, L., and Roux, J.T. (1980). Noradrenergic overactivity in chronic schizophrenia, *British Journal of Psychiatry*, **137**, 346–51.

Goodwin, D.W., and Guze, S.B. (1984). *Psychiatric Diagnosis*, 3rd edition, Oxford University Press, Oxford.

Gordon, E.B. (1968). Serial EEG studies in presenile dementia, *British Journal of Psychiatry*, **114**, 779–80.

Gordon, E.B., and Sim, M. (1967). The EEG in presenile dementia, *Journal of Neurology, Neurosurgery and Psychiatry*, **30**, 285–91.

Gorman, J.M., Levy, G.F., Liebowitz, M.R., et al. (1983). Effect of acute beta adrenergic blockade on lactate-induced panic, *Archives of General Psychiatry*, **40**, 1079–82.

Gorman, J., Liebowitz, M.R., Fyer, A.J., et al. (1985). Platelet MAO activity in patients with panic disorder, *Biological Psychiatry*, **20**, 852–8.

Gottesman, I.I. (1962). Differential inheritance of the psychoneuroses, *Eugenics Quarterly*, **9**, 223–7.

Gottesman, I.I., and Shields, J. (1967). A polygenic theory of schizophrenia, *Proceedings of the National Academy of Science*, **58**, 199–205.

Gottesman, I.I., and Shields, J. (1972). *Schizophrenia and Genetics: A Twin Study Vantage Point*, Academic Press, London.

Gowers, W.R. (1907). *The Borderland of Epilepsy*, Philadelphia, Maryland.

Gray, J.A. (1982). *The Neuropsychology of Anxiety*, Oxford University Press, Oxford.

Graybiel, A.M. (1984). Neurochemically specified subsystems in the basal ganglia. In D. Evered and M. O'Conner (Eds.), *Functions of the Basal Ganglia*, Pitman, London, pp. 114–43.

Green, A.R. (1986). Changes in GABA biochemistry and the seizure threshold. In S. Malitz and H.A. Sackheim (Eds.), *ECT*, Annals of the New York Academy of Sciences, Vol. 462, pp. 105–18.

Greenberg, D.B., and Brown, G.L. (1985). Mania resulting from brain stem tumour, *Journal of Nervous and Mental Diseases*, **173**, 434–6.

Greenwood, R., Bhalla, A., Gordon, A., and Roberts, J. (1983). Behaviour disturbances during recovery from herpes simplex encephalitis, *Journal of Neurology, Neurosurgery and Psychiatry*, **46**, 809–17.

Griesinger, W. (1867). *Mental Pathology and Therapeutics* (Translated by C. Lockhart Robertson and J. Rutherford), New Sydenham Society, London.

Grout, R., and Simmons, J. (1950). Loss of nerve cells in experimental cerebral concussion, *Journal of Neuropathology and Experimental Neurology*, **9**, 150–63.

Gudmundsson, G. (1966). Epilepsy in Iceland, *Acta Neurologica Scandinavica*, **43**, Suppl. 25, 1–124.

Guenther, W., and Breitling, D. (1985). Predominant sensory motor area left hemisphere dysfunction in schizophrenia measured by BEAM, *Biological Psychiatry*, **20**, 515–32.

Guenther, W., Breitling, D., Moser, E., Davous, P., and Petch, R. (1986). Brain mapping, rCBF and MRI measurements of motor dysfunction in Type 1 and Type 2 schizophrenic patients, 3rd International Symposium on *Cerebral Dynamics, Laterality and Psychopathology*, Abstract VI–1, Hakone, Japan.

Guerrant, J., Anderson, J., Fischer, A., Weinstein, M.R., Jaros, R.M., and Deskins, A. (1962). *Personality in Epilepsy*, Charles C. Thomas, Illinois.

428

Guillain, G. (1959). *J M Charcot — His Life, His Work*, Paul B. Hoeber, New York.

Gunn, J. (1977). *Epileptics in Prison*, Academic Press, London.

Gunne, L.M., Haggstrom, J.E., and Sjoquist, B. (1984). Association with persistant neuroleptic-induced dyskinesia of regional changes in brain GABA synthesis, *Nature*, **304**, 347–9.

Gur, R.E. (1977). Motoric laterality imbalance in schizophrenia, *Archives of General Psychiatry*, **34**, 33–7.

Gur, R.E. (1986). Regional brain dysfunction in schizophrenia, 3rd International Symposium on *Cerebral Dynamics, Laterality and Psychopathology*, Abstract V–7, Hakone, Japan.

Gur, R.E., Gur, R.C., Skolnick, B.E., and Reivich, M. (1983a). Regional brain abnormalities in schizophrenia, American Psychiatric Association Abstracts, New York, No. 18c.

Gur, R.E., Skolnick, B.E., Gur, R.C., Caroff, S., Rieger, W., Obrist, W.D., Younkin, D., and Reivich, M. (1983b). Brain function in psychiatric disorders. rCBF in medicated schizophrenics, *Archives of General Psychiatry*, **40**, 1250–4.

Gur, R.E., Skolnick, B.E., Gur, R.C., Carloff, S., Rieger, W., Obrist, W.D., Younkin, D., and Reivich, M. (1984). Brain function in psychiatric disorders, *Archives of General Psychiatry*, **41**, 695–702.

Gur, R.E., Gur, R.C., Skolnick, B., Caroff, S., Obrist, W.D., Reswick, S., and Reivich, M. (1985). Brain function in psychiatric disorders III. rCBF in unmedicated schizophrenics, *Archives of General Psychiatry*, **42**, 329–34.

Gustafson, L., and Risberg, J. (1979). Regional CBF measurements by the Xe^{133} inhalation technique in the differential diagnosis of dementia, *Acta Neurologica Scandinavica*, Suppl. 172, **60**, 546–7.

Hachinski, V.C., Iliff, L.D., Zilkha, E., DuBoulay, G.H., McAlister, V.L., Marshall, J., Ross-Russell, R.W., and Symon, L. (1975). Cerebral blood flow in dementia, *Archives of Neurology*, **32**, 632–7.

Hagberg, B., and Ingrar, D.H. (1976). Cognitive reduction in presenile dementia related to regional abnormalities of CBF, *British Journal of Psychiatry*, **128**, 209–22.

Hakola, H.P.A., and Iivanainen, M. (1978). Pneumoencephalographic and clinical findings of the XYY syndrome, *Acta Psychiatrica Scandinavica*, **58**, 360–6.

Hall, R.C.W. (1980). Depression. In R.C.W. Hall (Ed.), *Psychiatric Presentations of Medical Illness*, MTP Press, Lancaster, pp. 37–63.

Halonen, P.E., Rimon, R., Arohonka, K., and Jantti, V. (1974). Antibody levels to HSV 1; measles and rubella viruses in psychiatric patients, *British Journal of Psychiatry*, **125**, 461–5.

Hardy, J., Cowburn, R., Barton, A., *et al.* (1987). Glutamate deficits in Alzheimer's disease, *Journal of Neurology, Neurosurgery and Psychiatry*, **50**, 356–9.

Hare, E. (1979). Schizophrenia as an infectious disease, *British Journal of Psychiatry*, **135**, 468–70.

Harlow, J.M. (1868). Recovery from the passage of an iron bar through the head, *Publications of the Massachusetts Medical Society*, **2**, 329–46.

Harper, M., and Roth, M. (1962). Temporal lobe epilepsy and the phobia anxiety–depersonalisation syndrome, *Comprehensive Psychiatry*, **3**, 129–51, 215–26.

Harrison, R.M., and Taylor, D.(1976). Childhood seizures: a 25-year follow-up, *Lancet*, **i**, 948–51.

Harrison, W.M., Cooper, T.B., Stewart, J.W., *et al.* (1984). The tyramine challenge test as a marker for melancholia, *Archives of General Psychiatry*, **41**, 681–5.

Haug, J.O. (1962). Pneumoencephalographic studies in mental disease, *Acta Psychiatrica Scandinavica*, **38**, 1–114.

Hays, P. (1977). Electroencephalographic variants and genetic predisposition to schizophrenia, *Journal of Neurology, Neurosurgery and Psychiatry*, **40**, 753–5.

Healy, D., Carney, P.A., and Leonard, B.E. (1983). Monoamine related markers of depression: changes following treatment, *Journal of Psychiatric Research*, **17**, 251–60.

Heath, R.G. (1954). *Studies in Schizophrenia*, Harvard University Press, Cambridge.

Heath, R.G. (1962). Common characteristics of epilepsy and schizophrenia, *American Journal of Psychiatry*, **118**, 1013–26.

Heath, R.G. (1972). Pleasure and brain activity in man, *Journal of Nervous and Mental Diseases*, **154**, 3–18.

Heath, R.G. (1982). Psychosis and epilepsy: similarities and differences in the anatomic–physiologic substrate. In W.P. Koella and M.R. Trimble (Eds.), *Temporal Lobe Epilepsy, Mania and Schizophrenia and the Limbic System*, Karger, Basle, pp. 106–16.

Heath, R.G., Martens, S., Leach, B.E., Cohen. M., and Angel, C. (1957). Effect on behaviour in humans with the administration of taraxein, *American Journal of Psychiatry*, **14**, 114–20.

Heath, R.G., Dempesy, C.W., Fontana, C.J., and Myers, W.A. (1978). Cerebellar stimulation: effects on septal region, hippocampus and amygdala of cats and rats, *Biological Psychiatry*, **13**, 501–29.

Heaton, R.K., and Crowley, T.J. (1981). The effects of psychiatric disorders and their somatic treatments on neuropsychological test results. In S.B. Filskov and T. Boll (Eds.), *Handbook of Clinical Neuropsychology*, Wiley Interscience, New York, pp. 481–525.

Heimer, L., and Larsson, E. (1966). Impairment of mating behaviour in male rats following lesions in the pre-optic and anterior hypothalamic continuum, *Brain Research*, **3**, 248–63.

Heimer, L., Switzer, R.D., and van Hoesen, G.W. (1982). Ventral striatum and ventral pallidum, *Trends in Neurosciences*, **5**, 83–7.

Helmberg, G., and Gershon, S. (1961). Autonomic and psychic effects of yohimbine, *Psychopharmacologia*, **2**, 93–106.

Heninger, G.R., Charney, D.S., Sternberg, D.E. (1984). Serotinergic function in depression, *Archives of General Psychiatry*, **41**, 398–402.

Henriksen, G.F. (1973). Status epilepticus partialis with fear as a clinical expression: report of a case and ictal EEG findings, *Epilepsia*, **14**, 39–46.

Herbert, J. (1984). Behaviour and the limbic system with particular reference to sexual and aggressive interactions. In M.R. Trimble and E. Zarifian (Eds.), *Psychopharmacology of the Limbic System*, Oxford University Press, Oxford, pp. 51–67.

Hermann, B.P., and Riel, P. (1981). Interictal personality and behavioural traits in temporal lobe and generalized epilepsy, *Cortex*, **17**, 125–8.

Hermann, B.P., Dickmen, S., Swartz, M.S., and Karnes, W.E. (1982). Interictal psychopathology in patients with ictal fear: a quantitative investigation, *Neurology*, **32**, 7–11.

Hermann, B.P., and Whitman, S. (1984). Behavioural and personality correlates of epilepsy: a review, methodological critique, and conceptual model, *Psychological Bulletin*, **95**, 451–92.

Heston, L.L. (1966). Psychiatric disorders in foster home reared children of schizophrenic mothers, *British Journal of Psychiatry*, **112**, 819–25.

Heston, L.L., Mastri, A.R., Anderson, E., and White, J. (1981). Dementia of the Alzheimer type, *Archives of General Psychiatry*, **38**, 1085–90.

Hierons, R., Janota, I., and Corsellis, J.A.N. (1978). The late effects of necrotising encephalitis of the temporal lobes and limbic areas: a clinico-pathological study of 10 cases, *Psychological Medicine*, **8**, 21–42.

Hill, D. (1950). Psychiatry. In D. Hill and G. Parr (Eds.), *Electroencephalography*, MacDonald, London, pp. 319–63.

Hill, D. (1952). EEG in episodic psychotic and psychopathic behaviour, *Electroencephalography and Clinical Neurophysiology*, **4**, 419–42.

Hill, D. (1981). Historical Review. In E.H. Reynolds and M.R. Trimble (Eds.), *Epilepsy and Psychiatry*, Churchill Livingstone, Edinburgh, pp. 1–11.

Hillbom, E. (1960). After effects of brain injuries, *Acta Psychiatrica Neurologica Scandinavica*, **35**, Suppl. 142.

Himmelhoch, J., Pincus, J., Tucker, G., and Detre, T. (1970). Sub-acute encephalitis: behavioural and neurological aspects, *British Journal of Psychiatry*, **116**, 531–8.

Hoehn-Saric, R. (1982). Neurotransmitters in anxiety, *Archives of General Psychiatry*, **39**, 735–42.

Hokfelt, T., Johansson, O., Ljungdahl, A., Lundberg, J.M., and Schultzberg, M. (1980). Peptidergic neurones, *Nature*, **284**, 515–21.

Hollander, D., and Strich, S.J. (1970). Atypical Alzheimer's disease with congophilic angiopathy, presenting with dementia of acute onset. In G.E.W. Wolstenholm, and M. O'Connor (Eds.), *Alzheimer's Disease and Related Conditions*, Ciba Symposium, Churchill, London, pp. 105–24.

Hollister, L.E., Davis, K.L., and Berger, P.A. (1980). Subtypes of depression based on excretion of MHPG and response to nortriptyline, *Archives of General Psychiatry*, **37**, 1107–10.

Holsboer, F., Gerkoen, A., Stalla, G.K., and Muller, O.A. (1985). ACTH, cortisol and corticosterone output after ovine corticotropin-releasing factor challenge during depression and after recovery, *Biological Psychiatry*, **20**, 276–86.

432

Holzman, P.S., Soloman, C.M., Levin, S., and Waternaux, C.S. (1984). Pursuit eye movement dysfunctions in schizophrenia, *Archives of General Psychiatry*, **41**, 136–9.

Howard, R.C., Fenton, G.W., and Fenwick, P.B.C. (1984). The CNV, personality and antisocial behaviour, *British Journal of Psychiatry*, **144**, 463–74.

Huber, G. (1957). *Pneumoencephalographische und Psychopathalogische Bilder Bei Endogen Psychosen*, Springer Verlag, Berlin.

Hughes, J.R., and Hermann, B.P. (1984). Evidence for psychopathology in patients with rhythmic mid-temporal discharges, *Biological Psychiatry*, **19**, 1623–34.

Hunter, R., and MacAlpine, I. (1963), *Three Hundred Years of Psychiatry*, Oxford University Press, Oxford.

Hunter, R., and Jones, M. (1966). Acute lethargica type encephalitis, *Lancet*, **ii**, 1023–4.

Hunter, R., and MacAlpine, I. (1974). *Psychiatry for the Poor*, Dawsons, London.

Hutchings, B., and Mednick, S.A. (1975). Registered criminality in the adoptive and biological parents of registered male criminal adoptees. In R.R. Fieve, D. Rosenthal and H. Brill (Eds.), *Genetic Research in Psychiatry*, Johns Hopkins Press, Baltimore, pp. 105–16.

ILAE (1981). Proposal for revised clinical and electroencephalographic classification of epileptic seizures, *Epilepsia*, **22**, 489–501.

ILAE (1985). Proposal for classification of the epilepsies and epileptic syndromes, *Epilepsia*, **26**, 268–78.

Imlah, N.W. (1985). An evaluation of alprazolam in the treatment of reactive or neurotic depression, *British Journal of Psychiatry*, **14**, 515–9.

Ingvar, D.H., and Franzen, G. (1974). Distribution of cerebral activity in chronic schizophrenia, *Lancet*, **ii**, 1484–6.

Insel, T.R., Gillin, J.C., Moore, A., Mendelson, W.B., Lowenstein, R.J., and Murphy, D.L. (1982). The sleep of patients with obsessive compulsive disorder, *Archives of General Psychiatry*, **39**, 1372–7.

Insel, T.R., Donnelly, E.F., Lalakea, M.L., Alterman, I.S., and Murphy, D.L. (1983). Neurological and neuropsychological studies of patients with obsessive compulsive disorder, *Biological Psychiatry*, **18**, 741–51.

Insel, T.R., Mueller, E.A., Alterman, I., Linnoila, M., and Murphy, D.L. (1985). Obsessive–compulsive disorder and serotonin: is there a connection?, *Biological Psychiatry*, **20**, 1174–88.

Isaacson, R.L. (1982). *The Limbic System*, 2nd edition, Plenum Press, New York.

Itil, T.M. (1975). Digital computer period analysed EEG in psychiatry and psychopharmacology. In G. Dolee and H. Kunkel (Eds.), *Symposium of Mercksche Gesellschaft für Kunst und Wissenschaft*, Gustav Fischer, Stuttgart, pp. 289–307.

Iversen, L. (1983). Biochemical characterization of benzodiazepine receptors. In M.R. Trimble (Ed.), *Benzodiazepines Divided*, John Wiley and Sons, Chichester, pp. 79–84.

Iversen, S. (1977). Temporal lobe amnesia. In C. Whitty and O.L. Zangwill (Eds.), *Amnesia*, Butterfields, London, pp. 136–82.

Iversen, S. (1983). Where in the brain do benzodiazepines act? In M.R. Trimble (Ed.), *Benzodiazepines Divided*, John Wiley and Sons, Chichester, pp. 167–85.

Iversen, S.D., and Iversen, L. (1981). Substance P — a new CNS transmitter, *Hospital Update*, **May**, 497–506.

Iversen, S. (1984). Behavioural effects of manipulation of basal ganglia neurotransmitters. In D. Evered and M. O'Connor (Eds.), *Functions of the Basal Ganglia*, Pitman, London, pp. 183–95.

Jackman, H., Luchins, P., and Meltzer, H.Y. (1983). Platelet serotonin levels in schizophrenia: relationship to race and psychopathology, *Biological Psychiatry*, **18**, 887–902.

Jackson, J.H. (1874). On the nature of the duality of the brain, *Medical Press and Circular*, **i**, 19–63.

Jacobsen, C.F. (1935). Functions of the frontal association cortex, *Archives of Neurology and Psychiatry*, **33**, 558–69.

Jacoby, R., and Levy, R. (1980a). CT scanning and the investigation of dementia: a review, *Journal of the Royal Society of Medicine*, **73**, 366–9.

Jacoby, R., and Levy, R. (1980b). Computed tomography in the elderly. ii. Senile dementia, *British Journal of Psychiatry*, **136**, 256–69.

Jacoby, R., and Levy, R. (1980c). Computed tomography in the elderly. iii. Affective disorder, *British Journal of Psychiatry*, **136**, 270–5.

434

Jacoby, R.J., Levy, R., and Bird, J.M. (1981). Computed tomography and the outcome of affective disorder: a follow up study of elderly patients, *British Journal of Psychiatry*, **139**, 288–92.

Janota, I. (1981). Dementia, deep white matter damage and hypertension: Binswanger's disease, *Psychological Medicine*, **11**, 39–48.

Janowsky, D.S., Risch, S.C., Parker, D., Huey, L., and Judd, L. (1980). Increased vulnerability to cholinergic stimulation in affective disorder patients, *Psychopharmacology Bulletin*, **16**, 29–31.

Jaspers, K. (1963). *General Psychopathology* (Translated by J. Hoenig and M.W. Hamilton), Manchester University Press, Manchester.

Jennett, B. (1975). *Epilepsy after Non-missile Head Injuries*, Heinemann, London.

Jensen, I., and Larsen, J. (1979). Psychoses in drug resistant TLE, *Journal of Neurology, Neurosurgery and Psychiatry*, **42**, 948–54.

Jernigan, T.L., Zatz, L.M., Moses, J.A., and Berger, P.A. (1982). Computed tomography in schizophrenics and normal volunteers, *Archives of General Psychiatry*, **39**, 765–70.

Jeste, D.V., Lohr, J.B., and Karson, C.N. (1985). Neuronometric studies of cerebellum and hippocampus in schizophrenia and ageing. IV, *World Congress of Biological Psychiatry Abstracts*, p. 310, No. 414. 1.

Jimerson, D.C., Insel, T.R., Reus, V.I., and Kopin, I.J. (1983). Increased plasma MHPG in dexamethasone resistant depressed patients, *Archives of General Psychiatry*, **40**, 173–6.

Johannesson, G., Brun, A., Gustaffson, L., and Ingvar, D.H. (1977). EEG in presenile dementia related to cerebral blood flow and autopsy findings, *Acta Neurologica Scandinavica*, **56**, 89–103.

Johannsson, O., and Hokfelt, T. (1981). Nucleus accumbens: transmitter neurochemistry with special reference to peptide-containing neurones. In R.B. Chronister and J.F. De France (Eds.), *The Neurobiology of the Nucleus Accumbens*, Haer Institute, Brunswick, N.J., pp. 147–72.

Johnstone, E., Crow, T.J., Frith, C.D., *et al.* (1976). Cerebral ventricular size and cognitive impairment in chronic schizophrenia, *Lancet*, **ii**, 924–6.

Johnstone, E.C., Crow, T.J., and Mashiter, K. (1977). Anterior pituitary hormone secretion in chronic schizophrenia — an approach to neurohormonal mechanisms, *Psychological Medicine,* **7**, 223–8.

Johnstone, E.C., Crow, T.J., Frith, C.D., Stevens, M., Kreel, L., and Husband, J. (1978). The dementia of dementia praecox, *Acta Psychiatrica Scandinavica,* **57**, 305–24.

Johnstone, E.C., Crow, T.J., MacMillan, J.F., Owens, D.G.C., Bydder, G.M., and Steiner, R.E. (1986a). A MRI study of early schizophrenia, *Journal of Neurology, Neurosurgery and Psychiatry,* **49**, 136–9.

Johnstone, E.C., Owens, D.G.C., Crow, T.J., Colter, N., Lawton, C.A., Jagoe, R., and Kreel, L. (1986b). Hypothyroidism as a correlate of lateral ventricular enlargement in manic depressive and neurotic illness, *British Journal of Psychiatry,* **148**, 317–21.

Jones, E.G., and Powell, T.P.S. (1970). An anatomical study of converging sensory pathways within the cerebral cortex of the monkey, *Brain,* **93**, 793–820.

Judd, F.K., Norman, T.R., and Burrows, G.D. (1986). Pharmacological treatment of panic disorder, *International Clinical Psychopharmacology,* **1**, 3–16.

Judd, L.L., Risch, C., Parker, D.C., Janowsky, D.S., Segal, D.S., and Huey, L.Y. (1982). Blunted prolactin response, *Archives of General Psychiatry,* **39**, 1413–16.

Kafka, M.S., van Kammen, D., and Bunney, W.E. (1979). Reduced cAMP production in the blood platelets from schizophrenic patients, *American Journal of Psychiatry,* **136**, 5–8.

Kafka, M.S., van Kammen, D., Kleinman, J.E., *et al.* (1980). Alpha adrenergic receptor function in schizophrenia, affective disorders, and some neurological disease, *Communications of Psychopharmacology,* **4**, 477–86.

Kallmann, F. (1946). The genetic theory of schizophrenia, *American Journal of Psychiatry,* **103**, 309–22.

Kallmann, F. (1954). Genetic principles in manic-depressive psychosis. In J. Zubin and P. Hoch (Eds.), *Depression: Proceedings of the American Psychopathological Association,* Grune & Stratton, New York.

Kandel, E.R., and Schwartz, J.H. (1981). *Principles of Neural Science,* Elsevier, North Holland.

Kantor, J.S., Zitrin, C.M., and Zeldis, S.M. (1980). Mitral valve prolapse syndrome in agoraphobic patients, *American Journal of Psychiatry,* **137**, 467–9.

Karis, D., Fabini, M., and Donchin, E. (1984). *Cognitive Psychology*, **16**, 177–216.

Kathol, R.G., Noyes, R., Slyman, D.J., Crowe, R.R., Clancy, J., and Kerber, R.E. (1980). Propranolol in chronic anxiety disorders, *Archives of General Psychiatry*, **37**, 1361–5.

Kathol, R.G., Noyes, R., Slyman, D.J., *et al.* (1981). Propranolol in chronic anxiety disorders. In D.F. Klein and J. Rabkin (Eds.), *Anxiety, New Research and Changing Concepts*, Raven Press, New York, pp. 81–93.

Katona, C.L.E., Hale, A.S., Theodorus, S.L., Tunnicliffe, D.C., Horton, R.W., Paykel, E.S., and Kelly, J.S. (1985). Which depressives have blunted growth hormone responses to clonidine?, *Abstracts of the Autumn Quarterly Meeting of the Royal College of Psychiatrists*, pp. 6–7.

Katz, B., and Milendi, R. (1967). The timing of calcium action during neuromuscular transmission, *Journal of Physiology*, **189**, 535–44.

Kay, D.W.K., Foster, E.M., McKenchnie, A.A., and Roth, M. (1970). Mental illness and hospital use in the elderly: a random sample followed up, *Comprehensive Psychiatry*, **11**, 26–35.

Keitner, G.I., Brown, W.A., Qualls, C.B., Haier, R.J., and Barnes, K.T. (1985). Results of DST in psychiatric patients with and without weight loss, *American Journal of Psychiatry*, **142**, 246–8.

Kemali, D., Vacca, L., Marciano, F., Nolfe, G., and Iorio, G. (1981). CEEG findings in schizophrenics, depressives, obsessives, heroin addicts and normals, *Advances in Biological Psychiatry*, **6**, 17–28.

Kendell, R.E. (1969). The continuum model of depressive illness, *Proceedings of the Royal Society of Medicine*, **62**, 335–9.

Kendell, R.E. (1975). *The Role of Diagnosis in Psychiatry*, Blackwells, Oxford.

Kendler, K.S. (1983). Overview: a current prospective on twin studies of schizophrenia, *American Journal of Psychiatry*, **140**, 1413–25.

Kendler, K.S., and Robinette, C.D. (1983). Schizophrenia in the National Academy of Sciences, *American Journal of Psychiatry*, **140**, 1557–63.

Kendler, K.S., Gruenberg, A.M., and Strauss, T.S. (1981). An independent analysis of the Danish adoption study of schizophrenia, *Archives of General Psychiatry*, **38**, 973–87.

Kendrick, J.F., and Gibbs, F.A. (1957). Origin, spread and neuro-surgical treatment of the psychomotor type of seizure discharge, *Journal of Neurosurgery*, **14**, 270–84.

Keshavan, M.S., Kumar, Y.V., and Channabasavanna, S.M. (1979). A critical evaluation of infantile reflexes in neuro-psychiatric diagnoses, *Indian Journal of Psychiatry*, **21**, 267–70.

Kety, S.S. (1980). The syndromes of schizophrenia, *British Journal of Psychiatry*, **136**, 421–36.

Kety, S.S. (1983). Mental illness in the biological and adoptive relations of schizophrenic adoptees, *American Journal of Psychiatry*, **140**, 720–7.

Kety, S.S., and Schmidt, C.F. (1948). The nitrous oxide method for the quantitative determination of cerebral blood flow in man: theory procedure and normal values, *Journal of Clinical Investigation*, **27**, 476–83.

Kidger, T., Barnes, T.R.E., Trauer, T., and Taylor, P.J. (1980). Subsyndromes of tardive dyskinesia, *Psychological Medicine*, **10**, 513–20.

Kilpatrick, C., Burns, R., and Blumbergs, P.C. (1983). Identical twins with Alzheimer's disease, *Journal of Neurology, Neurosurgery and Psychiatry*, **46**, 421–5.

King, J.R., and Hullin, R.P. (1983). Withdrawal symptoms from lithium, *British Journal of Psychiatry*, **143**, 30–5.

Kinney, D.K., Wods, B.K., and Yurgelun-Todd, D. (1986). Neurologic abnormalities in schizophrenic patients and their families, *Archives of General Psychiatry*, **43**, 665–8.

Klapper, P.E., Cleator, G.M., and Longson, M. (1984). Mild forms of herpes encephalitis, *Journal of Neurology, Neurosurgery and Psychiatry*, **47**, 1247–50.

Klein, D.F., and Davis, J.M. (1969). *Diagnosis and Drug Treatment of Psychiatric Disorders*, Williams and Wilkins, Baltimore.

Kleinman, J.E., Karoum, F., Rosenblatt, J.E., et al. (1982a). Post mortem neurochemical studies in chronic schizophrenia. In E. Usdin and I. Hania (Eds.), *Biological Markers in Psychiatry and Neurology*, Pergamon Press, New York, pp. 67–76.

Kleinman, J.E., Weinberger, D.R., Rogal, A.D., Bigelow, L.B., et al. (1982b). Plasma prolactin concentrations and psychopathology in chronic schizophrenia, *Archives of General Psychiatry*, **39**, 655–7.

Kleinman, J.E., Reid, A., Lake, C.R., and Wyatt, R.J. (1985). Studies of norepinephrine in schizophrenia. In C.R. Lake and

438

M.G. Ziegler (Eds.), *The Catecholamines in Psychiatric and Neurologic Disorders*, Butterworths, London, pp. 285–312.

Kleist, K.K. (1969). Schizophrenic symptoms and cerebral pathology, *Journal of Mental Science,* **106**, 246–55.

Kligman, D., and Goldberg, D.A. (1975). Temporal lobe epilepsy and aggression, *Journal of Nervous and Mental Diseases,* **160**, 324–41.

Kline, N.S., Li, C.H., Lehmann, H.E., Lajha, A., Laski, E., and Cooper, T. (1977). Beta endorphin induced changes in schizophrenic and depressed patients, *Archives of General Psychiatry,* **34**, 1111–14.

Kling, A., Orbach, J., Schwartz, N.B., and Towne, J.C. (1960). Injury to the limbic system and associated structures in cats, *Archives of General Psychiatry,* **3**, 391–420.

Kluver, H., and Bucy, P.C. (1939). Preliminary analysis of functions of the temporal lobe in monkeys, *Archives of Neurology and Psychiatry,* **42**, 979–1000.

Ko, G.N., Elsworth, J.D., Roth, R.H., Rifkin, B.G., Leigh, H., and Redmond, E. (1983). Panic induced elevation of plasma MHPG levels in phobic anxious patients, *Archives of General Psychiatry,* **40**, 425–30.

Koehler, K., and Jakumeit, N. (1976). Sub-acute sclerosing panencephalitis presenting as Leonhard's speech-prompt catatonia, *British Journal of Psychiatry,* **129**, 29–31.

Koella, W. (1982). The functions of the limbic system — evidence from animal experimentation. In W. Koella and M.R. Trimble (Eds.), *Temporal Lobe Epilepsy, Mania, and Schizophrenia and the Limbic System*, Karger, Basel, pp. 12–39.

Kogeorgos, J., Fonagy, P., and Scott, D.F. (1982). Psychiatric symptom patterns of chronic epileptics attending a neurological clinic: a controlled investigation, *British Journal of Psychiatry,* **140**, 236–43.

Kojima, H., Yamada, S., Nakamura, J., *et al.* (1986). Brain morphological changes in chronical schizophrenia, 3rd International Symposium on *Cerebral Dynamics, Laterality and Psychopathology*, Abstract V-13, Hakone, Japan.

Kolakowska, T., Orr, M., Gelder, M., Heggie, M., Wiles, D., and Franklin, M. (1979). Clinical significance of plasma drug and prolactin levels during acute chlorpromazine treatment: a replication study, *Psychological Medicine,* **135**, 352–9.

Kolalowska, T., Williams, A.O., Jambor, K., and Ardern, M. (1985a). Schizophrenia with good and poor outcome, *British Journal of Psychiatry*, **146**, 348–57.

Kolakowska, T., Williams, A.O., Jambor, K., Ardern, M., Reveley, M.A., Jambor, K., Gewer, M.G., and Mandelbrote, B.M. (1985b). Schizophrenia with good and poor outcome, *British Journal of Psychiatry*, **146**, 229–46.

Kolvin, I., Ounsted, C., and Roth, M. (1971). Cerebral dysfunction and childhood psychosis, *British Journal of Psychiatry*, **118**, 407–14.

Kopelman, M.D. (1985). Multiple memory defecits in Alzheimer-type dementia, *Psychological Medicine*, **15**, 527–41.

Korpi, E.R., Kleinman, J.E., Goodman, S.I., Phillips, I., De Lisi, L., Linnoila, M., and Wyatt, R.J. (1986). Serotonin and 5-HIAA in brains of suicide patients, *Archives of General Psychiatry*, **43**, 594–600.

Kovelman, J.A., and Scheibel, A.B. (1984). A neurohistological correlate of schizophrenia, *Biological Psychiatry*, **19**, 1601–22.

Kraepelin, E. (1904). *Lectures on Clinical Psychiatry*, William Wood, New York.

Kraepelin, E. (1919). *Dementia Praecax*, E. and S. Livingstone, Edinburgh.

Kraepelin, E. (1923). *Psychiatrie*, Vol. 3, 8th edition, J. A. Barth, Leipzig.

Krauthammer, C., and Klerman, G.L. (1978). Secondary mania, *Archives of General Psychiatry*, **35**, 1333–9.

Kretchmer, E. (1936). *Physique and Character*, Miller, London.

Kringlen, E. (1965). Obsessional neurotics, *British Journal of Psychiatry*, **111**, 709–22.

Kringlen, E. (1967). *Heredity and Environment in the Functional Psychoses*, Heinemann, London.

Krishnan, K.R.R., Davidson, J.R.T., Rayasam, K., and Shope, F. (1984). The DST in borderline personality disorder, *Biological Psychiatry*, **19**, 1149–53.

Kristensen, O., and Sindrup, E.H. (1978). Psychomotor epilepsy and psychosis, *Acta Neurologica Scandinavica*, **57**, 361–70.

Lader, M.H. (1969). Psychophysiological aspects of anxiety. In M.H. Lader (Ed.), *Studies of Anxiety*, Headley Bros., Kent, pp. 53–61.

Laitinen, L.V. (1979). Emotional responses to subcortical electrical stimulation in psychiatric patients, *Clinical Neurology and Neurosurgery*, **81–83**, 148–57.

440

Lake, C.R., Sternberg, D.E., van Kammen, D.P., Ballenger, J.C., *et al.* (1980). Schizophrenia, elevated CSF norepinephrine, *Science*, **207**, 331–3.

Lake, C.R., Pickar, D., Ziegler, M.G., Lipper, S., Slater, S., and Murphy, D.L. (1982). High plasma norepinephine levels in patients with major affective disorders, *American Journal of Psychiatry*, **139**, 1315–16.

Lammertsma, A.A., Jones, T., Frackowiak, R.S.J., and Lenzi, G.U. (1981). A theoretical study of the steady-state model for measuring rCBF and oxygen utilisation using oxygen-15, *Journal of Computer Assisted Tomography*, **5**, 544–50.

Landolt, H. (1958). Serial electroencephalographic investigations during psychotic episodes in epileptic patients and during schizophrenic attacks. In Lorenz de Haas (Ed.), *Lectures on Epilepsy*, Elsevier, London, pp. 91–133.

Lange, J. (1929). *Verbrechen als Schicksal*, Thomas, Leipzig.

Largen, J.W., Smith, R.C., Calderon, M., *et al.* (1984). Abnormalities of brain structure and density in schizophrenia, *Biological Psychiatry*, **19**, 991–1014.

Larkin, E.P. (1985). The X-ray department and psychiatry, *British Journal of Psychiatry*, **146**, 62–5.

Larson, E.B., Mack, L.A., Watts, B., and Cromwell, L. (1981). CT in patients with psychiatric illness, *Annals of Internal Medicine*, **95**, 360–4.

Lauterbur, P.C. (1973). Image formation by induced local interactions: examples employing NMR, *Nature*, **242**, 190–1.

Lazare, A., Klerman, G.L., and Armor, D.J. (1970). Oral, obsessive and hysterical personality patterns, *Journal of Psychiatric Research*, **7**, 275–90.

Leckman, J.F., Gershon, E.S., Nichols, A.S., and Murphy, D.L. (1977). Reduced MAO activity in first degree relatives of individuals with bipolar affective disorders, *Archives of General Psychiatry*, **34**, 601–08.

Lee, T., and Seeman, P. (1980). Elevation of brain neuroleptic/dopamine receptors in schizophrenia, *American Journal of Psychiatry*, **137**, 191–7.

Le May, M., and Geschwind, N. (1975). Hemispheric differences in the brains of great apes, *Brain, Behaviour and Evolution*, **11**, 48–52.

Lennox, W.G., and Lennox, M. (1960). *Epilepsy and Related Disorders*, J. and A. Churchill, London.

Leonhard, K. (1957). *Aufteilung der Endogenen Psychosen*, Akademie Verlag, Berlin.

Leonhard, K. (1979). E. Robins (Ed.), *The Classification of Endogenous Psychoses* (Translated by R. Berman), Irvington, New York.

Leonhard, K. (1980). Contradictory issues in the origin of schizophrenia, *British Journal of Psychiatry*, **136**, 437–44.

Lerner, P., Goodwin, F.K., van Kammen, D.P., Post, R.M., *et al.* (1978). Dopamine beta hydrolase in the CSF of psychiatric patients, *Biological Psychiatry*, **13**, 685–94.

Levin, A.P., Liebowitz, M.R., Fyer, A.J., Gorman, J.M., and Klein, D.F. (1984). Lactate induction of panic: hypothesised mechanisms and recent findings. In J.C. Ballenger (Ed.), *Biology of Agoraphobia*, APA, Washington, pp. 81–98.

Levi Strauss, C. (1962). *The Savage Mind*, Weindenfeld & Nicolson.

Levy, A.B., Kurtz, N., and Kling, A.S. (1984). Association between cerebral ventricular enlargement and suicide attempts in chronic schizophrenia, *American Journal of Psychiatry*, **141**, 438–9.

Lewis, A. (1934). Melancholia: a clinical survey of depressive states, *Journal of Mental Science*, **80**, 277–378.

Lewis, A. (1970). Paranoia and paranoid: a historical perspective, *Psychological Medicine*, **1**, 2–12.

Lewis, A. (1971). 'Endogenous' and 'exogeneous' — a useful dichotomy, *Psychological Medicine*, **1**, 191–6.

Lewis, D.A., and McChesney, C. (1985). Tritiated imipramine binding distinguishes among subtypes of depression, *Archives of General Psychiatry*, **42**, 485–8.

Lewis, D.A., Campbell, M.J., Foote, S.L., Goldstein, M., and Morrison, J.H. (1986). The dopaminergic innervation of primate neocortex is widespread, yet regionally specific, *Society of Biological Psychiatry Abstracts*, p. 1, Washington, May 1986.

Leysen, J.E. (1984). Problems in in vitro receptor binding studies and identification and role of serotonin receptor sites, *Neuropharmacology*, **23**, 2B, 247–54.

Leysen, J., and Niemegeers, C.J.E. (1985). Neuroleptics. In A. Lagtha (Ed.), *Handbook of Neurochemistry*, Vol.9, Plenum, New York, pp. 331–61.

L'Hermitte, F. (1983). Utilization behaviour and its relation to lesions of the frontal lobes, *Brain*, **106**, 237–55.

442

Lidberg, L., Tuck, J.R., Åsberg, M., Scalia–Tomba, G., and Bertillson, L. (1985). Homicide, suicide and CSF 5-HIAA, *Acta Psychiatric Scandinavica*, **71**, 230–6.

Lieberman, J.A., Kane, J.M., Sarantakos, S., Cole, K., *et al.* (1985). Dexamethasone suppression tests in patients with obsessive–compulsive disorder, *American Journal of Psychiatry*, **142**, 747–51.

Liebowitz, M.R., Fyer, A.J., Gorman, J.M., *et al.* (1985). Specificity of lactate infusions in social phobia versus panic disorders, *American Journal of Psychiatry*, **142**, 947–50.

Lindy, D.C., Walsh, T., Roose, S.P., Gladis, M., and Glassman, A.H. (1985). The DST in Bulimia, *American Journal of Psychiatry*, **142**, 1375–6.

Linnoila, M., and Martin, P.R. (1983). Benzodiazepines and alcoholism. In M.R. Trimble (Ed.), *Benzodiazepines Divided*, John Wiley and Sons, Chichester, pp. 291–306.

Linnoila, M., Karoum, F., Rosenthal, N., and Potter, W.Z. (1983a). ECT and lithium carbonate, *Archives of General Psychiatry*, **40**, 677–80.

Linnoila, M., Virkkunen, M., Scheinin, M., *et al.* (1983b). Low CSF 5-HIAA concentration differentiates impulsive from non-impulsive violent behaviour, *Life Science*, **33**, 2609–14.

Lipsey, J.K., Robinson, R.G., Pearlson, G.D., Rao, K., and Price, T.R. (1985). The DST and mood following stroke, *American Journal of Psychiatry*, **142**, 318–22.

Lishman, A. (1978). *Organic Psychiatry*, Blackwell, Oxford.

Lloyd, K.G., Farley, I.J., Deck, J.H.N., Hornykiewicz, O. (1974). Serotoin and 5-HIAA in discrete areas of the brainstem of suicide victims and control patients, *Advances in Biochemical Psychopharmacology*, **11**, 387–97.

Longson, M. (1985). Herpes simples encephalitis. In W.B. Matthews and G. Glaser (Eds.), *Recent Advances in Neurology*, Churchill Livingstone, Edinburgh, pp. 123–40.

Lorenz, K. (1966). *On Aggression*, Methuen, London.

Lostra, F., Verbanc, P., Mendlewicz, J., and Vanderhaeghen, J.J. (1984). No evidence of antipsychotic effect of caerulin in schizophrenic patients free of neuroleptics, *Biological Psychiatry*, **19**, 877–9.

Luchins, D.J., Weinberger, D.R., and Wyatt, R.J. (1979). Schizophrenia: evidence for a subgroup with reversed asymmetry, *Archives of General Psychiatry*, **36**, 1309–11.

Luchins, D.J., Lewine, R.R.J., and Meltzer, H.Y. (1984). Lateral ventricular size, psychopathology and medication response in the psychoses, *Biological Psychiatry*, **19**, 29–44.

Luria, A.R. (1973). *The Working Brain*, Basic Books, New York.

Lycke, E., Norrby, R., and Roos, B.J. (1974). A serological study on mentally ill patients, *British Journal of Psychiatry*, **124**, 273–9.

Maas, J.W. (1975). Biogenic amines and depression, *Archives of General Psychiatry*, **32**, 1357–61.

Maas, J.W., Fawcett, J.A., and Dekirmenjian, H. (1972). Catecholamine metabolism, depressive illness and drug response, *Archives of General Psychiatry*, **26**, 252–62.

McCreadie, R.G., Dingwall, J.M., Wiles, D.H. and Heykants, J.J.P. (1980). Intermittant pimozide versus fluphenazine as maintainence therapy in chronic schizophrenia, *British Journal of Psychiatry*, **137**, 510–17.

McDonald, C. (1969). Clinical heterogeneity in senile dementia, *British Journal of Psychiatry*, **115**, 267–71.

MacDonald, R.T. (1982). Drug treatment of senile dementia. In D. Wheatley (Ed.), *Psychopathology of Old Age*, Oxford University Press, Oxford, pp. 113–37.

Mackay, A. (1979). Self poisoning — a complication of epilepsy, *British Journal of Psychiatry*, **134**, 277–82.

McGuffin, P. (1984a). Principles and methods of psychiatric genetics. In P. McGuffin, M.F. Shanks and R.J. Hodgson (Eds.), *The Scientific Principles of Psychopathology*, Grune and Stratton, London, pp. 155–72.

McGuffin, P. (1984b). Genetic influences on personality, neurosis and psychosis. In P. McGuffin, M.F. Shanks and R.J. Hodgson (Eds.), *The Scientific Principles of Psychopathology*, Stratton, London, pp. 191–228.

McGuffin, P., Farmer, A.E., and Yonace, A.H. (1981). HLA antigens and subtypes of schizophrenia, *Psychiatry Research*, **5**, 115–22.

McGuffin, P., Farmer, A.E., Gottesman, I.I., Murray, R.M., and Reveley, A.M. (1984). Twin concordance for operationally defined schizophrenia, *Archives of General Psychiatry*, **41**, 541–5.

McHenry, L.C. (1969). *Garrison's History of Neurology*, Charles C. Thomas, Illinois.

Mackay, A.V.P. (1980). Positive and negative schizophrenic symptoms and the role of dopamine, *British Journal of Psychiatry*, **137**, 379–86.

Mackay, A.V.P., Iversen, L.L., Rossor, M., Spokes, E., *et al.* (1982). Increased brain dopamine and dopamine receptors in schizophrenia, *Archives of General Psychiatry*, **39**, 991–7.

McKeon, J., McGuffin, P., and Robinson, P. (1984). Obsessive–compulsive neurosis following head injury: a report of four cases, *British Journal of Psychiatry*, **144**, 190–2.

MacLean, P.D. (1958). The limbic system with respect to self preservation and preservation of the species, *Journal of Nervous and Mental Diseases*, **127**, 1–11.

MacLean, P.D. (1970). The triune brain, emotion and scientific bias. In F.O. Schmidt and F.G. Worden (Eds.), *The Neurosciences, Second Study Program*, Rockefeller University Press, New York, pp. 336–49.

MacLean, P.D., and Ploog, D.W. (1962). Cerebral representation of penile erection, *Journal of Neurophysiology*, **25**, 29–55.

Mahendra, B. (1984). *Dementia*, MTP Press, Lancaster.

Makowski, L., Caspar, D.L.D., Phillips, W.C., and Goodenough, D.A. (1977). Gap junction structures, *Journal of Cell Biology*, **74**, 629–45.

Malamudl, D.N. (1975). Organic brain disease mistaken for psychiatric disorder. In D.F. Benson and D. Blumer (Eds.), *Psychiatric Aspects of Neurologic Disease*, Vol II, Grune & Stratton, New York, pp. 287–305.

Maletsky, B.M. (1978). Seizure duration and clinical effect in ECT, *Comprehensive Psychiatry*, **19**, 541–50.

Malitz, S., and Sackheim, H.A. (Eds.), (1986). *Electroconvulsive Therapy*, Annals of the New York Academy of Sciences, New York, p. 462.

Mann, A.H. (1973). Cortical atrophy and air encephalography: a clinical and radiological study, *Psychological Medicine*, **3**, 374–8.

Mann, D.M.A., Lincoln, J., Yates, P.O., Stamp, J.E., and Toper, S. (1980). Changes in monoamine containing neurones of the human CNS in senile dementia, *British Journal of Psychiatry*, **136**, 533–41.

Mann, J. (1979). Altered platelet MAO activity in affective disorders, *Psychological Medicine*, **9**, 729–36.

Mann, J.J., Stanley, M., McBride, A., and McEwan, B.S. (1986). Increased serotonin-2 and beta adrenergic receptor binding in the frontal cortices of suicidal victims, *Archives of General Psychiatry*, **43**, 954–9.

Mann, M.D. (1981). *The Nervous System and Behaviour*, Harper & Row, Philadelphia.

Manschreck, T.C., and Ames, D. (1984). Neurological features and psychopathology in schizophrenic disorders, *Biological Psychiatry*, **19**, 703–19.

Manschreck, T.C., Maher, B.A., Rucklos, M.E., and Vereen, D.R. (1982). Disturbed voluntary motor activity in schizophrenic disorder, *Psychological Medicine*, **12**, 73–84.

Marcus, J., Hans, S.L., Mednick, S.A., Schulsinger, F., and Michelsen, N. (1985). Neurological dysfunctioning in offspring of schizophrenics in Isreal and Denmark, *Archives of General Psychiatry*, **42**, 753–61.

Marsden, C.D., and Harrison, M.J.G. (1972). Outcome of investigation of patients with presenile dementia, *British Medical Journal*, **ii**, 249–52.

Masters, C.L., Harris, J.O., Gajdusek, D.C., Gibbs, C.J., Bernoulli, C., and Asher, D.M. (1979). Creutzfeld–Jakob disease: patterns of worldwide occurrence and significance of familial and sporadic clustering, *Annals of Neurology*, **5**, 177–88.

Mathew, R.J., Ho, B.T., Kralik, P., *et al.* (1980a). COMT and catecholamines in anxiety and relaxation, *Psychiatry Research*, **3**, 85–91.

Mathew, R.J., Meyer, J.S., Semchuk, K.M., Francis, D.J., Mortel, K., and Claghorn, J.L. (1980b). CBF in depression, *Lancet*, **i**, 1308.

Mathew, R.J., Duncan, G.D., Weinman, M.L., Barr, P.H., and Barr, D.L. (1982a). rCBF in schizophrenia, *Archives of General Psychiatry*, **39**, 1121–24.

Mathew, R.J., Ho, B.T., Khan, M.M., Perale, S.C., Weinman, M.L., and Claghorn, J.L. (1982b). True and pseudo-cholinesterases in depression, *American Journal of Psychiatry*, **139**, 125–7.

Mathew, R.J., Partain, C.L., Prakash, R., Kalkarni, M.V., Logan, T.P., and Wilson, W.H. (1985). A study of the septum pellucidum and corpus callosum in schizophrenia with MRI, *Acta Psychiatrica Scandinavica*, **72**, 414–21.

Maudsley, H. (1868). *The Physiology and Pathology of Mind*, 2nd edition, Macmillan and Co., London.

Maudsley, H. (1870). *Body and Mind*, Macmillan and Co., London.

Mayeux, R., Stern, Y., Cote, L., and Williams, J.B.W. (1984). Altered serotonin metabolism in depressed patients with Parkinson's disease, *Neurology,* **34**, 642–6.

Mazière, B., Comar, D., and Mazière, M. (1986). Pharmacokinetic studies using PET. In M.R. Trimble (Ed.), *New Brain Imaging Techniques and Psychopharmacology,* Oxford University Press, Oxford, pp. 63–76.

Meador-Woodruff, J.H., Grunhaus, L., Haskett, R.F., and Greden, J.F. (1986). Post-dexamethasone cortisol levels in major depressive disorder, *Society of Biological Psychiatry Abstracts,* No. 177, Washington, 7–11 May, 1986.

Melamed, E., Lavy, S., Siew, F., Bentin, S., and Cooper, G. (1978). Correlation between rCBF and brain atrophy in dementia, *Journal of Neurology, Neurosurgery and Psychiatry,* **41**, 894–9.

Meldrum, B.S. (1976). Neuropathology and pathophysiology. In J. Laidlaw and A. Richens (Eds.), *A Textbook of Epilepsy,* Churchill Livingstone, Edinburgh, pp. 314–54.

Meltzer, H.Y., and Fang, V.S. (1983). Cortisol determination and the DST, *Archives of General Psychiatry,* **40**, 501–5.

Meltzer, H.Y., Ross–Stanton, J., and Schlessinger, S. (1980). Mean serum creatine kinase activity in patients with functional psychoses, *Archives of General Psychiatry,* **37**, 650–5.

Meltzer, H.Y., Arora, R.C., Baber, R., and Tricou, B.J. (1981). Serotonin uptake in blood platelets of psychiatric patients, *Archives of General Psychiatry,* **38**, 1322–6.

Meltzer, H.Y., Kolakowska, T., Fang, V.S., *et al.* (1984). Growth hormone and prolactin response to apomorphine in schizophrenia and the major affective disorder, *Archives of General Psychiatry,* **41**, 512–9.

Mendlewicz, J., and Rainer, J.D. (1977). Adoption-studies supporting genetic transmission in manic depressive illness, *Nature,* **268**, 327–9.

Mendlewicz, J., and Youdim, M.B.H. (1983). L-deprenil — a selective MAOB inhibitor, in the treatment of depression: a double-blind evaluation, *British Journal Psychiatry,* **142**, 508–11.

Mendlewicz, J., Linkowski, P., and Wilmotte, J. (1980). Linkage between glucose-6-phosphate dehydrogenase deficiency and manic depressive psychosis, *British Journal of Psychiatry,* **137**, 337–42.

Mendlewicz, J., Charles, G., and Franckson, J.M. (1982). The dexamethasone suppression test in affective disorders: relationship to clinical and genetic subgroups, *British Journal of Psychiatry*, **141**, 464–70.

Mendlewicz, J., Kerkhofs, M., Hoffmann, G., and Linkowski, P. (1984). DST and REM sleep in patients with major depressive disorder, *British Journal of Psychiatry*, **145**, 383–8.

Merskey, H., and Buhrich, N.A. (1975). Hysteria and organic brain disease, *British Journal of Medical Psychology*, **48**, 359–66.

Merskey, H., and Trimble, M.R. (1979). Personality, sexual adjustment and brain lesions in patients with conversion symptoms, *American Journal of Psychiatry*, **136**, 179–82.

Meyer, M.K., Shea, A., Hendrie, H.C., and Yoshimura, N.N. (1981). Plasma tryptophan and five other amino acids in depressed and normal subjects, *Archives of General Psychiatry*, **38**, 642–6.

Mialet, J.P., and Pichot, P. (1981). Eye tracking patterns in schizophrenia, *Archives of General Psychiatry*, **38**, 183–6.

Mindham, R.H.S., Marsden, C.D., and Parkes, J.D. (1976). Psychiatric symptoms during L-dopa therapy for Parkinson's disease and their relationship to physical disability, *Psychological Medicine*, **6**, 23–33

Mindham, R.H.S., Steele, C., Folstein, M.F., and Lucas, J. (1985). A comparison of the frequency of major affective disorder in Huntington's disease and Alzheimer's disease, *Journal of Neurology, Neurosurgery and Psychiatry*, **48**, 1172–74.

Mitchell-Heggs, N., Kelly, D., Richardson, A. (1976). Stereotactic limbic leucotomy: a follow up at 16 months, *British Journal of Psychiatry*, **128**, 226–40.

Modai, I., Apter, A., Golomb, A.M., and Wijsenbeek, H. (1979). Response to amitriptyline and urinary MHPG in bipolar depressed patients, *Neuropsychobiology*, **5**, 181–4.

Mogenson, G.J., Jones, D.L., and Yim, C.Y. (1980). From motivation to action: functional interface between the limbic system and the motor system, *Progress in Neurobiology*, **14**, 69–97.

Møller, S.E., Kirk, L., and Honoré, P. (1979). Free and total plasma tryptophan in endogenous depression, *Journal of Affective Disorders*, **1**, 69–76.

Money, J. (1975). Human behavioural cytogenetics: review of psychopathology in three syndromes — 47XXY: 47XYY and 45X, *The Journal of Sex Research*, **11**, 181–200.

Moniz, E. (1936). *Tentatives Operatroires dans le Traitment de Certaines Psychoses*, Masson, Paris.

Monroe, R. (1970). *Episodic Behaviour Disorders*, Harvard Press, Harvard.

Montigny, C.De, and Blier, P. (1985). Electrophysiological aspects of serotonin neuropharmacology. In A.R. Green (Ed.), *Neuropharmacology of Serotonin*, Oxford University Press, Oxford, pp. 181–92.

Morihisa, J.M., Duffy, F.H., and Wyatt, R.J. (1983). BEAM in schizophrenic patients, *Archives of General Psychiatry*, **40**, 719–28.

Morselli, P.L., Bossi, L., Henry, J.F., Zarifian, E., and Bartholini, G. (1980). On the therapeutic action of SL76002, a new GABA–mimetic agent, *Brain Research Bulletin*, **5** (Suppl. 2), 411–15.

Morstyn, R., Duffy, F.H., and McCarley, R.W. (1983). Altered P300 topography in schizophrenia, *Archives of General Psychiatry*, **40**, 729–34.

Mueller, P.S., Heninger, G.R., and MacDonald, R. (1969). Insulin tolerance test in depression, *Archives of General Psychiatry*, **21**, 587.

Munro, J.G., Hardiker, T.M., and Leonhard, D.P. (1984). The dexamethasone suppression test in residual schizophrenia with depression, *American Journal of Psychiatry*, **141**, 250–2.

Murphy, D.L., Brodie, H.K.H., Goodwin, F.R., *et al.* (1971). Regular induction of hypomania by L-dopa in bipolar manic depressive patients, *Nature*, **229**, 135–6.

Murphy, D.L., Belmaker, R., and Wyatt, R.J. (1974). Monoamine oxidase in schizophrenia and other behavioural disorders, *Journal of Psychiatric Research*, **11**, 221–47.

Murphy, D.L., Belmaker, R.H., Buchsbaum, M., Martin, N.F., Ciaranello, R., and Wyatt, R.J. (1977). Biogenic amine-related enzymes and personality variables in normals, *Psychological Medicine*, **7**, 149–57.

Murphy, D.L., Cohen, R.M., Siever, L.J., Roy, B., *et al.* (1983). Clinical and laboratory studies with selective MAOI drugs, *Modern Problems in Psychopharmacology*, **19**, 287–303.

Murray, R.M., Clifford, C., Fulker, D.W., and Smith, A. (1981). Does heredity contribute to obsessional traits and symptoms? In

T. Tsuang (Ed.), *Genetic Issues*, Neale Watson Press, New York.

Murray, R.M., Lewis, S.W., and Reveley, A.M. (1985). Towards an aetiological classification of schizophrenia, *Lancet*, **i**, 1023–26.

Myslobodsky, M., Mintz, M., and Tomer, R. (1979). Asymmetric reactivities of the brain and components of hemispheric imbalance. In J. Gruzelier and P. Flor-Henry (Eds.), *Hemisphere Asymmetries of Function in Psychopathology*, Elsevier, North Holland, pp. 125–48.

Naguib, M., and Levy, R. (1982). Prediction of outcome in senile dementia — a CT study, *British Journal of Psychiatry*, **140**, 263–7.

Nahorski, S.P. (1981). Identification and significance of beta adrenoceptor sub-types, *Trends in the Pharmacological Sciences*, **2**, 95–8.

Narabayashi, H. (1971). Stereotactic amygdalotomy for behavioural disorders of epileptic aetiology. In *Excerpta Medica International Congress*, Series No. 274, Excerpta Medica, Amsterdam, pp. 175–84.

Nasrallah, H.A., and Coffman, A. (1985). Computerized tomography in psychiatry, *Psychiatric Annals*, **15**, 239–46.

Nasrallah, H.A., McCalley-Whitters, M., and Jacoby, C.G. (1982a). Cortical atrophy in schizophrenia and mania: a comparative CT study, *Journal of Clinical Psychiatry*, **43**, 439–11.

Nasrallah, H.A., McCalley-Whitters, M., and Jacoby, C.G. (1982b). Cerebral ventricular enlargement in young manic males, *Journal of Affective Disorders*, **4**, 15–19.

Nasrallah, H.A., Olson, S.C., McCalley-Whitters, M., Chapman, S., and Jacoby, C.G. (1986a). Cerebral ventricular enlargement in schizophrenia, *Archives of General Psychiatry*, **43**, 157–9.

Nasrallah, H.A., Andreasen, N.A., Coffman, J.A., *et al.* (1986b). A controlled MRI study of corpus callosum thickness in schizophrenia, *Biological Psychiatry*, **21**, 274–82.

Nauta, W.J.H. (1964). Some efferent connections of the prefrontal cortex in the monkey. In J.M. Warren and K. Akert (Eds.), *The frontal granular cortex and behaviour*, McGraw Hill, New York, pp. 397–407.

Nauta, W.J.H., and Domesick, V.B. (1982). Neural associations of the limbic system. In A. Beckman (Ed.), *The Neural Basis of Behaviour*, Spectrum Inc., New York, pp. 175–206.

Naylor, G.J., McNamee, H.B., and Moody, J.P. (1970). Erythrocyte sodium and potassium in depressive illness, *Journal of Psychosomatic Research*, **14**, 173–7.

Naylor, G.J., Dick, D.A.T., and Dick, E.G. (1976). Erythrocyte membrane cation carrier, relapse rate of manic depressive illness and response to lithium, *Psychological Medicine*, **6**, 257–63.

Naylor, G.J., Smith, A.H.W., Bryce-Smith, D., and Ward, N.I. (1984). Tissue vanadium levels in manic depressive illness, *Psychological Medicine*, **14**, 767–72.

Neal, J.B. (1942). *Encephalitis*, H.K. Lewis, London.

Nesse, R.M., Cameron, O.G., Curtis, G.C., McCann, D.S., and Huber-Smith, M.J. (1984). Noradrenergic function in patients with anxiety, *Archives of General Psychiatry*, **41**, 771–6.

Newmark, M.E., and Penry, J.K. (1980). *Genetics of Epilepsy: A Review*, Raven Press, New York.

Nielsen, H., and Kristensen, O. (1981). Personality correlates of sphenoidal EEG foci in temporal lobe epilepsy, *Acta Neurologica Scandinavica*, **64**, 289–300.

Nieto, D., and Escobar, A. (1972). Major psychoses. In J. Minkler (Ed.), *Pathology of the Nervous System*, Vol. 3, McGraw-Hill, New York, pp. 2654–63.

Ninan, P.T., van Kammen, D.P., Scheinin, M., *et al.* (1984). CSF 5-HIAA levels in suicidal schizophrenic patients, *American Journal of Psychiatry*, **141**, 566–9.

Noyes, R., Clancy, J., Crowe, R., Hoenk, P.R., and Slymen, D.J. (1978). The familial prevalence of anxiety neurosis, *Archives of General Psychiatry*, **35**, 1057–59.

Nyback, H., Walters, J.R., Aghajanian, G.K., *et al.* (1975). Tricyclic antidepressants: effect on the firing rate of noradrenergic neurones, *European Journal of Pharmacology*, **32**, 302–12.

Nyirö, J., and Jablonsky, A. (1929). Einige daten zur Prognose der Epilepsie: mit besondere Rücksicht auf die Konstitution, *Psychiatrische Neurologische Wochenschrift*, **31**, 547–9.

O'Keefe, J., and Nadel, L. (1978). *The Hippocampus as a Cognitive Map*, Oxford University Press, Oxford.

Olajide, D., and Lader, M. (1984). Depression following withdrawal from long-term benzodiazepine use: a report of four cases, *Psychological Medicine*, **14**, 937–40.

Oldendorf, W.H. (1980). *The Quest for an Image of the Brain*, Raven Press, New York.

Olds, J., and Milner, P. (1954). Positive reinforcement produced by electrical stimulation of septal area and other regions of rat

451

brain, *Journal of Comparative and Physiological Psychology*, **47**, 419–27.

Oon, M.C.H., Murray, R.M., Brockington, I.F., Rodnight, R., and Birley, J.L.T. (1975). Urinary DMT in psychiatric patients, *Lancet*, **ii**, 1146–7.

Oppenheimer, D.R. (1968). Microscopic lesions in the brain following head injury, *Journal of Neurology, Neurosurgery and Psychiatry*, **31**, 299–306.

Oreland, L., von Knorring, L., von Knorring, A.L., and Bohman, M. (1984). Studies on the connection between alcoholism and low platelet MAO. In S. Parvez *et al.* (Eds.), *Alcohol, Nutrition and the Nervous System*, International Science Press, Utrecht.

Ottosson, J.O. (1960). Experimental studies in the mode of action of ECT, *Acta Pychiatrica Scandinavica*, **35**, Suppl. 135, 1–141.

Ounsted, C., and Lindsay, J. (1981). The long-term outcome of temporal lobe epilepsy in childhood. In E.H. Reynolds and M.R. Trimble (Eds.), *Epilepsy and Psychiatry*, Churchill Livingstone, Edinburgh, pp. 185–215.

Owen, F., Crow, T.J., Poulter, M., Cross, A.J., Longden, A., and Riley, G.J. (1978). Increased dopamine-receptor sensitivity in schizophrenia, *Lancet*, **ii**, 223–5.

Owen, F., Bourne, R.C., Crow, T.J., Fadhli, A.A., and Johnstone, E.C. (1981). Platelet MAO in acute schizophrenia: relationship to symptomatology and neuroleptic medication, *British Journal of Psychiatry*, **139**, 16–22.

Owen, F., Bourne, R.C., Poulter, M., Crow, T.J., Paterson, S.J., and Kosterlitz, H.W. (1985a). Tritated etorphine and naloxone binding to opiod receptors in caudate nucleus in schizophrenia, *British Journal of Psychiatry*, **146**, 507–9.

Owens, D.G.C., Johnstone, E.C., Bydder, G.M., and Kreel, L. (1980). Unsuspected organic disease in chronic schizophrenia demonstrated by computed tomography, *Journal of Neurology, Neurosurgery and Psychiatry*, **43**, 1065–9.

Owens, D.G.C., Johnstone, E.C., Crow, T.J., Frith, C.D., Jagoe, J.R., and Kreel, L. (1985b). Lateral ventricular size in schizophrenia: relationship to the disease process and its clinical manifestations, *Psychological Medicine*, **15**, 27–41.

Palmer, A., Sims, N.A., Bowen, D.M., Neary, D., *et al.* (1984). Monoamine metabolite concentrations in lumbar CSF of patients with histologically verified Alzheimer's disease, *Journal of Neurology, Neurosurgery and Psychiatry*, **47**, 481–4.

Pandurangi, A.K., Dewan, M.J., Lee, H., et al. (1984). The ventricular system in chronic schizophrenic patients, British Journal of Psychiatry, **144**, 172–6.

Pandurangi, A.K., Dewan, M.J., Boucher, M., et al. (1986). A comprehensive study of chronic schizophrenic patients, Acta Psychiatrica Scandanavica, **73**, 161–71.

Pandy, G.N., Dysken, M.W., Garter, D.L., and Davis, J.M. (1979). Beta adrenergic receptor function in affective illness, American Journal of Psychiatry, **136**, 675–8.

Papez, J.W. (1937). A proposed mechanism of emotion, Archives of Neurology and Psychiatry, **38**, 725–33.

Pare, C.M.B. (1985). The present state of MAOI, British Journal of Psychiatry, **146**, 576–84.

Pare, C.M.B., Hallestrom, C., Kline, N., and Cooper, T.B. (1982). Will amitriptyline prevent the 'cheese' reaction of mono-amine–oxidase inhibitors, Lancet, **ii**, 183–6.

Parnas, J., Mednick, S.A., and Moffitt, T.E. (1981). Perinatal complications and adult schizophrenia, Trends in Neurosciences, **4**, 262–4.

Parnavelas, J.G. (1984). Transmitters and neuronal types in the visual cortex. In The Cerebral Cortex, Brain Research Association Abstracts, Cardiff, June 1984.

Paul, M.I., Cramer, H., and Bunney, W.E. (1971a). Urinary adenosine 3,5 monophosphate in the switch process from depression to mania, Science, **171**, 300–5.

Paul, M.I., Cramer, H., and Goodwin, F.K. (1971b). Urinary cyclic AMP excretion in depression and mania, Archives of General Psychiatry, **24**, 327–33.

Paykel, E.S. (1974). Life stress and psychiatric disorder. In B.S. Dohrenwend and B.P. Dohrenwend (Eds.), Stressful Life Events: Their Nature and Effects, John Wiley and Sons, Chichester, pp. 135–49.

Paykel, E.S., and Hollyman, J.A. (1984). Life events and depression — a psychiatric view, Trends in Neurosciences, **7**, 475–80.

Paykel, E.S., Klerman, G.L., and Prusoff, B.A. (1976). Personality and symptom pattern in depression, British Journal of Psychiatry, **129**, 327–34.

Pearce, J., and Miller, E. (1973). Clinical Aspects of Dementia, Baillière Tindall, London.

Pearlson, G.D., and Verloff, A.E. (1981). CT scan changes in manic-depressive illness, Lancet, **ii**, 470.

Peet, M., Middlemiss, D.N., and Yates, R.A. (1981). Propranolol in schizophrenia, *British Journal of Psychiatry*, **138**, 112–17.

Perez, M.M., and Trimble, M.R. (1980). Epileptic psychosis — diagnostic comparison with process schizophrenia, *British Journal of Psychiatry*, **137**, 245–9.

Perez, M.M., Trimble, M.R., Reider, I., and Murray, N. (1984). Epileptic psychosis, a further evaluation of PSE profiles, *British Journal of Psychiatry*, **146**, 155–63.

Perris, C. (1974). A study of cycloid psychosis, *Acta Psychiatrica Scandinavica*, **1974**, Suppl. 253

Perris, H., von Knorring, L., Oreland, L., and Perris, C. (1984). Life events and biological vulnerability, *Psychiatry Research*, **12**, 111–20.

Perry, E.K., and Perry, R.H. (1980). The cholinergic system in Alzheimer's disease. In P.J. Roberts (Ed.), *Biochemistry of Dementia*, John Wiley and Sons, Chichester, pp. 135–83.

Perry, E.K., and Perry, R.H. (1982). Neurotransmitter and neuropeptide systems in Alzheimer-type dementia. In S. Hoyer (Ed.), *The Ageing Brain*, Springer-Verlag, Berlin.

Perry, E.K., Marshall, E.F., Blessed, G., Tomlinson, B.E., and Perry, R.H. (1983). Decreased imipramine binding in the brains of patients with depressive illness, *British Journal of Psychiatry*, **142**, 188–92.

Phelps, M.E., and Mazziotta, J.C. (1983). Human sensory stimulation and deprivation as demonstrated by PET. In W.D. Heiss and M.E. Phelps (Eds.), *Positron Emission Tomography of the Brain*, Springer-Verlag, Berlin, pp. 139–52.

Pichot, P. (1983). *A Century of Psychiatry*, Roger Da Costa, Paris.

Pickar, D., Labarca, R., Linnoila, M., *et al.* (1984). Neuroleptic induced decrease in plasma HVA and antipsychotic activity in schizophrenic patients, *Science*, **225**, 954–6.

Pisani, F., Narbone, M.C., Fazio, A., *et al.* (1984). Increased serum carbamazepine levels by viloxazine in epileptic patients, *Epilepsia*, **25**, 482–3.

Pitts, F., and McClure, J.N. (1967). Lactate metabolism in anxiety neurosis, *New England Journal of Medicine*, **227**, 1329–36.

Pollin, W., Allen, M.G., Hoffer, A., Stabenall, J.R., and Hrubec, Z. (1969). Psychopathology in 15,909 pairs of veteran twins, *American Journal of Psychiatry*, **126**, 597–610.

Pond, D. (1957). Psychiatric aspects of epilepsy, *Journal of the Indian Medical Profession*, **3**, 1441–51.

Pond, D.A., and Bidwell, B.H. (1959). A survey of epilepsy in 14 general practices, *Epilepsia*, **1**, 285–99.

Post, R.M., and Goodwin, F.K. (1975). Time dependent effects of phenothiazines on dopamine turnover in psychiatric patients, *Science*, **190**, 488–9.

Post, R.M., and Goodwin, F.K. (1978). Approaches to brain amines in psychiatric patients, *Handbook of Psychopharmacology*, **13**, 147–85.

Post, R.M., and Uhde, T.W. (1986). Anticonvulsants in non-epileptic psychosis. In M.R. Trimble and T.G. Bolwig (Eds.), *Aspects of Epilepsy and Psychiatry*, John Wiley and Sons, Chichester, pp. 177–212.

Post, R.M., Gordon, E.K., Goodwin, F.K., and Bunney, W.E. (1973). Central norepinephrine metabolism in affective illness: MHPG in the CSF, *Science*, **179**, 1002–3.

Post, R.M., Fink, E.D., Carpenter, W.T., and Goodwin, F.K. (1975). Cerebrospinal fluid amine metabolites in acute schizophrenia, *Archives of General Psychiatry*, **32**, 1063–9.

Post, R.M., Jimerson, D.C., Ballenger, J.C., Lake, R., Wade, T.W., and Goodwin, F.K. (1985). CSF norepinephrine and its metabolites in manic depressive illness. In R.M. Post and J.C. Ballenger (Eds.), *Neurobiology of Mood Disorders*, Williams and Wilkins, Baltimore, pp. 539–51.

Post, R.M., Rubinow, D.R., Uhde, T.W., Ballenger, J.C., and Linnolla, M. (1986). Dopaminergic effects of carbamazepine, *Archives of General Psychiatry*, **43**, 392–6.

Prange, A., Wilson, I., Lynn, C.W., *et al.* (1974). L-tryptophan in mania: contribution to a permissive hypothesis of affective disorder, *Archives of General Psychiatry*, **30**, 52–62.

Prange, A.J., Loosen, P.T., Wilson, I.C., Meltzer, H.Y., and Fang, V.S. (1979). Behavioural and endocrine responses of schizophrenic patients to TRH, *Archives of General Psychiatry*, **36**, 1086–93.

Price, J. (1968). The genetics of depressive disorder. In A. Coppen and A. Walk (Eds.), *British Journal of Psychiatry Special Publication*, No. 2, pp. 37–54.

Price, J.L. (1981). The efferent projections of the amygdaloid complex in the rat, cat and monkey. In Y. Ben-Ari (Ed.), *The Amygdaloid Complex*, Elsevier, North Holland, pp. 121–32.

Procci, W.R. (1976). Schizoaffective psychosis: fact or fiction, *Archives of General Psychiatry*, **33**, 1167–78.

Pudenz, R.H., and Sheldon, C.H. (1946). The lucite calvarium — a method for direct observation of the brain, *Journal of Neurosurgery*, **3**, 487–505.

Quitkin, F., Rifkin, A., and Klein, D.F. (1976). Neurological soft signs in schizophrenia and character disorders, *Archives of General Psychiatry*, **33**, 845–53.

Rabkin, J.G., Steward, J., and Klein, D.F. (1985). Overview on the relevance of the DST to differential diagnosis. In R.M.A. Hirschfeld (Ed.), *Clinical Utility of the Dexamethasone Suppression Test*, NIH, Maryland, pp. 12–33.

Racine, R.J., and McIntyre, D. (1986). Mechanisms of kindling. In B. Doane and K.E. Livingston (Eds.), *The Limbic System: Functional Organisation and Clinical Disorders*, Raven Press, New York, pp. 109–21.

Randrup, A., Munkvad, I., Fog, R., Gerlach, J., *et al.* (1975). Mania, depression and brain dopamine. In L. Valzelli (Ed)., *Current Development in Psychopharmacology*, Spectrum Publications, New York, Vol. 2, pp. 207–48.

Rangel Guerra, R.A., Perez-Payan, H., Minkoff, L., and Todd, L.E. (1983). NMR in bipolar affective disorders, *American Journal of Neuroradiology*, **4**, 229–32.

Rao, V.A.R., Bishop, M., and Coppen, A. (1980). Clinical state, plasma levels of haloperidol and prolactin: a correlation study in chronic schizophrenia, *British Journal of Psychiatry*, **137**, 518–21.

Rapopport, S.R., and Webb, W.B. (1950). An attempt to study intellectual deterioration by premorbid and psychotic testing, *Journal of Consulting Psychology*, **14**, 95–8.

Rasmussen, S.A. (1984). Lithium and tryptophan augmentation on clomipramine resistant obsessive compulsive disorder, *American Journal of Psychiatry*, **141**, 1283–5.

Reiman, E.M., Raicle, M.E., Butler, F.K., Herscovitch, P., and Robins, E. (1984). A focal brain abnormality in panic disorder, *Nature*, **310**, 683–5.

Reisine, T.D., Rossor, M., Spokes, E., *et al.* (1980). Opiate and neuroleptic receptor alterations in human schizophrenic brain tissue. In G. Pepeu, M.J. Kumar and S.J. Enna (Eds.), *Receptors for Neurotransmitters and Peptide Hormones*, Raven Press, New York, pp. 443–50.

Reveley, A.M., and Reveley, M.A. (1983). Aqueduct stenosis and schizophrenia, *Journal of Neurology, Neurosurgery and Psychiatry*, **46**, 18–22.

Reveley, M.A., and Reveley, A.M. (1986). Left cerebral hemisphere hypodensity in schizophrenia, 3rd International Symposium on *Cerebral Dynamics Laterality and Psychopathology*, Abstract VI–Z, Hakone, Japan.

Reveley, M.A., Glover, V., Sandler, M., and Coppen, A. (1981). Increased platelet MAO activity in affective disorders, *Psychopharmacology*, **73**, 257–60.

Reveley, A.M., Reveley, M.A., Clifford, C.A., and Murray, R.M. (1982). Cerebral ventricular size in twins discordant for schizophrenia, *Lancet*, **i**, 540–1.

Reveley, M.A., Reveley, A.M., Clifford, C.A., and Murray, R.M. (1983). Genetics of platelet MAO activity in disconcordant schizophrenic and normal twins, *British Journal of Psychiatry*, **142**, 560–5.

Reynolds, E.H. (1975). Chronic antiepileptic toxicity: a review, *Epilepsia*, **16**, 319–52.

Reynolds, E.H. (1976). Neurological aspects of folate and vitamin B12 metabolism, *Clinics in Haematology*, **5**, 661–96.

Reynolds, E.H. (1981). Biological factors in psychological disorders associated with epilepsy. In E.H. Reynolds and M.R. Trimble (Eds.), *Epilepsy and Psychiatry*, Churchill Livingstone, Edinburgh, pp. 264–90.

Reynolds, E.H. (1986). Antiepileptic drugs and personality. In M.R. Trimble and T. Bolwig (Eds.), *Aspects of Epilepsy and Psychiatry*, John Wiley, New York, pp. 89–98.

Reynolds, E.H., and Stramentinoli, G. (1983). Folic acid, SAM and affective disorder, *Psychological Medicine*, **13**, 705–10.

Reynolds, E.H., Carney, M.W.P., and Toone, B.K. (1984). Methylation and mood, *Lancet*, **iii**, 196–7.

Reynolds, G.P. (1983). Increased concentrations and lateral asymmetry of amygdala dopamine in schizophrenia, *Nature*, **305**, 527–9.

Reynolds, G.P., Riederer, P., Jellinger, K., and Gabriel, E. (1981). Dopamine receptors and schizophrenia: the neuroleptic drug problem, *Neuropharmacology*, **20**, 1319–20.

Richelson, E. (1986). The newer antidepressants: structures, pharmacokinetics, pharmacodynamics and proposed mechanism of action, *Psychopharmacology Bulletin*, **20**, 313–23.

Richens, A. (1976). *Drug Treatment of Epilepsy*, Henry Kimpton, London.

Rickles, W.H. (1969). UCLA conference: clinical neurophysiology, *Annals of Internal Medicine*, **71**, 619–45.

Riding, B.E.J., and Munroe, A. (1975). Pimozide in mono-symptomatic psychosis. Lancet, **ii**, 400–1.

Rieder, R.O., Mann, L.S., Weinberger, D.R., van Kammen, D.P., and Post, R.M. (1983). CT scans in patients with schizophrenia, schizo-affective and bipolar affective disorder, *Archives of General Psychiatry,* **40**, 735–9.

Riese, W. (1953). *The Conception of Disease,* Philosophical Library, New York.

Riese, W. (1954). Hughlings Jackson's doctrine of consciousness: sources, versions and elaborations, *Journal of Nervous and Mental Diseases,* **120**, 330–7.

Riese, W. (1959). *A History of Neurology,* M.D. Publications, New York.

Riley, G.J., and Shaw, D.M. (1976). Total and non-bound tryptophan in unipolar illness, *Lancet,* **ii**, 1249.

Rimon, R., Roos, B-E., Rakkolainen, V., and Alanen, Y. (1971). The content of 5-HIAA and HVA in the CSF of patients with acute schizophrenia, *Journal of Psychosomatic Research,* **15**, 375–8.

Rimon, R., Liira, J., Kampman, R., and Hyyppa, M. (1981). Prolactin levels in CSF of patients with chronic schizophrenia, *Neuropsychobiology,* **7**, 87–93.

Roberts, G.W., Polak, J.M., and Crow, T.J. (1984). Peptide circuitry of the limbic system. In M.R. Trimble and E. Zarifian (Eds.), *Psychopharmacology of the Limbic System,* Oxford University Press, Oxford, pp 226–43.

Roberts,G.W., Colter, N., Lofthouse, R., Brown, R., and Crow, T.J. (1985). Is there gliosis in the brain of schizophrenics? IV, *World Congress of Biological Psychiatry Abstracts,* p. 6, No. 105–2.

Roberts, J.K.A. (1984). *Differential Diagnosis in Neuropsychiatry,* John Wiley and Sons, Chichester.

Roberts, J.K.A., and Lishman, W.A. (1984). The use of the CAT brain scanner in clinical psychiatry, *British Journal of Psychiatry,* **145**, 152–8.

Roberts, M.A., and Caird, F.I. (1976). Computerized tomography and intellectual impairment in the elderly, *Journal of Neurology, Neurosurgery and Psychiatry,* **39**, 986–9.

Robertson, G., and Taylor, P. (1985). Some cognitive correlates of schizophrenic illnesses, *Psychological Medicine,* **15**, 81–98.

Robertson, M.M. (1986). Ictal and interictal depression in patients with epilepsy. In M.R. Trimble and T. Bolwig (Eds.), *Aspects of*

458

Epilepsy and Psychiatry, John Wiley and Sons, Chichester, pp. 211–32.

Robertson, M.M., and Trimble, M.R. (1982). Major tranquillisers as antidepressants, *Journal of Affective Disorders*, **4**, 173–93.

Robertson, M.M., and Trimble, M.R. (1983). Depressive illness in patients with epilepsy: a review, *Epilepsia*, **24**, Suppl. 2, S109–S116.

Robins, A.H. (1976). Depression in patients with Parkinsonism, *British Journal of Psychiatry*, **128**, 141–5.

Robinson, R.G., and Szetela, B. (1981). Mood change following left hemisphere brain injury, *Annals of Neurology*, **9**, 447–53.

Robinson, R.G., Starr, L.B., and Price, T.R. (1984). A two year longitudinal study of mood disorders following stroke, *British Journal of Psychiatry*, **144**, 256–62.

Rodin, E., and Schmaltz, S. (1983). Folate levels in epileptic patients. In M. Parsonage *et al.* (Eds.), *Advances in Epileptology: The 14th Epilepsy International Symposium*, Raven Press, New York, pp. 143–53.

Rodin, E.A., and Schmaltz, S. (1984). The Bear–Fedio inventory and temporal lobe epilepsy, *Neurology*, **34**, 591–6.

Rogers, D. (1986). The intellectual disorder of psychiatric illness (Unpublished data).

Ron, M.A., Acker, W., and Lishman, W.A. (1979a). Dementia in chronic alcoholism. In J. Obiols *et al.* (Eds.), *Biological Psychiatry Today*, Elsevier, North Holland, pp. 1446–50.

Ron, M.A., Toone, B.K., Garralda, M.E., and Lishman, W.A. (1979b). Diagnostic accuracy in presenile dementia, *British Journal of Psychiatry*, **134**, 161–8.

Roos, R.P., Davis, K., and Meltzer, H.Y. (1985). Immunoglobulin studies in patients with psychiatric diseases, *Archives of General Psychiatry*, **42**, 124–8.

Rose, F.C., and Symonds, C.P. (1960). Persistent memory defect following encephalitis, *Brain*, **83**, 195–212.

Rosen, J., Silk, K.R., Rice, H.E., and Smith, C.B. (1985). Platelet alpha-2 adrenergic dysfunction in negative symptom schizophrenia, *Biological Psychiatry*, **20**, 539–45.

Rossor, M.N. (1981). Parkinson's disease and Alzheimer's disease as disorders of the isodendritic core, *British Medical Journal*, **283** (ii), 1588–90.

Rossor, M.N., Iversen, L.L., Mountjoy, C.Q., Roth, M., *et al.* (1980). AVP and ChAT in brains of patients with Alzheimer-type senile dementia, *Lancet*, **ii**, 1367–8.

Rossor, M.N., Iversen, L.L., Reynolds, G.P., Mountjoy, C.Q., and Roth, M. (1984). Neurochemical characteristics of early and late onset types of Alzheimer's disease, *British Medical Journal*, **288** (i), 961–4.

Rosvold, H.E., Mirsky, A.F., and Pribram, K.H. (1954). Influence of amygdalectomy on social behaviour in monkeys, *Journal of Comparative and Physiological Psychology*, **47**, 173–80.

Roth, M. (1977). The borderlands of anxiety and depressive states. In H.N. Van Praag and J. Bruinvels (Eds.), *Neurotransmission and Disturbed Behaviour*, Bohn, Scheltema and Holkema, Utrecht, pp. 209–57.

Routtenberg, A. (1979). Participation of brain stimulation reward substrates in memory: anatomical and biochemical evidence, *Federation Proceedings*, **38**, 2446–53.

Roy, A. (1977). Hysterical fits previously diagnosed as epilepsy, *Psychological Medicine*, **7**, 271–3.

Roy, A., Ninan, P., Mazonson, A., *et al.* (1985a). CSF monoamine metabolites in chronic schizophrenic patients who attempt suicide, *Psychological Medicine*, **15**, 335–40.

Roy, A., Pickar, D., Linnoila, M., and Potter, W.Z. (1985b). Plasma norepinephrine levels in affective disorders, *Archives of General Psychiatry*, **42**, 1181–5.

Roy, A., Pickar, D., Douillet, P., Karoum, F., and Linnoila, M. (1986a). Urinary monoamines and monamine metabolites in sub-types of unipolar depressive disorder and normal controls, *Psychological Medicine*, **16**, 541–6.

Roy, A., Pickar, D., Linnoila, M., Doran, A.R., and Paul, S.M. (1986b). CSF monoamine and metabolite levels and the DST in depression, *Archives of General Psychiatry*, **43**, 356–60.

Roy-Byrne, P., Uhde, T.W., Gold, P.W., Rubinow, D., and Post, R.M. (1985a). Neuroendocrine abnormalities in panic disorder, *Psychopharmacology Bulletin*, **21**, 546–50.

Roy-Byrne, P., Bierer, L.M., and Uhde, T.W. (1985b). The DST in panic disorder, *Biological Psychiatry*, **20**, 1237–40.

Rubinow, D.R., Gold, P.W., Post, R.M., Ballenger, J.C., and Cowdry, R.W. (1985). Somatostatin in patients with affective illness and normal volunteers. In R.M. Post and J.C. Ballenger (Eds.), *Neurobiology of Mood Disorders*, Williams and Wilkins, Baltimore, pp. 369–87.

Rudorfer, M.V., Hwu, H., and Clayton P.J. (1982). DST in primary depression: significance of family history and psychosis, *Biological Psychiatry*, **17**, 41–8.

Rush, A.J., Giles, D.E., Roffwarg, H.P., and Parker, C.R. (1982). Sleep EEG and DST findings in out patients with unipolar major depressive disorders, *Biological Psychiatry,* **17**, 327–41.

Rutter, M., Graham, P., and Yule, W. (1970). A neuropsychiatric study in childhood, *In Clinics in Developmental Medicine,* Vol.35, Heinemann, London.

Rydin, E., Schalling, D., and Åsberg, M. (1982). Rorschach rating in depressed and suicidal patients with low levels of 5-HIAA in CSF, *Psychiatry Research,* **7**, 229–43.

Sabelli, H.C., Fawcett, J., Gusovsky, F., Javaid, J., Edwards, J. and Jeffries, H. (1983). Urinary phenyl acetate: a diagnostic test for depression, *Science,* **220**, 1187–88.

Sachar, E.J., Hellman, L., Roffwarg, H., *et al.* (1973). Disrupted 24 hour patterns of cortisol secretion in psychotic depression, *Archives of General Psychiatry,* **28**, 19–24.

Sacks, O. (1973). *Awakenings,* Duckworth, London.

St Clair, D.M., Blackwood, D.H.R., and Christie, J.E. (1985). P3 and other long latency auditory evoked potentials in presenile dementia, Alzheimer-type and the alcoholic Korsakoff syndrome, *British Journal of Psychiatry,* **147**, 702–6.

Saleem, P.T. (1984). Dexamethasone Suppression Test in depressive illness: its relation to anxiety symptoms, *British Journal of Psychiatry,* **144**, 181–4.

Saletu, B. (1982). Pharmaco-EEG profile of typical and atypical antidepressants. In E. Costa and G. Racagni (Eds.), *Typical and Atypical Antidepressants: Clinical Practice,* Raven Press, New York, pp. 257–68.

Saletu, B., Grunberger, J., and Rajna, P. (1983). Pharmaco-EEG profiles with antidepressants, *British Journal of Clinical Pharmacology,* **15**, 369S–384S.

Sandler, M. (1983). Benzodiazepines: studies on a possible endogenous ligand. In M.R. Trimble (Ed.), *Benzodiazepines Divided,* John Wiley and Sons, Chichester, pp. 139–47.

Sandler, M., Bonham Carter, S., Cuthbert, M.F., and Pare, C.M.B. (1975). Is there an increase in monoamine oxidase activity in depressive illness?, *Lancet,* **i**, 1045–8.

Sandler, M., Ruthven, C.R., Goodwin, B.L., Field, H., and Matthews, R. (1978). Phenylethylamine overproduction in aggressive psychopaths, *Lancet,* **ii**, 1269–70.

Sargant, W., and Slater, E. (1944). *An Introduction to Physical Methods of Treatment in Psychiatry,* Livingstone, Edinburgh.

Sawyer, C.H. (1957). Triggering of the pituitary by the CNS. In P. Bullock (Ed.), *Physiological Triggers*, Waverly Press, Baltimore, pp. 164–74.

Scatton, B. and Zivkovic, B. (1984). Neuroleptics and the limbic system. In M.R. Trimble and E. Zarifian (Eds.), *Psychopharmacology of the Limbic System*, Oxford University Press, Oxford, pp. 174–97.

Schatzberg, A.F., Rothschild, A.J., Gershon, B., Lerbinger, J.E., and Schildkraut, J.J. (1985). Toward a biochemical classification of depressive disorders, *British Journal of Psychiatry*, **146**, 633–7.

Scher, M., Krieger, J.N., and Juergens, S. (1983). Trazadone and priapism, *American Journal of Psychiatry*, **140**, 1362–3.

Schildkraut, J.J., and Kety, S.S. (1967). Biogenic amines and emotion, *Science*, **156**, 21–30.

Schildkraut, J.J., Orsulak, P.J., Schatzberg, A.F., and Rosenbaum, A.H. (1984). Urinary MHPG in affective disorders. In R.M. Post and J.C. Ballenger (Eds.), *Neurobiology of Mood Disorders*, Williams & Wilkins, Baltimore, pp. 519–628.

Schneider, K. (1957). Primary and secondary symptoms in schizophrenia. In S.R. Hirsch and M. Shepherd (Eds.), *Themes and Variations in European Psychiatry*, John Wright, Bristol (1974), pp. 40–6.

Schneider, K. (1959). *Clinical Psychopathology* (Translated by M.W. Hamilton and E.W. Anderson), Grune & Stratton, New York.

Schooler, C., Zahn, T.P., Murphy, D.I., and Buchsbaum, M.S. (1978). Psychological correlates of monoamine oxidase activity in normals, *Journal of Nervous and Mental Disease*, **166**, 177–86.

Schriner, L., and Kling, A. (1956). Rhinencephalon and behaviour, *American Journal of Physiology*, **184**, 486–90.

Schulz, S.C., Koller, M.M., Kishore, P.R., Hamer, R.M., Gehl, J.J., and Friedel, R.O. (1983). Ventricular enlargement in teenage patients with schizophrenia spectrum disorders, *American Journal of Psychiatry*, **140**, 1592–5.

Schwartz, J.H. (1981). Chemical basis of synaptic transmission. In E.R. Kandel and J.H. Schwartz (Eds.), *Principles of Neural Science*, Elsevier, North Holland, pp. 106–20.

Schwartz, M.F., Bauman, J.E., and Masters, W.H. (1982). Hyperprolactinaemia and sexual disorders in men, *Biological Psychiatry*, **17**, 861–76.

462

Sedvall, G.C., and Wode-Helgodt, B. (1980). Aberrant mono-amine metabolite in CSF and family history of schizophrenia, *Archives of General Psychiatry*, **37**, 1113–6.

Serafetinides, E.A. (1965). Aggressiveness in TLE, and its relation to cerebral dysfunction and environmental factors, *Epilepsia*, **6**, 33–42.

Shagass, C. (1972). *Evoked Brain Potentials in Psychiatry*, Plenum Press, New York.

Shagass, C., Roemer, R.A., Straumanis, J.J., and Amadeo, M. (1979). Evoked potential evidence of lateralised hemispheric dysfunction in the psychoses. In J. Gruzelier and P. Flor-Henry (Eds.), *Hemisphere Asymmetries of Function in Psychopathology*, Elsevier, North Holland, pp. 293–316.

Shagass, C., Roemer, R.A., Straumanis, J.J., and Josiassen, R.C. (1981). Differentiation of depressive and schizophrenic psychoses by evoked potentials, *Advances in Biological Psychiatry*, **6**, 173–9.

Shagass, C., Roemer, R.A., Straumanis, J.J., and Josiassen, R.C. (1984). Distinctive somatosensory evoked potential features in obsessive–compulsive disorder, *Biological Psychiatry*, **19**, 1507–24.

Shaw, D.M., Camps, F.E., and Eccleston, E.G. (1967). 5-Hydroxytryptamine in the hind-brains of depressive suicides, *British Journal of Psychiatry*, **113**, 1407–11.

Shaw, D.M., Tidmarsh, S.F., Johnson, A.L., *et al.* (1978). Multi-compartmental analysis of amino acids. ii. Tryptophan in affective disorders, *Psychological Medicine*, **8**, 487–94.

Shaw, D.M., Kellam, A.M.P., and Mottram, R.F. (1982). *Brain Sciences in Psychiatry*, Butterworths, London.

Shear, M.K., Devereux, R.B., Kramer-Fox, R., Mann, J., and Frances, A. (1984). Low prevalence of mitral valve prolapse in patients with panic disorder, *American Journal of Psychiatry*, **141**, 302–3.

Sheppard, G., Manchandra, R., Gruzelier, J., Hirsch, S.R., Inse, R., Frackowiak, R., and Jones, T. (1983). O-15 PET scanning in predominantly never-treated acute schizophrenic patients, *Lancet*, **ii**, 1448–52.

Sherman, B., Pfohl, B., and Winokur, G. (1984). Circadian analysis of plasma cortisol levels before and after dexamethasone administration in depression patients, *Archives of General Psychiatry*, **41**, 271–5.

Sherrington, C. (1947). *The Integrative Action of the Nervous System*, Cambridge University Press, Cambridge.

Sherwin, I. (1982). The effect of the location of an epileptogenic lesion on the occurrence of psychosis in epilepsy. In W. Koella and M.R. Trimble (Eds.), *Temporal Lobe Epilepsy, Mania, and Schizophrenia and the Limbic System*, Karger, Basel, pp. 81–97.

Shibasaki, J., Barrett, G., Halliday, E., and Halliday, A.M. (1980). Components of the movement-related cortical potential and their scalp topography, *Electroencephalograpy and Clinical Neurophysiology*, **49**, 213–26.

Shields, J. (1954). Personality differences and neurotic traits in normal twin schoolchildren, *Eugenics Review*, **45**, 213–46.

Shields, J. (1962). *Monozygotic Twins Brought up Apart and Brought up Together*, Oxford University Press, London.

Shopsin, B., Friedman, E., and Gershon, S. (1976). Parachlorophenylalanine reversal of tranylcypramine effects in depressed patients, *Archives of General Psychiatry*, **33**, 811–19.

Shorvon, S.D., and Reynolds, E.H. (1982). Early prognosis of epilepsy, *British Medical Journal*, **ii**, 1699–701.

Shrikhande, S., Hirsch, S.R., Coleman, J.C., Reveley, M.A., and Dayton, R. (1985). Cytomegalovirus and schizophrenia, *British Journal of Psychiatry*, **146**, 503–6.

Siegel, A., Edinger, H., and Dotto, M. (1975). Effects of electrical stimulation of the lateral aspects of the pre-frontal cortex upon attack behaviour in cats, *Brain*, **93**, 473–84.

Siegel, R.E. (1973). *Galen on Psychology, Psychopathology and Function and Diseases of the Nervous System*, Karger, Basel.

Siesjo, B.K. (1978). *Brain Energy Metabolism*, John Wiley and Sons, Chichester.

Siever, L.J., and Coursey, R.D. (1985). Biological markers for schizophrenia and the biological high-risk approach, *Journal of Nervous and Mental Disease*, **173**, 4–16.

Siever, L.J., and Uhde, T.W. (1984). New studies and perspectives on the noradrenergic receptor system in depression: effects of the alpha-2 adrenergic agonist clonidine, *Biological Psychiatry*, **19**, 131–56.

Siever, L.J., Insel, T.R., Jimerson, D.C., Lake, C.R., Uhde, T.W., Aloi, J., and Murphy, D.L. (1983). Growth hormone response to clonidine in obsessive-compulsive patients, *British Journal of Psychiatry*, **142**, 184–7.

Siever, L.J., Kafka, M.S., Targum, S., and Lake, C.R. (1984). Platelet alpha-2 adrenergic binding and biochemical responsiveness in depressed patients and controls, *Psychiatry Research*, **11**, 287–302.

Silfverskiöld, P., Gustafson, L., Ingvar, D.H., and Risberg, J. (1985). RCBF in manic psychosis, Abstracts: XII International Symposium on *CBF and Metabolism*, Lund, June 1985, p. 224.

Silfverskiöld, P., Gustafson, L., Risberg., J., and Rosen, I. (1986). Acute and late effects of ECT. In S. Malitz and H.A. Sackheim (Eds.), *ECT*, Annals of the New York Academy of Sciences, Vol. 462, pp. 236–48.

Sim, M. (1979). Early diagnosis of Alzheimer's disease. In A. Glen and L.J. Whalley (Eds.), *Alzheimer's Disease*, Churchill Livingstone, Edinburgh, pp. 78–85.

Slade, A.P., and Checkley, S.A. (1980). A neuroendocrine study of the mechanism of action of ECT, *British Journal of Psychiatry*, **137**, 217–21.

Slater, E. (1936). The inheritance of manic depressive insanity, *Proceedings of the Royal Society of Medicine*, **29**, 981–90.

Slater, E. (1943). The neurotic constitution, *Journal of Neurology and Psychiatry*, **6**, 1–16.

Slater, E., and Beard, A.W. (1963). The schizophrenia-like psychoses of epilepsy, *British Journal of Psychiatry*, **109**, 95–150.

Slater, E., and Glithero, E. (1965). A follow up of patients diagnosed as suffering from hysteria, *Journal of Psychosomatic Research*, **9**, 9–13.

Slater, E., and Roth, M. (1960). *Clinical Psychiatry*, 1st edition, Ballière Tindall and Cassell, London.

Slater, E., and Roth, M. (1969). *Clinical Psychiatry*, 3rd edition, Baillière Tindall and Cassell, London.

Slater, E., and Slater, P. (1944). A heuristic theory of neurosis, *Journal of Neurology and Psychiatry*, **7**, 49–55.

Small, J.G. (1970). Small sharp spikes in a psychiatric population, *Archives of General Psychiatry*, **22**, 277–84.

Small, J.G., Small, I.F., Milstein, V., and Moore, D.F. (1975). Familial associations with EEG variants in manic depressive disease, *Archives of General Psychiatry*, **32**, 43–8.

Small, J.G., Milstein, V., Klapper, M.H., Kellams, J.J., Miller, M.J., and Small, I.F. (1986). ECT for manic episodes. In S. Malitz and H.A. Sackheim (Eds.), *ECT*, Annals of the New York Academy of Sciences, Vol. 462, pp. 37–49.

Smith, D.A., and Lantos, P.L. (1983). A case of combined Pick's disease and Alzheimer's disease, *Journal of Neurology, Neurosurgery and Psychiatry,* **46**, 675–7.

Smith, J.S., and Kiloh, L.G. (1981). The investigation of dementia, *Lancet,* **i**, 824–7.

Smith, R.G., Baumgartner, R.N., Calderon, M., Ravichandran, G.K., Peters, I.O., and Schoolar, J.C. (1985). *NMR Studies of Schizophrenia,* APA Abstracts, p. 116, No. 66D, Dallas, 1985.

Smythe, G.E., and Stern, K. (1938). Tumours of the thalamus — a clinico pathological study, *Brain,* **61**, 339–74.

Smythies, J.R. (1976). Recent progress in schizophrenia research, *Lancet,* **ii**, 136–9.

Smythies, J.R. (1983). The transmethylation and one-carbon cycle hypothesis of schizophrenia, *Psychological Medicine,* **13**, 711–14.

Snyder, S. (1980). Brain peptides as neurotransmitters, *Science,* **209**, 976–83.

Snyder, S.H., Banerjee, S.P., Yamamura, H.I., and Greenberg, D. (1974). Drugs, neurotransmitters and schizophrenia, *Science,* **184**, 1243–53.

Sokoloff, L.M., Reivich, C., Kennedy, M.H., *et al.* (1977). The 14C deoxyglucose method for the measurement of local cerebral glucose utilisation, *Journal of Neurochemistry,* **28**, 897–916.

Sorensen, B., Kragh-Sorensen, P., Larsen, N.E., *et al.* (1978). The practical significance of nortriptyline plasma control, *Psychopharmacology,* **59**, 35–9.

Sourander, P., and Sjögren, H. (1970). The concept of Alzheimer's disease and its clinical implications. In G. Wolstenholme and M. O'Connor (Eds.), *Ciba Symposium: Alzheimer's Disease and Related Conditions,* Churchill, London, pp. 11–36.

Spar, J.E., and Gerner, R. (1982). Does the DST distinguish dementia from depression?, *American Journal of Psychiatry,* **139**, 238–40.

Spiegel, R., and Aebi, H-J. (1981). *Psychopharmacology: An Introduction,* John Wiley and Sons, Chichester.

Stafford-Clarke, D., and Taylor, F.H. (1949). Clinical and EEG studies of prisoners charged with murder, *Journal of Neurology, Neurosurgery and Psychiatry,* **12**, 325–30.

Standage, K.F., and Fenton, G.W. (1975). Psychiatric symptoms profiles of patients with epilepsy: a controlled investigation, *Psychological Medicine,* **5**, 152–60.

Stanley, M., and Mann, J.J. (1983). Increased serotonin-2 binding sites in frontal cortex of suicide victims, *Lancet*, **i**, 214–16.

Stein, L., and Wise, C.D. (1971). Possible aetiology of schizophrenia: progressive damage to the noradrenergic reward system by 6 OH-dopamine, *Science*, **171**, 1032–6.

Stengel, E. (1949). The borderlands of neurology and psychiatry, *Journal of Mental Science*, **95**, 416–47.

Stephan, H. (1975). Allocortex. In W. Bargmann (Ed.), *Handbuch der mikroskopischer Anatomie der Menschen*, Springer, Berlin.

Stern, R.S., and Cobb, J.P. (1978). Phenomenology of obsessive compulsive neurosis, *British Journal of Psychiatry*, **132**, 233–9.

Sternberg, D.E., Charney, D.S., Heninger, G.R., *et al.* (1982). Impaired presynaptic regulation of NE in schizophrenia, *Archives of General Psychiatry*, **39**, 285–9.

Stevens, J.R. (1973). An anatomy of schizophrenia, *Archives of General Psychiatry*, **29**, 177–89.

Stevens, J.R. (1978). Disturbances of ocular movements and blinking in schizophrenia, *Journal of Neurology, Neurosurgery and Psychiatry*, **41**, 1024–30.

Stevens, J.R. (1979). All that spikes is not fits. In C. Shagass, S. Gershon and A.J. Friedhoff (Eds.), *Psychopathology and Brian Dysfunction*, Raven Press, New York, pp. 183–98.

Stevens, J.R. (1982). Neuropathology of schizophrenia, *Archives of General Psychiatry*, **39**, 1131–9.

Stevens, J.R. (1986). Epilepsy and psychosis: neuropathological studies of six cases. In M.R. Trimble and T. Bolwig (Eds.), *Aspects of Epilepsy and Psychiatry*, John Wiley and Sons, Chichester, pp. 117–45.

Stevens, J.R., and Hermann, B.P. (1981). Temporal lobe epilepsy, psychopathology and violence: the state of the evidence, *Neurology*, **31**, 1127–32.

Stevens, J.R., and Livermore, A. (1978). Kindling in the mesolimbic dopamine system: animal model of psychosis, *Neurology*, **28**, 36–46.

Stevens, J.R., and Livermore, A. (1982). Telemetered EEG in schizophrenia: spectral analysis during abnormal behaviour episodes, *Journal of Neurology, Neurosurgery and Psychiatry*, **45**, 385–95.

Stevens, J.R., Langloss, J.M., Albrecht, P., Yolken, R., and Wang, Y.W. (1984). A search for cytomegalovirus and herpes viral antigen in brains of schizophrenic patients, *Archives of General Psychiatry*, **41**, 795–801.

Stevens, M., Crow, T.J., Bowman, M.J., and Coles, E.C. (1978). Age disorientation in schizophrenia, *British Journal of Psychiatry*, **133**, 130–6.

Stores, G. (1977). Behavioural disturbance and type of epilepsy in children attending ordinary schools. In J.K. Penry (Ed.), *Epilepsy: The 8th International Symposium*, Raven Press, New York, pp. 245–9.

Struve, F.A., and Willner, A.E. (1983). Cognitive dysfunction and tardive dyskinesia, *British Journal of Psychiatry*, **143**, 597–600.

Struve, F.A., Saraf, K.R., Arko, R.S., Klein, D.F., and Becka, D.R. (1979). Relationships between paroxysmal electroencephalographic dysrythmia and suicide ideation and attempts in psychiatric patients. In C. Shagass, S. Gershon and A.J. Friedhoff (Eds.), *Psychopathology and Brian Dysfunction*, Raven Press, New York, pp. 199–221.

Stuss, D.T., and Benson, D.F. (1984). Neuropsychological studies of the frontal lobes, *Psychological Bulletin*, **95**, 3–28.

Sulser, F. (1984). Regulation and function of noradrenaline receptor systems in brain, *Neuropharmacology*, **23** (2B), 255–61.

Swanson, L.W. (1978). The anatomical organisation of the septo-hippocampal projections. In K. Elliott and J. Whelan (Eds.), *Functions of the Septo-hippocampal System*, Ciba Foundation Symposium and Series 58, London, pp. 25–43.

Sydenham, T. (1740). *The Whole Works*, 11th edition, J. Pechey, Ware, London.

Symonds, C. (1962). The schizophrenia-like psychoses of epilepsy — discussion, *Proceedings of the Royal Society of Medicine*, **55**, 311.

Syvalahti, E.K.G., Sako, E., Scheinin, M., Pihlajanki, K., and Hietala, J. (1986). Effects of intravenous and subcutaneous administration of apomorphine on the clinical symptoms of chronic schizophrenics, *British Journal of Psychiatry*, **148**, 204–8.

Szasz, T.S. (1976). Schizophrenia: the sacred symbol of psychiatry, *British Journal of Psychiatry*, **129**, 308–16.

Takahashi, S., Kondo, H., and Kato, N. (1975). Effect of L-5HTP on brain monoamine metabolism and evaluation of its clinical effect in depressed patients, *Journal of Psychiatric Research*, **12**, 177–87.

Talairach, J., Bancaud, J., Geier, S., Bordas-Ferrer, M., Bonis, A., Szikla, G., and Risu, M. (1973). The cingulate gyrus and human behaviour. *Electroencephalography and Clinical Neurophysiology*, **34**, 45–52.

Tamminga, C., Smith, R.C., Chang, S., Naraszti, J.S., and Davis, J.M. (1976). Depression associated with oral choline, *Lancet*, **2**, 905.

Tamminga, C.A., Schaffer, M.H., Smith, R.C., and Davis, J.M. (1977). Schizophrenic symptoms improve with apomorphine, *Science*, **200**, 567–8.

Targum, S.D., Rosen, L., and Capodanno, A.E. (1983a). The dexamethasone suppression test in suicidal patients with unipolar depression, *American Journal of Psychiatry*, **140**, 877–9.

Targum, S.D., Rosen, L.N., De Lisi, L.E., Weinberger, D.R., and Citrin, C.M. (1983b). Cerebral ventricular size in major depressive disorder: association with delusional symptoms, *Biological Psychiatry*, **18**, 329–36.

Taube, S.L., Kirstein, L.S., Sweeney, D.R., Heninger, G.R., and Maas, J.W. (1978). Urinary MHPG and psychiatric diagnosis, *American Journal of Psychiatry*, **135**, 78–82.

Taylor, D.C. (1975). Factors influencing the occurrence of schizophrenia-like psychosis in patients with TLE, *Psychological Medicine*, **5**, 249–54.

Taylor, J. (1958). *Selected Writings of John Hughlings Jackson*, Staples Press, London.

Taylor, M.A., and Abrams, R. (1984). Cognitive impairment in schizophrenia, *American Journal of Psychiatry*, **141**, 196–201.

Taylor, P., and Fleminger, J.J. (1980). ECT for schizophrenia, *Lancet*, **i**, 1380–3.

Temkin, O. (1971). *The Falling Sickness*, Johns Hopkins Press, Baltimore.

Tennant, C., Bebbington, P., and Hurry, J. (1981). The role of life events in depressive illness: is there a substantial causal relation?, *Psychological Medicine*, **11**, 379–89.

Teuber, H.L. (1964). The riddle of frontal lobe function in man. In J.M. Warren and K. Akert (Eds.), *The Frontal-Granular Cortex and Behaviour*, McGraw-Hill, New York, pp. 410–44.

Thaker, G.K., Tamminga, C.A., Alphs, L.D., Lafferman, J., Ferraro, T.N., and Hare, T.A. (1987). Brain GABA abnormality in tardive dyskinesia, *Archives of General Psychiatry*, **44**, 522–31.

Thompson, P.J., and Trimble, M.R. (1982a). Anticonvulsant drugs and cognitive functions, *Epilepsia*, **23**, 531–44.

Thompson, P.J., and Trimble, M.R. (1982b). Non-MAOI antidepressant drugs and cognitive function: a review, *Psychological Medicine*, **12**, 539–48.

Thoren, P., Åsberg, M., Cronholm, B., Jörestedt, L., and Traskman, L. (1980a). Clomipramine treatment of obsessive–compulsive disorder. i. Controlled clinical trial, *Archives of General Psychiatry*, **37**, 1281–5.

Thoren, P., Åsberg, M., Bertilsson, L., Mellstrom, B., Sjoquist, F., and Traskman, L. (1980b). Clomipramine treatment of obsessive compulsive disorder. ii. Biochemical aspects, *Archives of General Psychiatry*, **37**, 1289–94.

Tienari, P. (1963). Psychiatric illness in identical twins, *Acta Psychiatrica Scandinavica*, **391**, Suppl. 171.

Tienari, P. (1971). Schizophrenia and monozygotic twins. In K.A. Achte (Ed.), *Psychiatrica Fennica*, Helsinki, pp. 97–104.

Todes, C.J., and Lees, A.J. (1985). The premorbid personality of patients with Parkinson's disease, *Journal of Neurology, Neurosurgery and Psychiatry*, **48**, 97–100.

Todrick, A., and Tait, A.C. (1969). The inhibition of human platelet 5HT uptake by tricyclic antidepressive drugs, *Journal of Pharmacy and Pharmacology*, **21**, 751–62.

Tomlinson, B.E. (1982). Plaques, tangles and Alzheimer's disease, *Psychological Medicine*, **12**, 449–59.

Toone, B. (1981). Psychoses of epilepsy. In E.H. Reynolds and M.R. Trimble (Eds.), *Epilepsy and Psychiatry*, Churchill Livingstone, Edinburgh, pp. 113–37.

Toone, B.K., Dawson, J., and Driver, M. (1982a). Psychoses of epilepsy. A radiological evaluation, *British Journal of Psychiatry*, **140**, 244–8.

Toone, B.K., Garralda, M.E., and Ron, M.A. (1982b). The psychosis of epilepsy and the functional psychoses: a clinical and phenomenological comparison, *British Journal of Psychiatry*, **141**, 256–61.

Torgersen, S. (1979). The nature and origin of common phobic fears, *British Journal of Psychiatry*, **134**, 343–51.

Träskman, L., Tybring, G., Åsberg, M., Bertilsson, L., Lantto, O., and Schalling, D. (1980). Cortisol in the CSF of depressed and suicidal patients, *Archives of General Psychiatry*, **37**, 761–7.

Treffert, D.A. (1964). The psychiatric patient with an EEG temporal lobe focus, *American Journal of Psychiatry*, **120**, 765–71.

470

Trimble, M.R. (1978a). Serum prolactin in epilepsy and hysteria, *British Medical Journal*, **2**, 1682.

Trimble, M.R. (1978b). Non-MAOI antidepressants and epilepsy, *Epilepsia*, **19**, 241–50.

Trimble, M.R. (1980). New antidepressant drugs and the seizure threshold, *Neuropharmacology*, **19**, 1227–8.

Trimble, M.R. (1981a). *Neuropsychiatry*, John Wiley and Sons, Chichester.

Trimble, M.R. (1981b). *Post-traumatic Neurosis*, John Wiley and Sons, Chichester.

Trimble, M.R. (1981c). Hysteria and other non-epileptic convulsions. In E.H. Reynolds and M.R. Trimble (Eds.), *Epilepsy and Psychiatry*, Churchill Livingstone, Edinburgh, pp. 92–112.

Trimble, M.R. (1985a). New brain imaging techniques and psychiatry. In K. Granville-Grossman (Ed.), *Recent Advances in Clinical Psychiatry*, Churchill Livingstone, Edinburgh, pp. 225–44.

Trimble, M.R. (1985b). Post-traumatic stress disorder. In C. Figley (Ed.), *Trauma and Its Wake*, Brunner Mazel, New York, pp. 5–14.

Trimble, M.R. (1986a). *New Brain Imaging Techniques and Psychopharmacology*, Oxford Unversity Press, Oxford.

Trimble, M.R. (1986b). PET in epilepsy. In M.R. Trimble and T. Bolwig (Eds.), *Aspects of Epilepsy and Psychiatry*, John Wiley and Sons, Chichester, pp. 147–60.

Trimble, M.R. (1986c). Hysteria, hystero-epilepsy and epilepsy. In M.R. Trimble and E.H. Reynolds (Eds.), *What is Epilepsy?*, Churchill Livingstone, Edinburgh, pp. 192–205.

Trimble, M.R. (1986d). Recent contributions of benzodiazepines to the management of epilepsy, *Epilepsia*, **27**, Suppl. 1.

Trimble, M.R. (1986e). Hypergraphia. In M.R. Trimble and T. Bolwig (Eds.), *Aspects of Epilepsy and Psychiatry*, John Wiley and Sons, Chichester, pp. 75–87.

Trimble, M.R., and Cummings, J.L. (1981). Neuropsychiatric disturbances following brain stem lesions, *British Journal of Psychiatry*, **138**, 56–9.

Trimble, M.R., and Meldrum, B.S. (1979). Monoamines, epilepsy, and schizophrenia. In J. Obiols *et al.* (Eds.), *Biological Psychiatry Today*, Elsevier, Amsterdam, pp. 470–5.

Trimble, M.R., and Perez, M.M. (1980). Psychosocial functioning in adults. In B. Kulig *et al.* (Eds.), *Epilepsy and Behaviour*, Swets and Zeitlinger, Amsterdam, pp. 118–26.

Trimble, M.R., and Reynolds, E.H. (1976). Anticonvulsant drugs and mental symptoms: a review, *Psychological Medicine*, **6**, 169–78.

Trimble, M.R., and Reynolds, E.H. (1984). Neuropsychiatric toxicity of anticonvulsant drugs. In W.B. Matthews (Ed.), *Recent Advances in Clinical Neurology*, Churchill Livingstone, Edinburgh, pp. 261–80.

Trimble, M.R., and Reynolds, E.H. (1986). *'What is Epilepsy?'* Churchill Livingstone, Edinburgh.

Trimble, M.R., and Robertson, M.M. (1983). Flupenthixol in depression, *Journal of Affective Disorders*, **5**, 81–9.

Trimble, M.R., and Robertson, M.M. (1986). The psychopathology of tics. In C. D. Marsden (Ed.), *Movement Disorders*, Vol. 2, Butterworths, Kent, pp. 406–220.

Trimble, M.R., and Thompson, P. (1985). Neuropsychiatric aspects of epilepsy. In I. Grant and K. Adams (Eds.), *Neuropsychological Assessment of Neuropsychiatric Disorders*, Oxford University Press, Oxford, pp. 321–48.

Trimble, M.R., Corbett, J.A., and Donaldson, J. (1980). Folic acid and mental symptoms in children with epilepsy, *Journal of Neurology, Neurosurgery and Psychiatry*, **43**, 1030–4.

Tucker, G., Detre, T., Harrow, M., and Glaser, G.H. (1965). Behaviour and symptoms of psychiatric patients and the EEG, *Archives of General Psychiatry*, **12**, 278–86.

Tucker, G.J., and Silberfarb, P.M. (1978). Neurologic dysfunction in schizophrenia: significance for diagnostic practice. In H.S. Akiskal and W.L. Webb (Eds.), *Psychiatric Diagnosis: Exploration of Biological Predictors*, Spectrum, New York, pp. 453–62.

Tuke, D.H. (1894). Imperative ideas, *Brain*, **17**, 179–97.

Tuke, D.H. (1982). *A Dictionary of Psychological Medicine*, J. and A. Churchill, London.

Turner, S.W., Toone, B.K., and Brett-Jones, J.R. (1986). Computerized tomographic scan changes in early schizophrenia — preliminary findings, *Psychological Medicine*, **16**, 219–25.

Tyrer, P. (1976). Towards rational therapy with MAOI, *British Journal of Psychiatry*, **128**, 354–60.

Tyrer, P.J., and Lader, M.H. (1974). Response to propranolol and diazepam in somatic and psychic anxiety, *British Medical Journal*, **2**, 14–16.

Tyrer, P.J., Owen, R., and Dawling, S. (1983). Gradual withdrawal of diazepam after long-term therapy, *Lancet*, **i**, 1402–6.

472

Tyrer, S.P., Delves, H.T., and Weller, M.P.I. (1979). CSF copper in schizophrenia, *American Journal of Psychiatry,* **136**, 937–9.

Tyrrell, D.A.J., Crow, T.J., Parry, R.P., Johnstone, E., and Ferrier, I.N. (1979). Possible virus in schizophrenia and some neurological disorders, *Lancet,* **i**, 842–4.

Uhde, T.W., Boulenger, J-P., Vittone, B., Siever, L.J., and Post, R.M. (1985). Human anxiety and noradrenergic function. In P. Pichot *et al.* (Eds.), *Psychiatry; The State of the Art,* Vol. 2, Plenum, New York, pp. 693–8.

Uhlenhuth, E.H., and Paykel, E.S. (1973). Symptom configuration and life events, *Archives of General Psychiatry,* **28**, 744–8.

Ungerstedt, U. (1971). Stereotaxic mapping of the monoamine pathways in the rat brain, *Acta Physiologica Scandinavica,* **197**, Suppl.367, 1–48.

Uytdenhoef, P., Portelange, P., Jaquy, J., Charles, G., Linkowski, P., and Mendlewicz, J. (1983). RCBF and lateralised hemisphere dysfunction, *British Journal of Psychiatry,* **143**, 128–32.

Valenstein, E., and Heilman, K.M. (1979). Emotional disorders resulting from lesions of the CNS. In K.M. Heilman and E. Valenstein (Eds.), *Clinical Neuropsychology,* Oxford University Press, New York, pp. 413–38.

Van Hoesen, G.U. (1982). The parahippocampal gyrus, *Trends in Neurosciences,* **5**, 345–9.

van Kammen, D.P., Sternberg, D.E., Hare, T.A., Walters, R.N., and Bunney, W.E. (1982). CSF levels of GABA in schizophrenia, *Archives of General Psychiatry,* **39**, 91–7.

van Kammen, D.P., Mann, L.S., Sternberg, D.E., *et al.* (1983). Dopamine beta-hydrolase activity and HVA in spinal fluid of schizophrenics with brain atrophy, *Science,* **220**, 974–7.

Van Praag, H.M. (1977a). Significance of biochemical parameters in the diagnosis, treatment and presentation of depressive disorders, *Biological Psychiatry,* **12**, 101–31.

Van Praag, H. (1977b). The significance of dopamine for the mode of action of neuroleptics and the pathogenesis of schizophrenia, *British Journal of Psychiatry,* **130**, 463–74.

Van Praag, H.M. (1980a). Central monoamine metabolism in depressions. 1. Serotonin and related compounds, *Comprehensive Psychiatry,* **21**, 30–43.

Van Praag, H. (1980b). Central monoamine metabolism in depressions. 11. Catecholamines and related compounds, *Comprehensive Psychiatry,* **21**, 44–54.

Van Praag, H. (1985). Depression, suicide and serotonin metabolism in the brain. In R.M. Post and J.C. Ballenger (Eds.), *Neurobiology of Mood Disorders*, Williams and Wilkins, Baltimore, pp. 601–18.

Van Praag, H.M., van den Burg, W., Bos, E., and Dols, L. (1974). 5HTP in combination with clomipramine in 'therapy resistant' depression, *Psychopharmacologia*, **38**, 267–9.

Van Praag, H.M., Verhoeven, W.M.A., van Ree, J.M., and de Wied, D. (1982). Treatment of schizophrenic psychoses with gamma type endorphins, *Biological Psychiatry*, **17**, 83–98.

van Wielink, P.S., Leysen, J.E. (1983). Choice of neuroleptics on the basis of in vitro pharmacology, *Journal of Drug Research*, **8**, 1984–97.

von Economo, C. (1931), *Encephalitis lethargica* (Translated by K.O. Newman), Oxford University Press, Oxford.

Victor, M., Adams, R.D., and Collins, G.H. (1971), *The Wernicke–Korsakoff Syndrome*, Davis, Philadelphia.

Volkow, N.D., Brodie, J.D., Wolf, A., and Gomez-Mont, F., *et al.* (1985). Differences in patterns of brain metabolism between normals and schizophrenics. XII International Symposium on *Cerebral Blood Flow and Metabolism*, Ronneby, Lund, Abstracts Q 304–5.

Waddington, J.L. (1985). Further anomalies in the dopamine receptor supersensivity hypothesis of tardive dyskinesia, *Trends in Neurosciences*, **8**, 200.

Walinder, J., Skott, A., Carlsson, A., Nagy, A., and Roos, B. (1976). Potentiation of the antidepressant action of clomipramine by tryptophan, *Archives of General Psychiatry*, **33**, 1384–9.

Walter, W.G., Cooper, R., Aldridge, V.J., McCallum, W.C., and Winter, A.L. (1964). Contingent negative variation, *Nature*, **203**, 380–4.

Walzer, S., Wolff, P.H., and Bowen, D., *et al.* (1978). A method for the longitudinal study of behavioural development in infants and children: the early development of XXY children, *Journal of Child Psychology and Psychiatry*, **19**, 213–29.

Waxman, S.G., and Geschwind, N. (1975). The interictal behaviour syndrome of temporal lobe epilepsy, *Archives of General Psychiatry*, **32**, 1580–6.

Wegner, J.T., Catalano, F., Gibralter, J., Kane, J.M. (1985). Schizophrenics with tardive dyskinesia, *Archives of General Psychiatry*, **42**, 860–5.

Weinberger, D.R., Fuller-Torrey, E., Neophytides, A.N., and Wyatt, J. (1979). Lateral cerebral ventricular enlargement in chronic schizophrenia, *Archives of General Psychiatry*, **36**, 735–9.

Weinberger, D., and Wyatt, R.J. (1980). Schizophrenia and cerebral atrophy, *Lancet*, **i**, 1130.

Weinberger, D.R., Wagner, R.L., and Wyatt, R.J. (1983). Neuropathological studies of schizophrenia: a selective review, *Schizophrenia Bulletin*, **9**, 193–212.

Weinberger, D.R., Berman, K.F., and Zec, D.F. (1986). Physiologic dysfunction of dorsolateral prefrontal cortex in schizophrenia, *Archives of General Psychiatry*, **43**, 114–24.

Weiner, R.D. (1986). Electrical dosage, stimulus parameter and electrode placement, *Psychopharmacology Bulletin*, **22**, 499–502.

Weingartner, H., and Silberman, S. (1985). Cognitive changes in depression. In R.M. Post and J. Ballenger (Eds.), *Psychobiology of Mood Disorders*, Williams and Wilkins, Baltimore, pp. 121–35.

Wells, C.E. (1979). Pseudodementia, *American Journal of Psychiatry*, **136**, 895–900.

Whalley, L.J., Christie, J.E., Brown, S., and Arbuthnott, G.W. (1984). Schneider's first rank symptoms of schizophrenia: an association with increased growth hormone response to apomorphine, *Archives of General Psychiatry*, **41**, 1040–3.

Whalley, L.J., Borthwick, N., Copolov, D., Dick, H., Christie, J.E., Fink, G. (1986). Glucocorticoid receptors and depression, *British Medical Journal*, **292**, 859–61.

White, L.E. (1981). Development and morphology of human nucleus accumbens. In R.B. Chronister and J.F. De France (Eds.), *The Neurobiology of the Nucleus Accumbens*, Haer Institute, Brunswick, New Jersey, pp. 198–209.

Whitlock, F.A. (1967). The aetiology of hysteria, *Acta Psychiatrica Scandinavica*, **43**, 144–62.

Whitlock, F.A. (1982). The neurology of affective disorder and suicide, *Australian and New Zealand Journal of Psychiatry*, **16**, 1–12.

Whitlock, F.A., and Evans, L.E.J. (1978). Drugs and depression, *Drugs*, **15**, 53–71.

Whytt, R. (1765). *Observations on the Nature, Causes and Cure of Those Disorders Which Have Been Called Nervous, Hypochondriac or Hysteric, to Which Are Prefixed Some Remarks on the Sympathy of the Nerves*, 3rd edition, Becket and Du Hondt, Edinburgh.

Widerlov, E., Linstrom, L.H., Besev, G.. *et al.* (1982). Subnormal CSF levels of neurotensin in a subgroup of schizophrenic patients, *American Journal of Psychiatry*, **139**, 1122–6.

Wiesel, F., Fyro, B., Nyback, H., Sedvall, G., and Wode-Helgodt, B. (1982). Relationship in healthy volunteers between secretion of monoamine metabolites in urine and family history of psychiatric morbidity, *Biological Psychiatry*, **17**, 1403–13.

Wieser, H.G. (1983). *Electroclinical Features of the Psychomotor Seizure*, Gustav Fischer, Stuttgart.

Will, R.G., and Matthews, W.B. (1984). A retrospective study of Creutzfeld–Jakob disease in England and Wales, *Journal of Neurology, Neurosurgery and Psychiatry*, **47**, 134–40.

Williams, D. (1956). The structure of emotions reflected in epileptic experiences, *Brain*, **79**, 29–67.

Williams, D. (1969). Neural factors related to habitual aggression, *Brain*, **92**, 503–20.

Willner, P. (1983). Dopamine and depression: a review of recent evidence, *Brain Research Reviews*, **6**, 225–36.

Wilson, M.D. (1969). *The Essential Descartes*, Mentor, London.

Wilson-Barnett, J., and Trimble, M.R. (1985). An investigation of hysteria using the IBQ, *British Journal of Psychiatry*, **146**, 601–8.

Winblad, B., Bucht, G., Gottfries, C-G., and Roos, B.E. (1979). Monoamines and monamine metabolites in brains from demented schizophrenics, *Acta Psychiatrica Scandinavica*, **60**, 17–28.

Wing, J.K., Cooper, J.E., and Sartorius, N. (1974). *Description and Classification of Psychiatric Symptoms*, Cambridge University Press, Cambridge.

Winokur, A., Amsterdam, J., Caroff, S., *et al.* (1982). Variability of hormonal responses to a series of neuro-endocrine challenges in depressed patients, *American Journal of Psychiatry*, **139**, 39–44.

Winokur, G. (1977). Delusional disorder, *Comprehensive Psychiatry*, **18**, 511–21.

Winokur, G. (1982). The development and validity of familial subtypes in primary unipolar depression, *Pharmaco-psychiatrica*, **15**, 142–6.

Winokur, G., Clayton, P., and Reich, T. (1959). *Manic-Depressive Illness*, C.V. Mosby, St Louis.

Winokur, G., and Tanna, V.L. (1969). Possible role of X-linked dominant factor in manic depressive disease, *Diseases of the Nervous System*, **30**, 87–94.

Winslow, R.S., Stillner, V., Coons, D.J., and Robinson, M.W. (1986). Prevention of acute dystonic reactions in patients beginning high-potency neuroleptics, *American Journal of Psychiatry*, **143**, 706–10.

Wirz-Justice, A. (1977). Theoretical and therapeutic potential of indolamine precursors in affective disorders, *Neuropsychobiology*, **3**, 199–233.

Wolf, P., and Trimble, M.R. (1985). Biological antagonism and epileptic psychosis, *British Journal of Psychiatry*, **146**, 272–6.

Wolpert, L. (1984). DNA and its message, *Lancet*, **ii**, 853–6.

Wood, P.L., Suranyi-Cadotte, B., Schwartz, G., and Nair, N.P.V. (1983). Platelet 3H-imipramine binding and red blood cell choline in affective disorders, *Biological Psychiatry*, **18**, 715–20.

Woods, B.T., and Short, M.P. (1985). Neurological dimensions of psychiatry, *Biological Psychiatry*, **20**, 192–8.

World Health Organisation (1973). Report of the international pilot study of schizophrenia, W.H.O., Geneva.

Wyatt, R.J., Termini, B.A., and Davis, J. (1971). Biochemical and sleep studies of schizophrenia: a review of the literature 1960–1970, *Schizophrenia Bulletin*, **4**, 10–66.

Yadalam, K.G., Jain, A.K., and Simpson, G. (1985). Mania in two sisters with similar cerebellar disturbance, *American Journal of Psychiatry*, **142**, 1067–9.

Yakovlev, P. (1948). Motility, behaviour and the brain, *Journal of Nervous and Mental Disease*, **107**, 313–35.

Young, S.W. (1984). *Nuclear Magnetic Resonance Imaging*, Raven Press, New York.

Zaleski, M.B., Dubiski, S., Niles, E.G., and Cunningham, R.K. (1983). *Immunogenetics*, Pitman, London.

Zemlan, F.P., Hitzemann, R.J., Hirschowitz, J., and Garver, D.L. (1985). Down regulation of central dopamine receptors in schizophrenia, *American Journal of Psychiatry*, **142**, 1334–7.

Zielinski, J.J. (1974). *Epidemiology and Medical–Social Problems of Epilepsy in Warsaw*, Warsaw Psychoneurological Institute, Warsaw.

Zilboorg, G. (1941). *A History of Medical Psychology*, W.W. Norton, New York.

Index

478

485

homovanilic acid (HVA) 79, 189,
209, 212, 213, 214, 223, 237, 238,
252, 265, 325, 372, 375, 393
homozygote 57
horseradish peroxidase 89
Hounsfield units 134, 135
human immunodeficiency virus
(HIV) 336
human leucocyte antigen
(HLA) 58
markers 203
studies 245, 291
Hunter 18, 28
Huntington's chorea 171, 218,
229, 230, 273, 276, 324, 334, 345
Husserl 29
hydergine 348
hydrazines 355, 356
hydrocephalus 335, 338–40, 342,
343, 345
normal pressure 125, 169, 339
hydrophobia 158
5-hydroxyindole acetic acid
(5-HIAA) 78, 188, 189, 252,
264–5, 266, 276, 325, 359
hydroxylation 353, 364
5-hydroxytryptophan (5-HTP) 78,
247, 261
hypergraphia 192, 197, 299, 300,
301, 303
hypermetamorphosis 155, 193
hyperphagia 113, 164
hyperprolactinaemia 366
hyperreligiosity 192
hypersomnia 171
hypertension 296, 331, 334, 343,
356, 358, 359, 390
hyperthyroidism 211
hypnosis 16
hypocalcaemia 291
hypochondriasis 44, 267, 318, 332,
357
'hypofrontality' 225, 226, 227, 272,
273
hypoglycaemia 291, 296
hypomagnesaemia 291
hypoparathyroidism 211
hypophyseal portal system 77, 98
hypopituitarism 255

hyposexuality 193
hypothalamus 78–82, 87, 89–91,
96, 98–101, 102, 107, 110, 113,
115, 118, 120, 171, 172, 211, 216,
217, 218, 260, 262, 263, 266, 381,
402, 403
hypothyroidism 211, 272, 341, 390
hypoxia 291
hysteria 3, 15, 44, 177, 178, 179,
181, 194, 195, 295, 344

'iatrochemists' 4
'iatromechanists' 4
ibuprofen 390
imipramine 21, 75, 185, 247, 248,
249, 252, 343, 359, 361, 363, 369,
370
binding sites 248, 249, 266
immunoglobulin, oligoclonal 125
implanted electrode studies 303
imprinting 54
indalpine 366
indolamines 204
indomethacin 390
infantile spasms 289, 296, 396
inhibitory postsynaptic potentials
(IPSP) 66–7, 75
initial slope index (ISI) 145
innate releasing mechanisms 54
insomnia 118, 372
insula 155
insulin 19, 218, 261, 262
coma 21
internal capsule 104, 111
interpeduncular nucleus 74, 89,
102
inversion recovery 143
ionization 351
ionophores 68, 69
iprindole 249, 367
ischaemic attacks
transient 296
vertebrobasilar 295
isocarboxazid 357
isocarboxide 356
'isodendritic core' 326
isoniazid 356
isoprenaline 181
isoxsuprine 348

492

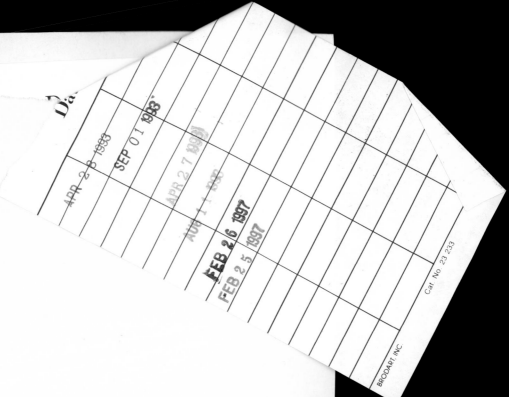

Da...

APR 2 8 1993
SEP 01 1993
APR 2 7 1994
AUG 1 1 1995
FEB 2 6 1997
FEB 2 5 1997

BRODART, INC.   Cat. No. 23 233

DRAKE MEMORIAL LIBRARY
WITHDRAWN
THE COLLEGE AT BROCKPORT